# Introduction to

# DENTAL

# MATERIALS

**Richard van Noort** BSc, DPhil, MIPSM
Senior Lecturer
School of Clinical Dentistry
Department of Restorative Dentistry
University of Sheffield
UK

**M Mosby**

London  Baltimore  Bogotá  Boston  Buenos Aires  Caracas  Carlsbad, CA  Chicago  Madrid  Mexico City  Milan  Naples, FL  New York  Philadelphia  St. Louis  Sydney  Tokyo  Toronto  Wiesbaden

Copyright © 1994 Times Mirror International Publishers Limited

Published in 1994 by Mosby, an imprint of Times Mirror International Publishers Limited

Printed by Grafos SA Arte Sobre Papel, Spain

ISBN 0 7234 1963 9

For full details of all Times Mirror International Publishers Limited titles, please write to Times Mirror International Publishers Limited, Lynton House, 7–12 Tavistock Square, London WC1H 9LB, England.

A CIP catalogue record for this book is available from the British Library.

**Library of Congress Cataloging-in-Publication Data:** applied for

| | |
|---|---|
| **Project Manager:** | Jonathan Brenchley |
| **Cover Design:** | Pete Wilder |
| **Illustration:** | Jenni Miller |
| **Production:** | Mike Heath |
| **Index:** | Anita Reid |
| **Publisher:** | Claire Hooper |

# CONTENTS

# PREFACE

There is scarcely a restorative dental procedure that does not make use of a dental material in one way or another, and so, without adequate materials, very little can be accomplished in the practice of restorative dentistry.

Restorative dental materials include metals (e.g. base and noble metals, amalgams and gold alloys), ceramics and glasses (e.g. gypsum compounds, investment refractories for casting and porcelain), polymers (e.g. impression materials and denture base resins), and composites, which are combinations of materials.

From 1900, advances in dental materials were extremely rapid, and, if anything, are speeding up with the passing of every decade. Many of the materials in use today will be superceded by new materials within a very short space of time. Indeed, many of the materials learnt about as an undergraduate will be obsolete by the end of a career in dental practise, so a course on dental materials must provide the dentist with the necessary knowledge to make the best use of a material, to realise its limitations, and to assess the potential of new materials. The development of these skills requires that the dentist has more than a superficial knowledge of the materials in question.

The science of dental materials is derived from the sciences of biology, chemistry and physics, but is impossible to draw distinct divisions between these separate sciences when applied to dental materials as they are so interwoven. In order to be a successful dental practitioner, it is necessary to have an appreciation of the biological, chemical and physical principles that form the foundation of the clinical application of dental materials. It is not enough simply to know how a material should be used. It is vital to understand the reasons for the way in which it is used, as this avoids abuse and misuse of the dental materials, a goal which, in the long run, will be of benefit to the patient.

The book is set out in three sections, each covering a different aspect of dental materials science:

- *Section I, Basic Science for Dental Materials* – This section describes the structure of materials and provides the necessary terminology used in the description of their behaviour.
- *Section II, Clinical Dental Materials* – This section deals with those materials commonly used in the dental surgery. The composition, chemistry, handling characteristics and properties appropriate to their clinical use are discussed.
- *Section III, Laboratory and Related Dental Materials* – Those materials the dentist should know about as used by dental technicians are described in this section. A sound knowledge of the materials available and how they are used will help towards developing an understanding of the work of the dental technician and assist in communicating to the dental technician specific requirements for the patient.

The process of learning never ceases, and should be continued by reading around the subject as this will help you to gain greater insight into the use and abuse of dental materials (see the Further Reading sections at the ends of the chapters).

The aim of this text book is to produce informed practitioners who not only know what should be done and how it should be done, but also *why* it should be done.

R. van Noort

# I
# BASIC SCIENCE FOR DENTAL MATERIALS

This section addresses the relationship between the microstructure and the properties of materials.

In order to understand why different materials should have different properties and what these properties mean in relation to their use, it is necessary to understand something about the science of materials.

As this book is not intended for would-be materials scientists but rather for dentists with a good foundation in dental materials, only those aspects of the behaviour of materials that are pertinent to dental applications will be considered.

The questions to be addressed in this section will be:
- What are the microstructural features of materials?
- How do we describe the behaviour of different materials?

# I.I

# BIOMATERIALS, BIOCOMPATIBILITY AND BIOMECHANICS

## Biomaterials

The dental restorative materials described in this textbook are a special subgroup of what are more generally described as biomaterials. When a material is placed in, or in contact with the human body, it is generally referred to as a biomaterial. A biomaterial may be defined as a non-living material designed to interact with biological systems.

The three main areas of use of biomaterials are:

- Dental restorative materials, e.g. metallic and composite filling materials, and casting alloys and ceramics for fixed and removable intra-oral prostheses.
- Structural implants, e.g. oral and maxillo-facial implants and joint prostheses.
- Cardiovascular implants, e.g. catheters, prosthetic heart valves and blood vessels, and dialysis and oxygenator membranes.

In this book, we will only concern ourselves with dental restorative materials. A great deal of space is devoted to two important aspects of their use: their composition and their characteristic properties. There are also the considerations of biocompatibility and biomechanics, which must be kept in mind in biological applications.

## Biocompatibility

When a biomaterial is placed in contact with the tissues and fluids of the human body, there is invariably some form of interaction between the material and the biological environment. This interaction forms the subject of biocompatibility.

A material may be said to be *biocompatible* when it has the quality of being non-destructive in the biological environment. It is important to appreciate that this interaction works both ways. That is, the material may be affected in some way by the biological environment, and, equally, the biological environment may be affected by the material.

The biological reactions can take place either at a local level or far removed from the site of contact (i.e. systemically). The latter is a very important consideration, because it may not always be readily apparent that clinical symptoms such as dermatological, rheumatic or neural reactions could be associated with a biomaterial. Both the patient and the dental personnel are exposed to these interactions and the potential risks, with the patient being the recipient of the restorative materials and the dental personnel handling many of the materials on a daily basis.

Possible interactions between dental restorative material and the biological environment include:

- Post-operative sensitivity.
- Toxicity.
- Corrosion.
- Hypersensitivity/allergy.

Post-operative sensitivity is a local reaction to a restorative procedure. It is often associated with the placement of filling materials, where there is an adverse pulpal reaction following the operative procedure. Although at one time this was thought to be due to a lack of biocompatibility of the restorative material itself, it has now become well accepted that a significant role is played by the ingress of bacteria down the gap between the restorative material and the tooth tissues. If the restorative material were able to provide a hermetic seal, which would prevent bacterial ingress, then post-operative sensitivity from this source would be far less likely. A pulpal reaction could still arise if the restorative material itself were found to be toxic to the pulp. Prevention of bacterial invasion has become an important consideration in the development of adhesive restorative materials.

Some materials have a distinctly positive effect on the pulp: for example, calcium hydroxide induces secondary dentine formation by the pulp. This highlights that the requirement for a biomaterial to be biocompatible is not that it is inert in the biological environment (i.e. that it elicits no reaction), but that it should ideally induce a response that is both appropriate to the situation and highly beneficial.

Corrosion is a negative interaction between the biological environment and the biomaterial. One of the better known dental examples of this is the corrosion of dental amalgams. This corrosion causes discoloration of the tooth tissues and has been implicated in the common observation of marginal breakdown of amalgam restorations. Composite restorative materials are known to discolour in the mouth due to the corrosive action of the environment, and this causes many to be replaced when the aesthetics become unacceptable. The corrosive effects of the biological environment on the casting alloys used in the construction of fixed and removable intra-oral prostheses are also a matter of concern. When a material is susceptible to corrosion in the biological environment it tends to release large amounts of corrosion products into the local bio-

logical tissues; this may cause an adverse reaction either locally or systemically.

Some patients can develop allergic or hypersensitive reactions to even very small quantities of metals such as mercury, nickel and cobalt, that may be released due to the corrosion process. Hence it is important that biomaterials are highly resistant to corrosion.

Mercury, of course is known to be highly toxic when present in sufficient quantities, and this has recently led to calls from some quarters for its use to be banned altogether.

From the above, it should be clear that it is very important for the dentist to know the composition and chemistry of the materials to be used in the oral cavity and how these materials may interact with the biological environment.

# Biomechanics

Whereas biocompatibility is concerned with the safety aspects and with the biological and chemical interactions between the biomaterial and the biological environment, there are other matters with enormous implications for the performance of dental restorative materials, such as how well the materials used are able to withstand the forces generated either from the action of mastication, occlusion, or a variety of other sources such as polymerisation shrinkage or thermal contraction and expansion.

The function of dental structures such as fillings, crowns and bridges depends, therefore, not only on the materials' properties but also on the quality of the design employed.

How materials behave in real structures is known as mechanics. Engineers have used this approach in the design of buildings, bridges, cars, etc. For example, from a knowledge of material properties and the design of a concrete beam, it is possible to calculate whether the beam will support the load of the structure above it. Similarly, it is possible to design long-span suspension bridges which do not collapse under the weight of traffic.

When mechanics is applied to biomaterials, it is called *biomechanics*; it is the application of the principles of engineering to the human body.

A dental restorative example where the considerations of biomechanics are important is fracture of the restoration. This problem arises with dental amalgams in particular; careful consideration of both the limitations of this restorative material and of how these limitations affect the design of cavities can avoid many potential failures. Fracture of a ceramic segment from a metal–ceramic restoration may be due to excessive loads arising from an occlusal interference; this may be avoided by a modified design.

Similarly, the failure of an adhesive bond between a restoration and the tooth may be due to material properties, such as polymerisation shrinkage, giving rise to excessive interfacial stresses. Persistent adhesive failure of a resin-bonded bridge may be due to an inadequate design that is unable to resist the loads applied. Such a problem would not be resolved merely by recementing the bridge in place, and an alternative approach would have to be considered.

When two surfaces come into contact, there is a tendency for one of the surfaces to cause removal of material from the other surface. This is the process of *wear*, and it continues to be a problem with composite restorative materials. A major contribution to the wear process is the load applied. It is also important to know how this load causes damage to the material. Restorations should be designed so as to minimise this problem, and should not be used in circumstances in which the material is unsuitable.

These are all examples of interaction between material properties and structural design, and it is this which forms the subject of biomechanics.

# Summary

The main objective of good design in restorative dentistry is to avoid failure of the restoration. However, it should be appreciated that failure can come in many guises. Some failures may be due to lack of aesthetics. A clear example of this is the discoloration of composite restorative materials, and this points to a lack of chemical stability in the biological environment. A material may need to be removed because it elicits an allergic reaction or corrodes excessively. These are aspects of the biocompatibility of the material.

Equally, a restoration may fail mechanically because it fractures or shows excessive wear, possibly because the design was poor or because the material was used in circumstances unsuited for its properties.

Thus the clinical performance of dental restorations depends on:

- Appropriate material selection, based on a knowledge of their properties.
- The optimum design of the restoration.
- A knowledge of how the material will interact with the biological environment.

All these aspects of the biocompatibility and biomechanics of dental materials will be covered where appropriate.

# Further Reading

Smith D. C. (1982) The biocompatibility of dental materials. Chapter 1 in *Biocompatibility of Dental Materials, Vol. 1*, Smith D. C. and Williams D. F. (Eds.) CRC Press, Boca Raton

Waters N. E. (1992) Dental biomechanics and the dental curriculum. J. Dent. **20**, 195–198

# A HISTORICAL PERSPECTIVE

## Introduction

Poor dentition is often thought of as being a modern day problem, arising as a consequence of an overindulgence in all things considered – naughty, but nice! At first glance, the diet of years gone by, consisting of raw meat, fish, rye bread and nuts, would be considered better for the dentition than the cooked food and high sugar intake foods consumed today.

However, the food wasn't washed as diligently then as it is now, meaning that it contained grit in the form of sand, flint and shells, which had the effect of wearing away the grinding surfaces of the teeth. The surface protective layer of enamel is only thin, and the underlying dentine is worn away rapidly.

Eventually, the pulp is exposed and will be invaded by bacteria, which, before long, will cause the formation of an abscess, leaving no other recourse than to have the offending tooth extracted. The problems this presented were formidable, and we will return to these at a later stage.

Thus, the loss of teeth is by no means a new problem, and has been with man for time *in memorium*.

## The Etruscans (1000–600 B.C.)

For some of the earliest records of the treatment of dental disease, one has to go back well before the time of Christ. While much is lost with the passage of time, the Etruscans did leave behind a legacy of some very high quality dentistry.

The Etruscans were a people that came from the near East and established themselves in the leg of Italy. They were the forebears of the Romans (upon whom they had a great influence), and laid the basis for the formation of the Roman Empire. The quality of their craftsmanship was outstanding. Their skills were put to good use, as they fashioned artificial teeth from cadaver teeth using gold to hold the tooth in place. Gold had the two advantages of being aesthetically acceptable, and of being one of the few metals available to them with the necessary malleability for the production of intricate shapes.

The Romans must have inherited at least some of their interest in teeth, as made evident by one of their articles of law of the Twelve Tables which states that:

'To cause the loss of a tooth of a free man will result in a fine of 300 As'.

More remarkable, perhaps, is the fact that the slaves too were offered some protection, but in their case the fine was only 100 As. Although no physical evidence remains that false teeth were worn, it may be inferred from the written records that this was the case, such as presented by Horace (65 B.C.) who wrote of 'witches being chased and running so fast that one lost her teeth', and later still by Martial (40–100 A.D.), who refers to ivory and wooden teeth.

# The Dark Ages

Little is known of what happened in dentistry from Martial's time until the 16th century, and this period must be considered as being the 'Dark Age of Dentistry'. We owe our patron saint of dental diseases, Saint Apollonia, to this period. She was 'encouraged' to speak ungodly words by having her teeth extracted or else be burnt on the pyre. She chose to burn! This did leave the church with somewhat of a dilemma, because suicide was not allowed, but in this case the problem was overcome by considering this as divine will.

There are odd records scattered about throughout this period showing that toothache was a persistent problem. For example, one important person was known to pad out her face with cloth in order to hide the loss of teeth, whenever there was an important function to attend. This was none other than Queen Elizabeth I. Then there was Louis XIV, the 'Sun King', who suffered terribly from toothache and had to make many momentous decisions, such as the revocation of the Edict of Nantes (in 1642), while suffering excruciating pain. Possibly this clouded his judgement.

# The First Dentures (18th Century)

In the 18th century, it became possible to produce reasonably accurate models of the mouth by the use of wax. These models were then used as templates from which ivory dentures were carved to the required shape. By the latter part of the 18th century, finely carved ivory teeth were being produced by various craftsmen who set up in business solely to supply false teeth to the rich. Of course, this type of dentistry was not available for the masses.

Lower dentures, made of ivory and inset with cadaver teeth, worked reasonably well and managed to stay in place without too much difficulty, especially if weighted with some lead. The difficulties really came to the fore with the upper denture, which refused to stay in place due both to the heavy weight and the poor fit. In order to overcome this problem, upper dentures were fashioned onto the lower denture by means of springs or hinges. This technique would ensure that the upper denture would always be pushed up against the roof of the mouth, but, as can be imagined, they were large, cumbersome and very heavy.

Clearly, the use of cadaver teeth could hardly have been hygienic. Similarly, ivory is slightly porous and thus presented an ideal substrate for the accumulation of bacteria. In fact, George Washington regularly soaked his dentures in port, ostensibly to overcome the bad taste and to mask the smell.

In 1728, Fauchard suggested that dentures should be made from porcelain instead of ivory inset with cadaver teeth, arguing that porcelain would be more attractive (as it could be coloured as required) and would be considerably more hygienic. What made this suggestion possible was the introduction into Europe of the secret of making porcelain by Father d'Entrecolle, a Jesuit priest who had spent many years in China. Given the problems of the high shrinkage of porcelain during firing, it is perhaps not surprising that we had to wait until 1744 for the first recorded case of a porcelain denture, made by a man called Duchateau.

# The Victorian Age

The Victorians frowned on the wearing of dentures as a terrible vanity, more so because all of these false teeth were absolutely useless for eating with! Nevertheless, false teeth were still worn extensively by the rich. The fact that they were non-functional, combined with Victorian prudishness, is said to lie behind the custom that developed during that time of eating in the bedroom just prior to going to dinner; a custom that insured against any possible disaster at the dinner table as well as making possible the romantic affectation that young ladies lived on air.

A number of important discoveries were made during the 19th century that were to have a profound effect on the treatment of dental disease. The first of these was made in about 1800 by a 'dentist' from Philadelphia by the name of James Gardette.

He had carved a full set of ivory dentures for a woman patient, and had delivered these to the woman saying that he did not have time to fit the springs there and then, but that he would return to do so as soon as he possibly could. (It was the custom in those days for the dentist to visit the patient!) As it turned out, it was some months before he returned to the woman patient, and he was astonished to find that on asking her to fetch the dentures, the woman replied that she had been wearing them ever since he had delivered them. She had found the dentures a little uncomfortable at first but had persevered, and, after a little while, had found them to be quite comfortable and had no need for the springs.

Upon examination of the dentures, he realised immediately that the retention of the dentures was due to a combination of a suction effect arising from the different pressure of the atmosphere and the fluid film, and the surface tension effects of the fluid. This retention was attained because of the close fit of the denture, so it was possible to do without springs altogether, if only the denture could be made to fit as closely as possible to the contours of the oral structures. Unfortunately, the production of close fitting dentures still presented a serious problem, which we will return to in a moment.

At this time, the extraction of diseased teeth presented a formidable problem, because there was no painless means of accomplishing the extraction. This situation was to change dramatically in 1844 due to the astuteness of a young dentist called Horace Wells, who discovered the anaesthetic effects of nitrous oxide, more commonly known as 'laughing gas'. One evening, he found himself present at a public entertainment on the amusing effects of laughing gas. A friend who subjected himself to the gas became very violent while under the influence,

and in the ensuing fracas stumbled and badly gashed his leg. He had no knowledge of this wound until Wells pointed to the bloodstained leg, upon which his friend responded that he had not felt a thing. Wells realised immediately the importance of this discovery, and the next day subjected himself to the removal of one of his own teeth with the aid of the gas. This turned out to be highly successful, and before long many sufferers of toothache had the offending teeth painlessly extracted.

Unfortunately, Wells did not live to see the benefit of his discovery for long, as he committed suicide three years later after becoming addicted to chloroform. As a consequence of Wells's discovery, there were many people who had their teeth painlessly extracted.

At that time, few were in the position of being able to afford dentures of either carved ivory or porcelain. Other techniques had been developed, whereby it was possible to obtain accurate impressions of the oral structures, and much of the ivory was replaced by swaged gold, beaten to a thin plate on a model. The fixing of the artificial teeth to the gold was a difficult and lengthy process, and, like dentures, was also expensive.

This situation was to change dramatically with the invention, by Charles Goodyear (in about 1850), of the process of vulcanisation. In this process, rubber was hardened in the presence of sulphur to produce a material called Vulcanite. This material was not only cheap but was also easy to work with; it could be moulded to provide an accurate fit to the model and hence to the oral structures. It did not take off as quickly as might have been expected however, because the Goodyear Rubber Company held all the patents on the process and charged dentists up to $100 a year to use it, with a royalty of $2 per denture on top of this. The situation changed when the patent expired in 1881, and cheap dentures could be made available to the masses of people in need of them.

Nowadays, Vulcanite has been replaced by acrylic resins, which came with the discovery of synthetic polymers, first made between the two World Wars. Also, wax has been superseded by a wide range of oral impression materials with far superior qualities; this has made possible the construction of very close fitting, complex prostheses.

## Tooth Conservation

If the 19th century was the time for tooth replacement, then the 20th century must be considered the time of tooth preservation. For example, in 1938, 60% of dental treatment was still concerned with the provision of dentures, but by 1976 this had dropped to 7%, with the rest consisting essentially of tooth preservation procedures.

Of course, the idea of preserving a decayed tooth was by no means new. As far back as the 11th century, Rhazes suggested that cavities in teeth could be filled with a mixture of alum, ground mastic and honey. Oil of cloves was promoted by Ambrose Pare (1562) to alleviate toothache, and Giovanni de Vigo (1460–1520) suggested the use of gold leaf to fill cavities. Pierre Fauchard (1728), considered by many to be the father of dentistry, discussed many aspects of dentistry, including operative and prosthetic procedures, and mentioned lead, tin and gold as possible filling materials.

However, there were a number of important gaps in the knowledge of the dentition that held back the development of conservative dental techniques.

There was a lack of understanding of the reasons for tooth decay, which was originally thought to be due to some evil spirit invading the tooth. Some thought it was due to a worm of sorts, and promoted various nasty tinctures with the objective of killing it.

The first serious conservative dental procedures did not come into use until the second half of the 19th century. By then, it was possible to work on people's teeth without causing severe pain and discomfort, thanks to the discovery of anaesthetics. This discovery made the use of the dental drill feasible.

The first such drill only became available in about 1870, but this is not too surprising, given that the drilling of teeth without an anaesthetic would have been unthinkable. Now that the preparation of teeth could be carried out, it was possible to undertake some more adventurous procedures than the wholesale extraction of decayed teeth.

## Crowns And Bridges

By the turn of the century, some highly advanced dental work was carried out in which badly broken-down teeth were reconstructed with porcelain crowns. This procedure was aided by the invention of a cement that would set in the mouth (i.e. zinc phosphate cement), and which is still widely used to this day. That this could give a great deal of satisfaction can be illustrated from the letters of President Roosevelt of the United States of America to his parents when still a young man:

'After lunch I went to the dentist, and am now minus my front tooth. He cut it off very neatly and painlessly, took impressions of the root and space, and is having the porcelain tip baked. I hope to have it put in next Friday, and in the meantime I shall avoid all society, as I talk with a lithp and look a thight.'

May 19, 1902

This was followed by a letter a week later in which he writes:

'My tooth is no longer a dream, it is an accomplished fact. It was put in on Friday and is perfect in form, colour, lustre, texture, etc. I feel like a new person and have already been proposed to by three girls.'

Obviously a delighted customer!

As is often the case with these rapid developments, there were to be some problems ahead. One of these was highlighted by an English physician, William Hunter, who accused what was then called 'American Dentistry' of contributing to the ill health of many of his patients. He had a number of patients with ailments he was at a loss to diagnose until he noticed the extensive restorative work in their mouths. These bridges and crowns appeared dirty, and were surrounded by unhealthy looking tissue, which would have been particularly bad, as oral hygiene was virtually non-existent. At that time, root canal treatment was unheard of, so the roots of teeth

**Table 1** Milestones in the history of dental materials.

| | |
|---|---|
| 600 B.C. | Etruscan gold bridge work |
| 1480 A.D. | First authentic record of gold fillings in human teeth by Johannes Arculanus, University of Bologna |
| 1500s | Ivory dentures began to be carved from wax models |
| 1728 | Fauchard proposed the use of porcelain |
| 1744 | Duchateau makes the first recorded porcelain denture |
| 1826 | Taveau of Paris suggests the use of silver and mercury to make a paste for filling teeth |
| 1839 | The first dental journal is published called the American Journal of Dental Science |
| 1840s | 'Amalgam war' – the use of silver amalgam is forbidden |
| 1850 | Charles Goodyear invented Vulcanite – sulphur hardened rubber |
| 1879 | The first cement to set in the mouth, zinc phosphate, is introduced |
| 1880s | Silicate cements developed |
| 1895 | G.V. Black publishes the first detailed study of the properties of amalgams |
| 1907 | W.H. Taggart of Chicago invented a practical method of casting gold inlays |
| 1950s | Introduction of acrylic resin for fillings and dentures |
| 1955 | Buonacore discovered the acid-etch technique for bonding to enamel |
| 1970 | Composites began to replace silicate cements |
| 1976 | Glass ionomer cements are invented by A. Wilson |
| 1978 | Light activated composites appear on the market |
| 1985 | Development of dentine bonding agents |

readily became infected. On many occasions, crowns and bridges would have been constructed on badly diseased teeth. He suggested that these crowns and bridges be removed and the teeth extracted, in response to which he received considerable objection from the patients because of the cost of the dental treatment. But, for those who agreed to have the bridgework removed, a significant number showed an immediate improvement in their health. This led Hunter to describe American Dentistry as 'mausoleums of gold over a mass of sepsis'. Consequently, teeth were blamed for all manner of illnesses that could not be readily diagnosed, and this led to many perfectly sound teeth being extracted unnecessarily.

Eventually, sanity prevailed with the introduction in 1913 of X-ray equipment by C. Edmund Kells. It could now be shown whether a tooth with a dead root was healthy or diseased. If healthy, it could be kept, and only if diseased would it be removed.

# Filling Materials

The middle of the 19th century saw the organisation of dentistry into a profession, and many dental societies came into existence, as well as numerous dental journals. One of the first acts of the American Society of Dental Surgeons was to forbid its members to use silver amalgam, resulting in the 'amalgam war'.

Amalgam is a mixture of silver, tin and mercury, and was one of the first filling materials used by the dental profession. However, many problems arose with the use of this material because of a lack of understanding of its qualities. It was not until the work of G. V. Black that some order was created out of the chaos.

He published two volumes on operative dentistry in 1895, which became the world standard for restorative dentistry. Until he had studied both the behaviour of amalgam in detail and how best to use it, amalgam did not have a very good reputation. Since then, however, and up until this very day, amalgam has became one of the most important restorative materials used by the dental profession.

It is a great credit to his intellect and ability that some of his philosophy is only now being challenged; especially in the light of what we know now compared to the turn of the century. It is a lesson the dental profession will have to learn over and over again as new materials are brought onto the market (see *Table 1*).

## Summary

As can be noted from the preceding discussion, there are numerous restorative techniques that the dentist needs to learn. In addition, dentists use a wide variety of different materials, some being hard and stiff and others being soft and flexible.

It is important that the dentist fully appreciates the various features of these materials, what it is that makes them so useful for dental applic-ations, and what their limitations are. Only then will the dentist be able to select the most appropriate material for a particular application.

## Further Reading

Greener E. H. (1979) Amalgam: yesterday, today and tomorrow. Oper. Dent. **4**, 24

Jacobsen P. H. (1980) The influence of dental materials on conservative dentistry. Dental Update **7**, 285–291

Little D. A. (1982) The relevance of prosthodontics and the science of dental materials to the practice of dentistry. J. Dent. **10**, 300–310

Phillips R. W. (1976) Future role of biomaterials in dentistry and dental education. J. Dent. Educ. **40**, 752–756

van Noort R. (1985) In defence of dental materials. Brit. Dent. J. **158**, 358–360

Williams H. A. (1976) The challenge tomorrow in dental care delivery. J. Dent . Educ. **40**, 587

Woodforde J. (1971) *The strange story of false teeth* Universal-Tandom Publ. Co., London

# ATOMIC BUILDING BLOCKS

## Introduction

All materials are built up from atoms and molecules, so it is not really surprising that there is a close relationship between the atomic basis of a material and its properties. Important in this context are the nature of the atoms and the ways in which they are arranged. The atoms combine to determine the microstructure of the solid, and, as a consequence, determine its properties. Therefore, if we are to understand the properties of materials we need to have an understanding of the way atoms can combine to make solids.

## Joining Atoms Together

When two atoms are brought together they may link to form a molecule; any bonds that form are called *primary bonds*. Alternatively, they may move apart and so retain their individual identity.

The controlling factor in bond formation is energy, and a bond will only form if it results in a lowering of the total energy of the atoms being joined, i.e., if the total energy of the molecule is less than the sum of the energies of the separate atoms, irrespective of the type of bond being formed. A simple way of visualising this, is the energy–separation diagram; it is arrived at by

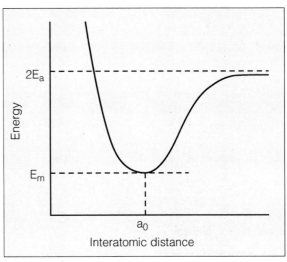

**1** Energy separation curve for two atoms, each of energy $E_a$.

considering what effect moving two atoms closer together will have on their total energy. A typical energy–separation curve is shown in **1**.

When the two atoms are far apart, the total energy is $2E_a$, where $E_a$ is the total energy of one atom. As they are brought closer together, the total energy begins to fall, until it reaches a minimum, $E_m$, at a distance $a_o$. Thereafter, as the atoms are brought more closely together, the total energy increases due to repulsion between their clouds of electrons As the atoms are brought even closer together their nuclei begin to

11

repel each other as well, but such proximity is not usually achived in normalcircumstances. Thus, we have attraction at long range, and repulsion at short range .

The conditions under which two atoms will bond together depends upon the atoms' electron configurations, which completely determine their chemical reactivity. The more stable the electron configuration, the less reactive the atom; the extremes of stability being the 'inert gases' such as argon, helium and neon, which are almost totally unreactive. Their near-inertness is caused by their having complete outermost electron orbitals, with no opportunity for more electrons to 'join' the atom, and no 'spare' or 'loose' electrons to leave the atom.

All atoms try to reach their lowest energy state, and this is tantamount to having a complete outermost electron orbital, as the inert gases have. The atoms of some elements have 'gaps' for electrons in their outermost orbits, whereas the atoms of other elements have 'spare' electrons in their outermost orbits. By combining with each other, these two different types of atoms can both achieve complete outermost orbitals. The formation of bonds, therefore, involves only the outermost *valence* electrons.

# Types Of Primary Bonds

There are three types of primary bonds: *covalent*, *ionic* and *metallic*.

## *Covalent Bonds*

The covalent bond is the simplest and strongest bond, and arises when atoms share their electrons so that each electron shell achieves an inert gas structure. The formation of such a bond for two hydrogen atoms is shown in **2**.

As the two atoms approach one another and the orbitals of the electrons begin to overlap, a molecular orbital is formed where the two electrons are shared between the two nuclei. Since the electrons will spend most of their time in the region where the orbitals overlap, the bond is highly directional.

## *Ionic Bonds*

An atom such as sodium would like to lose its single valence electron, as this would give it a

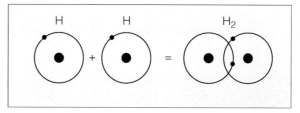

**2** Two hydrogen atoms combine through covalent bonding to form hydrogen gas.

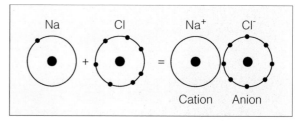

**3** Formation of an ionic bond between sodium and chlorine.

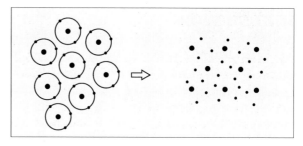

**4** Formation of a metallic bond, showing a cloud of electrons surrounding the nuclei.

configuration similar to that of neon. Naturally, it can not do so unless there is another atom nearby which will readily accept the electron.

Elements which can attain an inert gas structure by acquiring a single extra electron are fluorine, chlorine, bromine and iodine, collectively known as the halogens. Thus, if a sodium and chlorine atom are allowed to interact, there is a complete transfer of the valence electron from the sodium atom to the chlorine atom. Both attain an inert gas structure with sodium having a positive charge due to loss of a negative electron and chlorine a negative charge due to its acquisition of the extra electron. These two ions will be attracted to one another because of their opposite electrical charges, and there is a reduction in the total energy of the pair as they approach. This is shown in the model in **3**; such bonds are called ionic bonds.

An important difference between the covalent bond and ionic bond is that the latter is not directional. This is because ionic bonds are a result of the electrostatic fields that surround ions, and these fields will interact with any other ions in the vicinity.

## Metallic Bonds

The third primary bond is the metallic bond. It occurs when there is a large aggregate of atoms, usually in a solid, which readily give up the electrons in their valence shells. In such a situation, the electrons can move about quite freely through the solid, spending their time moving from atom to atom. The electron orbitals in the metallic bond have a lower energy than the electron orbitals of the individual atoms. This is because the valence electrons are always closer to one or other nucleus than would be the case in an isolated atom. The atoms are surrounded by a cloud of electrons as shown in **4.** Like the ionic bond, this bond is non-directional.

## Bond Energies

An important feature of a bond is the *bond energy*. This is the amount of energy that has to be supplied to separate the two atoms, and is equal to $2E_a - E_m$, as defined in **1.** Typical bond energies for each of the three types of bond are given in *Table 2*.

A general feature that can be seen from the bond energies is that the covalent bonds tend to be the strongest, followed by the ionic bonds, and then finally the metallic bonds. For the metallic bonds, there is a wide range of bond energies, with some approaching that of ionic bonds, and some being very low. Mercury has a very low bond energy, giving a bond that is not even strong enough to hold the atoms in place at room temperature, resulting in mercury's liquidity at this temperature.

# The Formation Of Bulk Solids

## Ionic Solids

Ions are surrounded by non-directional electrostatic fields, and it is possible that the positively and negatively charged ions can find positional arrangements that are mutually beneficial, from the point of view of reaching a lower energy. The ions can form a regular, three-dimensional network, with the example of sodium chloride being shown in **5.**

Ionic substances such as chlorides, nitrides and oxides of metals are the basic building blocks of a group of materials known as *ceramics,*

| Table 2 Typical bond energies for the three bond types. | | |
|---|---|---|
| Atoms bonded | Bond type | Bond energy (eV) |
| C–C | | 6.3 |
| C–F | | 5.6 |
| H–H | Covalent | 4.5 |
| H–O | | 4.4 |
| C–Cl | | 4.0 |
| Na–Cl | | 4.2 |
| K–Br | Ionic | 3.9 |
| Na–I | | 3.2 |
| Au–Au | | 2.3 |
| Cu–Cu | | 2.0 |
| Ag–Ag | Metallic | 1.8 |
| Pb–Pb | | 0.8 |
| Hg–Hg | | 0.2 |

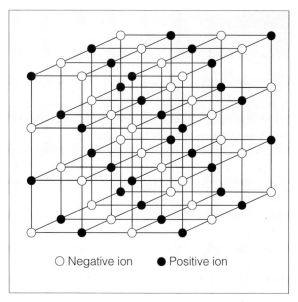

○ Negative ion    ● Positive ion

**5** Formation of a bulk solid, through the ionic bonding of sodium (●) and chlorine ions (○).

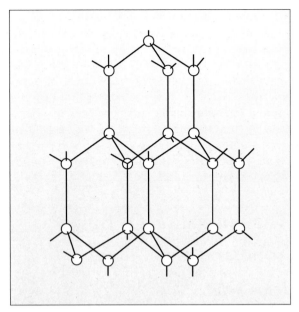

**6** The structure of diamond, showing the three-dimensional network built up from the tetrahedrally arranged bonds of carbon.

of which a rather special group are the *glasses* (see section I.IV). These materials are very stable because of their high ionic bond strengths.

## Metallic Solids

A similar arrangement to that of the ionic solids is possible with the metallic bond. In this case, there is no strong electrostatic attraction between the individual atoms (as there was between the ions in the ionic solids), as they are held together by the cloud of electrons; this cloud forms the basis of the *metals* which are discussed in section I.V.

## Covalent Solids

There are only a few instances in which atoms of the same element join by covalent bonds to form a solid; these are carbon, silicon and germanium. It is the directionality of the covalent bond that is the essential difference between it and the other two primary bonds. This directionality places severe constraints on the possible arrangements of the atoms.

An example of a covalently bonded solid is diamond, which is a form of carbon. Carbon has an arrangement of electrons in its outer shell such that it needs four more electrons to obtain a configuration similar to neon; in the case of diamond, it achieves this by sharing electrons with neighbouring carbon atoms. The direction of these bonds is such that they are directed towards the four corners of a tetrahedron with the carbon atom's nucleus at its centre. The three–dimensional structure of diamond can be built up as shown in **6**.

Covalent solids consisting of a single element tend to be very rare. Covalent bonds are more usually formed between dissimilar elements where each takes up an inert gas configuration. Once the elements have reacted to form these bonds, the created molecule becomes highly unreactive towards molecules of the same type, and does not provide a basis for the formation of a three-dimensional network.

The electron orbitals overlap and the electrons are shared, resulting in a filled orbital which is very stable. In this configuration, there are no partially filled orbitals available for further bonding by primary bonding mechanisms. Thus, covalently bonded elements result in stable molecules, and most elements which join by covalent bonding tend to be gases or liquids, e.g. water, oxygen and hydrogen. Of these examples, water will solidify at 0°C, and for this to be possible there must be some additional attraction between the water molecules; something must hold these molecules together, but it is not primary bonding.

## Secondary Bonding

A consequence of the sharing of electrons by two or more atomic nuclei is that the electrons will spend a disproportionately longer time in one particular position. The effect of this is that one end of the molecule may acquire a slight positive charge and the other end a slight negative charge, resulting in an electrical imbalance known as an *electric dipole*. These dipoles allow molecules to interact with one another, and to form weak bonds called *van der Waal's bonds*. The three main factors which contribute to these relatively weak interactions are:

- Interactions between permanent dipoles.
- Interactions between induced dipoles.
- Interactions between instantaneous dipoles.

The latter, known as the *London Dispersion Effect*, is completely general, and operates whenever two molecules, ions or atoms are in close contact. It is the result of an interaction between random motions of the electrons in the two species.

A special case of the dipole–dipole interaction is the hydrogen bond. The hydrogen atom can be imagined as a proton on the end of a covalent bond, but, unlike other atoms, the positive charge of the proton is not shielded by surrounding electrons. Therefore, it will have a positive charge and will be attracted to the electrons of atoms in other molecules. A necessary condition for the formation of a hydrogen bond is that an electronegative atom should be in the neighbourhood of the hydrogen atom, which is itself bonded to an electronegative atom. An example of this is ice, where there is an interaction between the hydrogen atom in one molecule and the oxygen atom in another molecule, shown schematically in **7**.

The bond strength is only about 0.4 eV, and is readily overcome by heating above 0°C. The hydrogen bond is important because it accounts for the extensive adsorption possible by organic molecules, including proteins, and is therefore considered essential to the life processes. Secondary bonding forms the basis of the molecular attraction in molecular solids.

## Molecular Solids

It is possible to create a wide variety of different molecules, some of which can be solid at room temperature. If the molecules are sufficiently large, they are bonded together due to numerous dipole–dipole interactions. The low bond strength means that such solids will have very low melting temperatures, and the upper limit for molecular solids is approximately 100°C.

The best way to appreciate how these solids are formed is through a group of molecules known as the linear alkanes. These are based on a straight chain of hydrocarbons, with the general formula $C_nH_{2n+2}$, where n can be any positive integer. The simplest of these is methane ($CH_4$) which has n=1. If we strip one of the hydrogen atoms from each of two methane molecules and join the molecules together through a carbon–carbon bond, we get ethane. We can continue to repeat this process and obtain very large molecules indeed (**8**).

Once the number of –$CH_2$– groups become very large, there is very little change in the

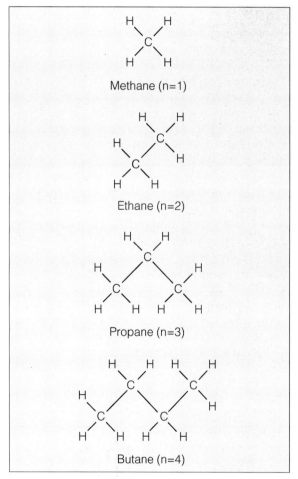

**7** Hydrogen bond formation in ice.

Methane (n=1)

Ethane (n=2)

Propane (n=3)

Butane (n=4)

**8** The first four members of the alkane family, which are straight-chain hydrocarbons, following the general formula $C_nH_{2n+2}$.

properties of these materials, which are known collectively as *polymethylene*. This name is derived from the word *poly* meaning *many* and the basic structural unit on which it is based, *methylene*. A material with this type of structure

15

is known as a *polymer* since it consists of many repeat units called *mers*. How polymers can form a variety of solid structures will be discussed in detail in section I.VI.

# The Structural Arrangement Of Atoms In Solids

Whereas the forces of attraction hold atoms close together, the mutual repulsion of the nuclei means that an equilibrium spacing is attained at which these forces balance. This interatomic spacing is presented as $a_o$ in **3**.

An external force is needed to move the atoms closer together or further apart. This interatomic spacing is the configuration of minimum energy, and in order to achieve this there is a tendency for the atoms to adopt a regular close-packed arrangement. If one considers atoms to be spheres, it is possible to use the analogy of ball bearings packed in a box. The densest packing of the ball bearings is obtained when they are arranged in a regular symmetrical manner as is shown in **9**. When atoms are arranged like this the material is said to be *crystalline*.

The important feature of a crystalline structure is that from the viewpoint of any atom in the structure, the arrangement of its neighbouring atoms is identical. Metals and ionic solids are usually crystalline at room temperature. Any solid in which there is no symmetry of the atoms is said to be *amorphous*.

## Crystal Structures

One of the simplest arrangements of atoms is the simple cube, in which the atoms occupy the eight corner positions.

Using the model of spheres for atoms again, this arrangement is shown in **10a**. Each sphere touches its nearest neighbour, such that the length of the side of the cube is equal to the diameter of the atom. If we consider a simple cube, containing only a portion of the atoms within it, as shown in **10b**, we get what is known as the *structural cell*. By stacking these structural cells one on top of the other, a whole three-dimensional solid can be built up.

Some of the space of the structural unit is not occupied by the atoms. The fraction of space occupied by the atoms is called the *packing factor* and is easily calculated.

If we assume that each side of the cube is of length a, then the volume of the structural cell is $a^3$. Correspondingly, the radius of each sphere must be a, and its volume will be given by $4/3 \pi a^3$. Each sphere actually only contributes 1/8 of its volume to the structural cell, but since there are eight such segments, the spheres within the cube occupy a total volume of $4/3 \pi a^3$. Thus, the packing factor for a simple cube is given by:

$$\text{packing factor} = \frac{\text{volume of atoms inside the cube}}{\text{volume of cube}}$$

$$= \frac{4}{3} \frac{\pi a^3}{(2a)^3}$$

$$= \frac{\pi}{6} = 0.54$$

This indicates that nearly 50% of the space is free.

It is in fact possible for other smaller atoms to occupy this free space without causing too much disruption to the crystalline structure, and this is something which we will return to later. Given the large amount of free space in this simple structure it is perhaps not surprising that there are other atomic arrangements where the packing factor is higher.

Two such arrangements that commonly occur in metals, are the body-centred cubic (BCC) and the face-centred cubic (FCC) configurations, which are shown in **11**. The packing factors for

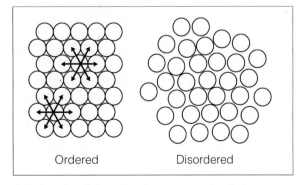

Ordered        Disordered

**9** Ordered and disordered arrangements of atoms.

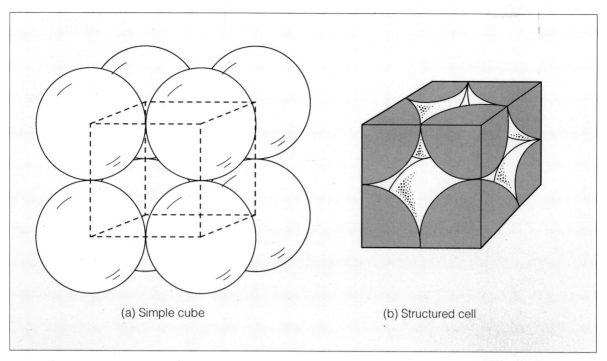

(a) Simple cube          (b) Structured cell

**10** The simple cubic structure (a) and its structural cell (b).

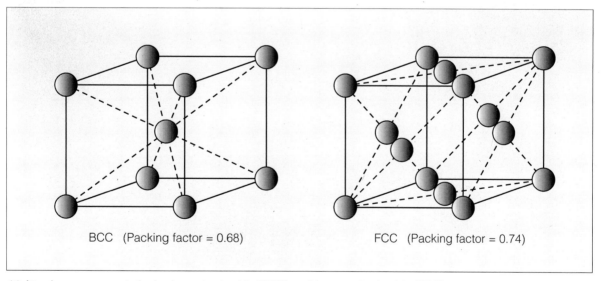

BCC   (Packing factor = 0.68)         FCC   (Packing factor = 0.74)

**11** Atomic arrangements for body-centred cubic (BCC) and face-centred cubic (FCC) structures.

these two structures are 0.68 and 0.74 for the BCC and FCC structures respectively. With these larger packing factors it is of course more difficult for smaller atoms to occupy the free space without upsetting the structure.

## Summary

In a sense it is not surprising to find that there are three main groups of solids based on the three types of primary bonding, namely:

- Ceramics – based on the ionic bond, which can exist in the crystalline and amorphous form, the latter being *glasses*.
- Metals – based on the metallic bond.
- Molecular solids – based on the covalent and secondary bonds, and including an important group of materials known as polymers.

There is one other important group of materials not as yet mentioned. These are the *composites*, which are based on a combination of two or more of the above solids.

There are many examples of composite materials, both natural and synthetic. Bone and dentine are natural composites, whose main constituents are collagen (a polymer), and apatite (a ceramic). Synthetic composites include glass fibre, reinforced polymers, and polymers containing ceramic particles. A dental example of the latter are the composite restorative materials discussed in section II.II.

# I.IV

# THE STRUCTURE OF CERAMICS

## Introduction

Ceramics are compounds of metallic elements, and non-metallic substances such as oxides, nitrides and silicates. Ceramics can appear as either crystalline or amorphous solids, the latter group being called glasses.

In ceramics, the negatively charged ions (*anions*) are often significantly different in size from the positively charged ions (*cations*). An example already considered is that of sodium chloride, which has a face-centred cubic structure.

The chlorine ions take up positions at the lattice points of the FCC arrangement, with the sodium ions adopting positions between the chlorine ions, in what are called *interstitial positions*. The sodium ions are able to do this because they are considerably smaller than the chlorine ions, and fit into the free space left between them. The exact lattice structure is shown in **12**. Another example of this type of structure is zinc oxide, which is widely used in dentistry. There are many other applications of ceramics in dentistry; they are used as fillers for composite resins, in glass-ionomer cements, and in investments and porcelains.

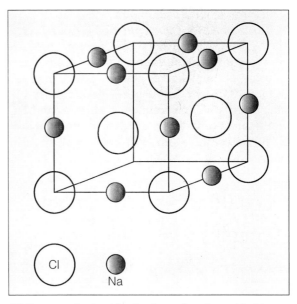

**12** Face-centred cubic structure of sodium chloride.

## Ceramic Raw Materials

Silica ($SiO_2$) forms the basis of many ceramics. Although it has a simple chemical formula, it is a versatile material and can exist in many different forms.

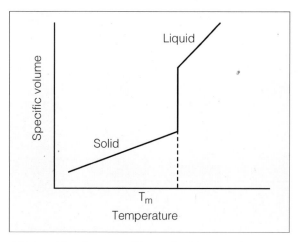

**13** Transition from a solid to a liquid, where $T_m$ is the melting temperature.

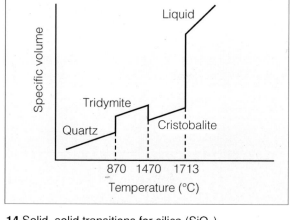

**14** Solid–solid transitions for silica ($SiO_2$).

Silica occurs as a crystalline material in the forms of quartz, crystobalite and tridymite, or as a glass as in the example of fused quartz.

It is the basis for the formation of many complex ceramic formulations, particularly in combination with aluminium oxide with which it forms alumino-silicate glasses, which are used in glass–ionomer cements. Similarly, feldspatic glasses are used in ceramic restorations, and are compounds containing oxides of aluminium and silicon in combination with potassium, sodium or calcium (e.g. $NaAlSi_3O_8$).

# Crystalline And Amorphous Ceramics

## Crystal Transitions

When a solid is heated it can undergo a number of transformations, the most easily recognisable of which is when the solid melts. This change of a crystal from solid to liquid is known as the *crystal melting transition*, and is accompanied by a change in the volume of the material. The volume can be monitored to allow one to detect such transformations.

A simple means of representing this change is to plot the specific volume of the material (i.e. the volume of a unit mass of the material) against the temperature. A curve such as that shown in **13** results, and at the melting point of

the crystal, there is a discrete (i.e. at a specific temperature) discontinuity in the specific volume.

The specific volume is effectively the inverse of the density. This specific volume–temperature curve shows that one effect of the melting of the crystal is an increase in the volume. This is not surprising when one thinks that this transition is one from an ordered crystalline structure to that of a disordered liquid; the packing density of the atoms in the liquid will be considerably less than that in the crystalline solid.

The specific volume–temperature curve for crystalline silica is as shown in **14**. In this example, there are a number of solid–solid transitions as well as the usual transition from solid to liquid. At room temperature, silica is in the form of quartz, but this changes into tridymite at 870°C. A further transformation takes place at 1471°C, where tridymite changes to crystobalite, and the crystobalite finally melts at 1713°C. Thus, it is possible to detect both solid–solid and solid–liquid transitions.

## Glass Transitions

When an amorphous solid such as a glass is heated, it does not show a discrete solid–liquid transition as the material is not crystalline. Instead, what happens is that at some point there is an increase in the rate of change of the specific volume as shown in **15**. The temperature at which this change in the slope of the specific volume occurs is known as the *glass transition*

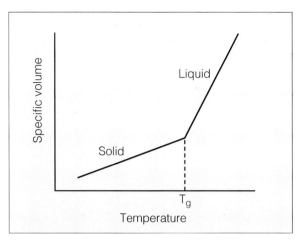

**15** The variation of specific volume with temperature for an amorphous solid.

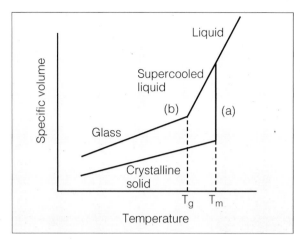

**16** Cooling curves for a material that can form a crystalline solid (a) or a glass (b).

*temperature*, $T_g$. This is generally (although not always) the case for molecular solids as well.

A consequence of this is that there is no *sudden* increase in the volume (and hence the unoccupied volume). Instead, there is a *gradual* increase in the volume, with the rate of increase becoming more rapid above the glass transition temperature.

The converse of this is that a liquid which cools without forming a crystalline structure will contain a large amount of unoccupied volume. Solids which are formed by moving through a glass transition rather than a crystal melting transition will be amorphous, and are referred to as *glasses*. Glasses are an important group of materials and warrant some special attention.

# The Formation Of A Glass

Given their regular shapes, atoms tend to form ordered structures. Small molecules, such as methane, are able to form crystal structures easily, and even some of the higher order linear alkanes can form crystalline structures if the molecule is regarded as a rigid rod. Once we get to larger, more complex molecules, however, regular arrangements become more difficult to achieve. Thus, large irregular molecules, have a high probability of forming a glass on solidification.

For crystal growth to occur *nuclei of crystallisation* must be present. These are usually in the

form of impurities, such as dust particles, that are virtually impossible to exclude. Thus, if there is any chance that the material can take up an ordered crystalline arrangement, it will usually do so.

Silica can form either glasses or crystalline solids, and their specific volume–temperature curves are shown in **16**. When crystallisation occurs on cooling (curve a), there is a sharp, discrete reduction in the specific volume. This contraction is due to 'configurational contraction', as there is a large increase in the packing fraction when changing from a disordered liquid to an ordered crystalline solid. Once this sharp contraction has been completed, the material continues to contract by normal thermal contraction.

If crystallisation did not occur, the material would follow curve b; the liquid continues to contract, partly by normal thermal contraction and partly by configurational contraction. The liquid takes up a less open structure, but there is no discrete jump in the specific volume. Below $T_m$, it forms an unstable *supercooled* liquid. This contraction continues as the temperature drops, until $T_g$, the glass transition temperature, is reached, whereupon the rate of contraction slows down markedly. At this point, the configurational contraction has stopped and only normal thermal contraction is taking place.

What happens at the glass transition temperature is that the supercooled liquid has become so viscous that configurational changes can no

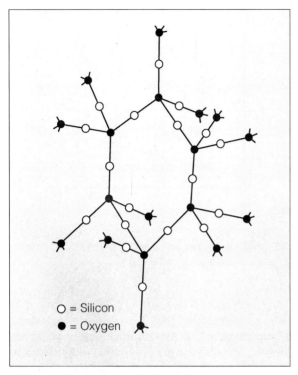

**17** Crystalline structure of cristobalite.

○ = Silicon
● = Oxygen

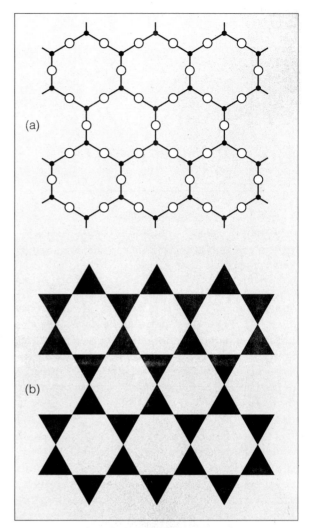

**18** Two-dimensional representation of crystalline silica: (a) position of atoms, (b) oxygen triangles.

longer take place, and the liquid structure has been frozen in. The temperature at which this occurs is not a sharply defined point, but is a range of temperatures of some 50°C, represented by the bend in the curve.

Once the supercooled liquid has cooled to below its glass transition temperature, it is now described as a *glass*. It is interesting to note that the viscosity at which this occurs is roughly the same for all glasses, about $10^{12}$ Pa, although the temperature at which this happens can vary from -89°C for glycerine to over 1500°C for pure silica glass. The distinction between a super-cooled liquid and a glass is that the latter has a viscosity greater than $10^{12}$ Pa.

The term *transformation temperature* is somewhat of a misnomer, since no transformation actually occurs at this temperature. The configurational changes are still taking place at temperatures below $T_g$, it is just that the rate of change is now so small, because of the high viscosity, that to all intents and purposes it has stopped. The transition temperature, i.e. the temperature at which a glass that is being cooled effectively ceases to undergo configurational changes, is sometimes referred to as the *fictive temperature* of the glass. It is the temperature below which there is no spontaneous tendency for the glass to become more dense.

The question is: '*What happens at $T_m$ that determines whether the crystal or glass forming route is followed?*'

When silica melts, it produces an extremely viscous liquid, which means that the molecules can only move past one another very slowly. This is not conducive to the formation of a crystalline solid, since crystallisation requires a substantial and rapid rearrangement of the molecules. Any crystal nuclei present will therefore tend to grow very slowly, especially given

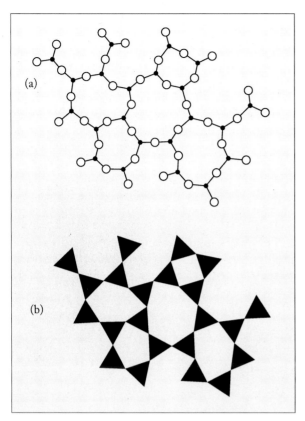

**19** Two-dimensional representation of a pure silica glass: (a) position of atoms, (b) oxygen triangles.

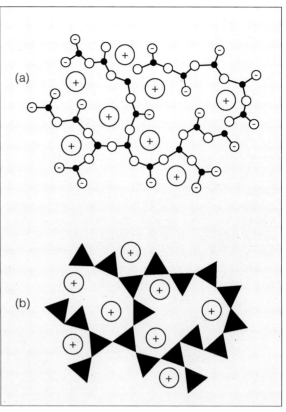

**20** Two dimensional representation of a mixed oxide glass: (a) position of atoms, (b) oxygen triangles.

the complex structure of crystalline silica which is similar to that of diamond. Thus, if the liquid is cooled quickly, the solid formed is likely to be a glass. The process of forming a glass is called *vitrification*.

## Glass Formers

The essential component that allows the formation of glass is silica, which can itself become either a glass or a crystalline solid on cooling. Cristobalite, one of the crystalline forms of silica, has a tetrahedron as its basic unit, with an oxygen atom at each corner and a silicon atom in the centre, as shown in **17**.

This is a rather complex structure to use when visualising the development of a glass, and the formation process can be understood more simply by considering a two-dimensional representation, in which one bond is missing from each of the atoms in the silica (**18**).

When molten silica is cooled rapidly, the crystalline structure does not have time to form so the silica solidifies as a glass, which is called fused quartz (**19**). The high melting point of this material, 1713°C makes it too expensive for general use. If certain metal oxides are mixed with the silica, the melting temperature is greatly reduced.

As an example, a composition of three-quarters silica and one-quarter sodium oxide will melt at only 1339°C. Such glasses are called *mixed oxide glasses* and their structure is shown in **20**. The metal atoms form positive ions that disrupt the oxygen tetrahedra such that not all of the oxygen atoms are shared. The silica plays the role of a *glass former* and the metal oxide acts as a *glass modifier*.

Oxides of titanium, zinc, lead and aluminium can all take part in the formation of the glassy network, and produce stiff network structures.

23

Soda (Na$_2$O) and lime (CaO) lower the viscosity, and thus the glass transition temperature, considerably, by causing extensive disruption of the network. This eases the production of the glass. Boric oxide (B$_2$O$_3$) is also capable of acting as a glass former, producing boron glasses.

Although it is possible to make glasses from mixtures of crystalline silica and metal oxides, this is an expensive approach. It is much cheaper to use naturally occurring minerals with the required glassy structure, because nature has already carried out the vitrification process.

At one time, only naturally occurring feldspars were used by manufacturers, and these were modified with other metallic oxides to produce fillers and dental porcelains with the required properties. Nowadays, many glasses are produced synthetically, as this allows greater control over the composition and properties.

# Devitrification

A small amount of crystallisation always occurs in the production of a glass, although the rate of the crystals' growth is very low.

When a glass begins to crystallise, the process is called *devitrification*. It may happen when the glass is kept at an elevated temperature for a long time, allowing some reorganisation of the molecules. The glass will tend to take on a translucent appearance, due to the scattering of light from the surfaces of the small crystals. This is the basis of the formation of glass ceramics (see section III.IV).

The process of heating a material to allow molecular or atomic rearrangement is called *annealing* and is important in many types of materials.

# I.V

# THE STRUCTURE OF METALS AND ALLOYS

## The Microstructure Of Metals

Metals consist of aggregates of atoms regularly arranged in a crystalline structure. Whereas so far we have considered the formation of single crystals, metals will not usually solidify (from what is known as the *melt*) as a single crystal, but are instead formed from a multitude of small crystals.

This happens because there are usually many *nuclei of crystallisation* scattered throughout the molten metal. Such nuclei may form when four atoms lose sufficient thermal energy, and become able to form a unit cell. These unit cells will grow as more metal atoms reach a low enough energy to join on, and hence crystal formation occurs. This process is known as homogeneous nucleation. It requires highly specialised equipment to grow a single crystal of metal from the entire melt.

More commonly, solidification is initiated by the presence of impurities in the melt. As the temperature drops below the melting point, metal atoms will deposit on these impurities and crystals begin to form. This process is known as heterogeneous nucleation. The crystals (or *grains*, as they are called) will continue to grow until all of the metal has solidified. During their growth they will begin to impinge on one another, giving rise to boundaries between the crystals

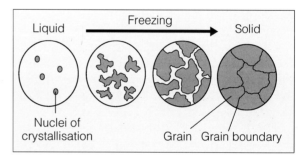

**21** Solidification of a metal.

where the atoms are irregularly arranged. This boundary is called the *grain boundary*, and is essentially a defect in the crystal structure of the metal.

The process of solidification of a metal is shown schematically in **21**. A fine grain size is usually desirable in a metal because it raises the yield stress, but the reason for this will not be considered now. One way in which to promote a finer grain size is rapid solidification, as used in the casting of dental gold alloys into an investment mould that is held at a temperature well below the melting temperature of the alloy. Alternatively, the presence of many nucleating sites will give rise to a fine grain size. This method is also employed in dental gold alloys by the addition of iridium. The iridium provides many sites for nucleation and acts as a grain refining ingredient.

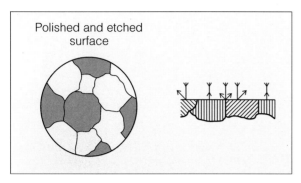

**22** Reflection of incident light from an etched metal surface.

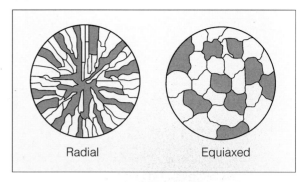

**23** Grain structures arising from different conditions at solidification.

It is very useful to be able to study the detailed structure of metals, in terms of the sizes of the crystals, their shape and their composition, because this information can tell us a lot about the properties of the metal and how it was made. Some idea of the structure can be obtained by examining the metal surface under a light-reflecting optical microscope.

Light is reflected from a polished metal surface, but the fraction of the incident light that is reflected from any region will depend on surface irregularities, as irregularities will cause the light to be scattered.

The action of chemicals on a polished surface (known as *etching*) can also reduce the amount of light reflected. A suitably chosen chemical will preferentially attack certain regions of the metal surface. These areas tend to be under high local stress, such as at the grain boundaries, where there is imperfect packing of the atoms. In effect, a groove is produced that will scatter the incident light and therefore show up as a dark line.

This effect is shown in **22** for a metal which has a very uniform grain structure. All the grains are of roughly the same size and shape; such a grain structure is described as *equiaxed*. Many other shapes and sizes of grains are possible, and these properties often depend on the methods employed during solidification. For example, if molten metal is poured into a mould with a square or circular cross-section that is held at a temperature well below the melting temperature of the metal, the grains could look something like that depicted in **23**. Crystal growth will have proceeded from the walls of the mould towards the centre.

Many metals are readily deformed, especially in their elemental (i.e. pure) form. This allows them to be shaped by hammering, rolling, pressing or drawing through a die. A large casting, known as an ingot, can thus be turned into any desired shape, be it a wing-panel for a car, the shell of a boat, or a wire.

When deformed in this way, the metal is said to be *wrought*. If we were to examine the microstructure of a wire under the optical microscope it would be seen to have a structure similar to that shown in **24**. The grains have been elongated in the direction of drawing, and have taken on a laminar structure. Thus, from looking at the microstructure of the metal we can gain a lot of information.

# Alloys

Elemental metals are not generally of much use, because of the severe limitations in their properties. Most metals in common use are a mixture of two or more metallic elements, sometimes with non-metallic elements included. They are usually produced by fusion of the elements above their melting temperatures. Such a mixture of two or more metals or metalloids is called an *alloy*. Two elements would constitute a *binary alloy* and a mixture of three is called a *ternary alloy*.

An alloy will often consist of a number of distinct solid phases, where a phase is defined as a structurally homogeneous part of the system that is separated from other parts by a definite physical boundary. Each phase will have its own distinct structure and associated properties.

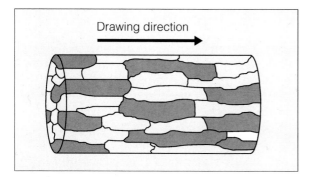

**24** Elongated grains of a metal drawn into a wire.

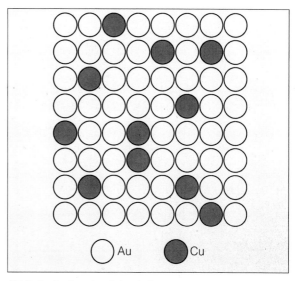

**25** Substitutional solid solution.

The commonly cited phases are the gas, liquid and solid phases, as these are markedly different from one another. A substance can exhibit several phases.

For example, water would be considered a single phase structure, whereas a mixture of water and oil would consist of two phases. Sand would be considered a single phase system, even though it is made up of lots of individual particles, since each particle of sand is identical.

A phase may have more than one component, as does saline for instance, which is an aqueous solution of sodium chloride. Similarly, phases in metals can consist of a mixture of metals. Copper can contain up to 40% zinc without destroying its FCC structure. Such a *solid solution*, as it is called, will satisfy some special conditions (see below).

# Solid Phases

When two different elements are mixed together, the resultant material can be a single-phase alloy or a multi-phase alloy. Which of these is formed depends on the solubility of the one element in the other, and this is governed by the crystalline nature of the elements, and their relative sizes.

There are essentially three different phases which can form in alloys; these are a pure metal, a solid solution or an inter-metallic compound. Of these, the solid solution and the inter-metallic compound require further description.

## Solid Solutions

A solid solution is a mixture of elements at the atomic level, and is analogous to a mixture of

liquids which are soluble in one another. There are two types of solid solutions: substitutional and interstitial.

### Substitutional Solid Solution

If the solute atom can substitute directly for the solvent atom at the normal lattice sites of the crystal, a substitutional solid solution of the two elements will be formed. This will only be possible if:

- The atoms have a similar valency.
- The atoms have the same crystal structure (e.g. FCC).
- The atomic sizes are within 15% of each other.

A dentally relevant example of such a system is a mixture of gold and copper (**25**).

Adding any amount of copper will always give a solid solution. Thus, a *substitutional solid solution* can be made to range from 100% gold to 100% copper. This is because the above conditions are met by these two metals (*Table 3*).

| Table 3 Properties of gold and copper. | | | |
|---|---|---|---|
| Element | Atomic diameter (Å) | Crystal structure | Valence |
| Au | 2.882 | FCC | 1 or 3 |
| Cu | 2.556 | FCC | 1 or 2 |

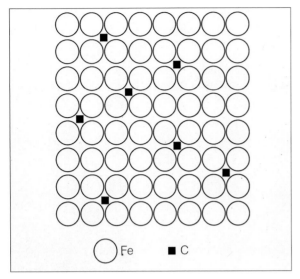

**26** Interstitial solid solution.

Other metals which readily form solid solutions with gold are platinum (2.775Å), palladium (2.750Å) and silver (2.888Å), all of which have a FCC crystal structure.

### Interstitial Solid Solution

As the name implies, an interstitial solid solution is achieved when the solute atoms are able to take up the space in between the solvent atoms. For this to occur, the solute atom must of course be much smaller than the solvent atom. In practice, the diameter of the solute atom must be less than 60% of the diameter of the solvent atom. This is illustrated for the example of a type of steel that contains a small amount of carbon in iron (**26**).

The interstitial space is usually very limited, and some distortion of the lattice will occur to accommodate the extra atoms. Other elements which readily form interstitial solid solutions are hydrogen, nitrogen and boron.

## *Inter-Metallic Compounds*

An inter-metallic compound is formed when two or more metals combine, forming a specific composition or stoichiometric ratio. Examples of metals with specific stoichiometric compositions are some of the phases in the alloy used in the production of a a dental amalgam; the alloy may contain regions of a Ag–Sn phase ($Ag_3Sn$), and a Cu–Sn phase ($Cu_6Sn_5$).

# Phase Diagrams

Alloys can consist of a wide number of different phases, depending on the composition and temperature, and a means of representing this graphically has been developed, in what is known as a *phase diagram*.

Such a diagram indicates the phases (including the liquid phase) that are present at any given temperature, for any given composition of the alloy.

## *Solid Solutions*

The simplest phase diagrams to understand are the binary phase diagrams.

An example of a phase diagram for such a simple system is shown in **27**. This phase diagram is for copper and nickel; the vertical axis represents the temperature, and the horizontal axis the composition. Copper and nickel are so close in characteristics that they readily substitute for one another in the crystal lattice, and form an example of a substitutional solid solution. Hence, throughout the compositional range from pure copper to pure nickel, only a single phase occurs.

Whereas one might expect the melting temperature of such an alloy to fall somewhere between that of pure copper and pure nickel, it is not immediately obvious why there should be region where there is a mixture of liquid and solid. The line which defines the transition from pure liquid to a mixture of liquid and solid is called the *liquidus* and the line which separates the mixture of solid and liquid from the solid is known as the *solidus*.

When a pure metal solidifies, the transformation from a liquid to solid takes place at a well defined discrete temperature; this is the characteristic melting temperature of the metal. If a temperature–time curve were constructed for such a metal as it cooled, it would look like **28**.

The plateau spans the period during which the metal is solidifying, and the liquidus and solidus are effectively one and the same point. The reason for this plateau is the release of energy (in the form of heat) during the solidification process, which maintains the metal at a constant temperature. This energy is called the *latent heat of fusion*.

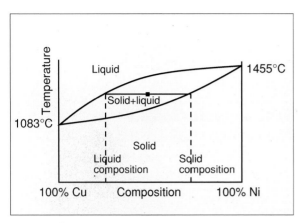

27 Equilibrium phase diagram for the Cu–Ni system, where a 50Cu:50Ni composition at 1300°C produces a mixture of a copper-rich liquid and a nickel-rich solid.

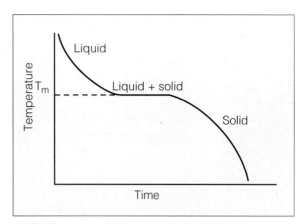

28 Cooling curve for a pure metal.

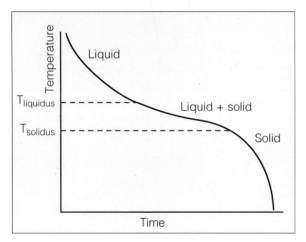

29 Cooling curve for an alloy.

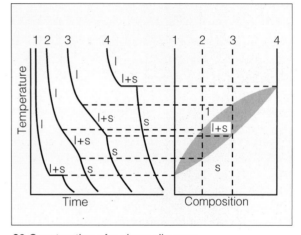

30 Construction of a phase diagram.

When two metals are mixed to form an alloy, the cooling curve looks quite different (29), as the alloy solidifies over a a range of temperatures. The liquidus and solidus are now separate points on the cooling curve.

The reason for the extended temperature range covering the transition from liquid to solid for an alloy of copper and nickel is that the copper and nickel atoms are not identical. As a consequence, in the region between the melting temperatures of the two metals, a copper-rich liquid and a nickel-rich solid are the most stable compounds.

For instance, for a 50:50 composition at 1300°C, solid nickel can not contain more than 37 w/o copper. Any copper atoms above the 37

w/o level will therefore appear in the liquid phase, mixed with the remaining nickel. Such a mixture of solid and liquid provides a lower free energy than a single phase alone.

In effect, the solidus and liquidus represent the limits of solubility, and it is these which form the basis of the phase diagram. By creating a series of the cooling curves shown in 29 for a range of compositions, it is possible to build up the phase diagram as shown schematically in 30.

As the temperature of the 50:50 composition is reduced, so the solubility of copper in nickel increases, until, at approximately 1220°C, all of the available copper can be dissolved in the nickel, and a single solid phase is the most stable configuration.

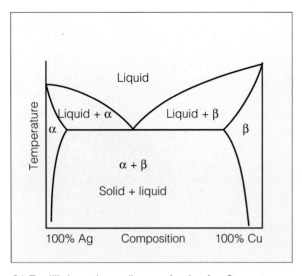

**31** Equilibrium phase diagram for the Ag–Cu system.

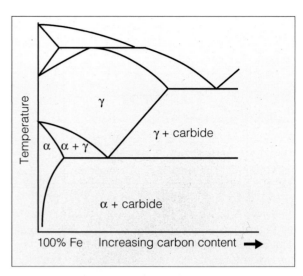

**32** Equilibrium phase diagram for the Fe–C system.

## *Partial Solid Solubility*

More usually, the components of materials are not sufficiently soluble to form a complete series of solid solutions. Examples of this are copper and silver, which are sufficiently different in atomic size that their atoms are only partially soluble in one another.

The phase diagram for this system is shown in **31**. For a wide range of compositions, the material will consist of two solid phases, one being silver rich and one being copper rich; by convention, these are called the α- and the β-phase, respectively. The α-phase consists of predominantly silver, with a small amount of copper dissolved in it, whereas the β-phase consists of copper with a small amount of silver dissolved in it.

At low concentrations of copper in silver, all of the copper is able to dissolve in the silver, and only a single phase exists. The maximum solubility of copper in silver is 8.8 w/o, and this occurs at a temperature of approximately 780°C.

At lower temperatures, the solubility of copper in silver decreases, and the excess copper separates out as the second, β-phase .

Similar behaviour occurs at the other end of the compositional range where the limited solubility of silver in copper also gives rise to the formation of a two phase structure.

An interesting and important feature of the phase diagram of the Ag–Cu system is the depression of the temperature of the liquidus at a composition of 72Ag:28Cu. At a temperature of 780°C, this composition of the alloy can exist as three phases: α, β and liquid. This is called the *eutectic point*, and the temperature at the intersection of the three phases is the *eutectic temperature*. The composition is called the *eutectic composition* of the alloy.

If a eutectic liquid is cooled, it changes directly into two solid phases, without an interposing state as a liquid–solid mixture, as occurs at all other compositions. This feature of some alloy systems can be utilised to form low melting temperature materials, such as solders.

In the same way that a eutectic involves the formation of two solid phases from a single liquid phase, such a transformation can also occur in solids.

The phase diagram of the Fe–C system, shown partially in **32**, is an example of this. For a composition of 0.8C:99.2Fe, the solid solution, γ, transforms to a solid solution of carbon in iron, α, and carbide (Fe$_3$C) at a temperature of 723°C. This is called a *eutectoid reaction*, and differs only from the eutectic in that all three phases are solids.

Such transformations as described (and it should be noted that there are others) are extremely important in determining the micro-structure, and, consequently, the properties of the alloy.

# Non-Equilibrium Conditions

It must be stressed that the phase diagrams described above are what are known as *equilibrium phase diagrams*. The material would have to be held at a set temperature for a considerable time to achieve the phase structure shown in such diagrams. In practice, the solidification and cooling rates of alloys do not allow the formation of an equilibrium phase structure.

Above, it was noted that for a composition of 50Cu:50Ni at 1300°C, a liquid phase rich in copper and a solid phase consisting of 63Ni:37Cu coexist. On rapid cooling, it is not possible for these liquid and solid phases to readjust their compositions, and some of the nickel rich solid will be retained. As the material continues to cool, so a composition richer in nickel will solidify, leaving the remaining liquid, and the subsequently formed solid richer in copper. The overall effect of this is that the solid will consist of a multitude of crystals with a wide range of compositions, all in the same phase. This formation of a solid with a non-uniform composition is known as *compositional segregation.*

In systems with multiple phases, the phase with the highest melting temperature will always be the first to solidify, followed by the phases with lower melting temperatures. As the first phase solidifies, it tends to form a lattice structure known as *dendrites*, as shown for a Co–Cr alloy in the scanning electron micrograph in **33**.

Compositional segregation can be eliminated, or reduced, by reheating the alloy to a temperature just below the solidus and holding it at that temperature for some time. This allows the atoms time to diffuse through the system and attain their equilibrium condition.

The process of heat treating an alloy is known as *annealing*, and if the intention is to achieve a homogeneous composition it is described as a *homogenisation anneal.*

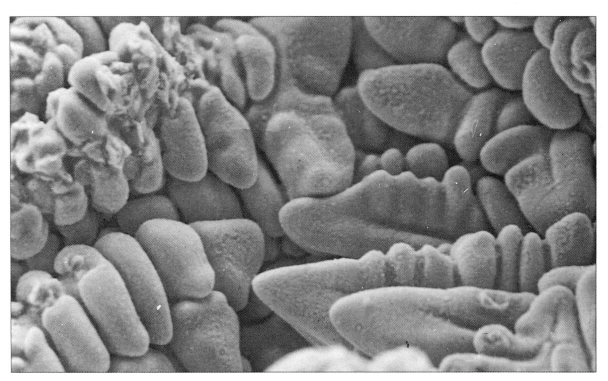

**33** Scanning electron microscope (SEM) micrograph of the coarse dendritic structure for a Co–Cr alloy.

# I.VI

## THE STRUCTURE OF POLYMERS

## Introduction

Plastics and rubbers, as they are generally called in everyday life, have the common property of being *polymers*. Polymers are long, chain molecules, consisting of many repeating units, as discussed already in section I.III. Polymers are not a 20th century invention, they are in fact older than man himself, and in one form or another are the basic constituents of every kind of living matter, whether plant or animal.

Examples of naturally occurring polymers are agar, cellulose, DNA, proteins, natural rubber, collagen and silk.

It is only relatively recently that we have begun to understand the structure of polymers and how to make them ourselves. Some examples of synthetic polymers, which are now everyday household names, are, PVC (polyvinyl chloride), polyethylene, nylon and polystyrene.

Originally, the synthetic polymers tended to be regarded as substitutes for existing natural polymers, such as rubber and silk.

Nowadays, such a wide variety of polymers can be produced that they have entered into every walk of life, satisfying needs that did not previously exist. Pertinent examples are medical applications, such as dialysis and oxygenator membranes, and dental applications such as filling materials.

The starting material for the production of a polymer is the *monomer*. In a material such as polyethylene, the repeating unit is a $CH_2$ group, with many of these units joined together to form a long chain (**34a**). The monomer from which this polymer is derived is ethylene (**34b**).

A polymer with a similar structure to polyethylene is polypropylene. It is formed by joining molecules of propylene (**35a**). Propylene differs from ethylene in having a methyl group ($CH_3$) replacing one of the hydrogen atoms, forming the polymer polypropylene (**35b**).

Polypropylene is slightly more complex than polyethylene, in that the arrangement of the methyl groups can vary so that they are:

- All on one side (*isotactic*).
- Alternate from side to side (*syndiotactic*).
- Switched from side to side in a random manner (*atactic*).

A number of polymers based on vinyl monomers are presented in *Table 4*.

It should be noted that the chemical routes by which these different polymers are made are quite different, and that it is not a simple matter of modification to form one from the other. Each polymer has its own characteristic repeating unit, or 'finger print', and this unit is the basis for the widely differing properties of the polymers.

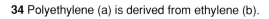

(α)

$$-C-C-C-C-$$

(b)

$$C=C$$

**34** Polyethylene (a) is derived from ethylene (b).

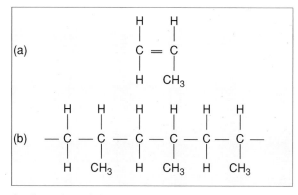

(a)

$$C=C$$

(b)

$$-C-C-C-C-C-C-$$

**35** Propylene (a) polymerises to give polypropylene (b).

**Table 4** Some monomers and their polymers.

| Name | Monomer | Polymer |
|------|---------|---------|
| Polyvinylchloride | H H<br>\| \|<br>C = C<br>\| \|<br>H Cl | H H H H H H H H<br>\| \| \| \| \| \| \| \|<br>— C — C — C — C — C — C — C — C —<br>\| \| \| \| \| \| \| \|<br>H Cl H Cl H Cl H Cl |
| PTFE | F F<br>\| \|<br>C = C<br>\| \|<br>F F | F F F F F F F F<br>\| \| \| \| \| \| \| \|<br>— C — C — C — C — C — C — C — C —<br>\| \| \| \| \| \| \| \|<br>F F F F F F F F |
| Polypropylene isotactic | H H<br>\| \|<br>C = C<br>\| \|<br>H CH₃ | H H H H H H H H<br>\| \| \| \| \| \| \| \|<br>— C — C — C — C — C — C — C — C —<br>\| \| \| \| \| \| \| \|<br>H CH₃ H CH₃ H CH₃ H CH₃ |
| Polyacrylic acid | H H<br>\| \|<br>C = C<br>\| \|<br>H C=O<br>\|<br>H | H H H H H H H H<br>\| \| \| \| \| \| \| \|<br>— C — C — C — C — C — C — C — C —<br>\| \| \| \| \| \| \| \|<br>H C=O H C=O H C=O H C=O<br>\| \| \| \|<br>H H H H |
| Polymethylmethacrylate | H CH₃<br>\| \|<br>C = C<br>\| \|<br>H C=O<br>\|<br>O<br>\|<br>CH₃ | H CH₃ H CH₃ H CH₃ H CH₃ H CH₃<br>\| \| \| \| \| \| \| \| \| \|<br>— C — C — C — C — C — C — C — C —<br>\| \| \| \| \| \| \| \| \| \|<br>H C=O H C=O H C=O H C=O H C=O<br>\| \| \| \|<br>O O O O<br>\| \| \| \|<br>CH₃ CH₃ CH₃ CH₃ |

CH₃ ... (figure)

$$\begin{array}{ccccc} & CH_3 & & CH_3 & & CH_3 \\ & | & & | & & | \\ -O- & Si & -O- & Si & -O- & Si- \\ & | & & | & & | \\ & CH_3 & & CH_3 & & CH_3 \end{array}$$

**36** The structure of polydimethylsiloxane.

The most common polymers are those made from the organic compounds of carbon, but polymers can also be made from inorganic compounds, based on silica ($SiO_2$).

Silicon, being four-valent like carbon, provides the opportunity to form the backbone for the polymer, together with oxygen. An example of a silicone polymer is polydimethylsiloxane (**36**).

When a polymer is formed from a single species of monomer, it is called a *homopolymer*; when different species are included, it is called a *heteropolymer*.

# Mechanisms Of Polymerisation

The monomers shown in *Table 4* all have a double bond in common, which is opened up to allow the monomer to bond to a neighbouring monomer. This process of preparing polymers from monomers is called *polymerisation*. There are two ways in which this may be achieved: *addition* and *condensation*.

## *Addition Polymerisation*

Definition: *Addition polymerisation* occurs when a reaction between two molecules (either the same, to form a *homopolymer*, or dissimilar, to form a *heteropolymer*) produces a larger molecule without the elimination of a smaller molecule (such as water).

This type of reaction takes place for vinyl compounds, which are reactive inorganic compounds containing carbon–carbon double bonds (see *Table 4*). The process of addition polymerisation to produce these polymers involves four stages:

- Activation.
- Initiation.
- Propagation.
- Termination.

**Activation**

The polymerisation of a vinyl compound requires the presence of *free radicals* (•). These are very reactive chemical species that have an odd (unpaired) electron. The process of producing free radicals is described as *activation*. Activation occurs, for instance, in the decomposition of a peroxide.

The peroxide commonly used in dental materials is benzoyl peroxide. Under appropriate conditions, a molecule of benzoyl peroxide can yield two free radicals:

$$C_6H_5COO\text{-}OOCH_5C_6 \rightarrow 2\,(C_6H_5COO\bullet)$$

This in turn can decompose to form other free radicals:

$$C_6H_5COO\bullet \rightarrow C_6H_5\bullet + CO_2$$

Such chemical species, known as *initiators*, are able to initiate vinyl polymerisation, as described later, and are designated as R•.

Before initiation occurs, however, the benzoyl peroxide needs to be activated. This activation is achieved by the decomposition of the peroxide, due to the use of an *activator*, such as:

- *Heat* – When heated above 65°C, the benzoyl peroxide decomposes, as shown above. This is the method used in the production of acrylic resin denture bases (see section III.II).
- *Chemical compounds* – The benzoyl peroxide can also be activated when brought into contact with a tertiary amine such as n, n dimethyl-p-toluidine. This method is employed in cold-cured acrylic resins, used, for example, in denture repairs, temporary restorations, orthodontic appliances and special trays (see section III.II). The same method is also used in chemically-cured composite restorative materials, which consist of a base paste containing the tertiary amine activator and a catalyst paste contain-

ing the benzoyl peroxide initiator (see section II.II).

- *Light* –Yet another method for the creation of free radicals is employed by light-activated composites; these rely on either ultraviolet light or visible light as the activator of the polymerisation reaction. In these instances, other initiators than benzoyl peroxide are employed.

Other forms of free radical production include the use of ultraviolet light in conjunction with a benzoin methyl ether, and visible light with an α-diketone and an amine (see section II.II).

### Initiation

The free radicals can react with a monomer such as ethylene and *initiate* the polymerisation process as follows:

$$
R\bullet \; + \;
\begin{array}{c} H \;\; H \\ | \;\; | \\ C = C \\ | \;\; | \\ H \;\; H \end{array}
\;\; \rightarrow \;\;
\begin{array}{c} H \;\; H \\ | \;\; | \\ R - C - C\bullet \\ | \;\; | \\ H \;\; H \end{array}
$$

### Propagation

The free radical is transferred to the monomer, which can in turn react with another monomer:

$$
\begin{array}{c} H \;\; H \\ | \;\; | \\ R - C - C\bullet \\ | \;\; | \\ H \;\; H \end{array}
+
\begin{array}{c} H \;\; H \\ | \;\; | \\ C = C \\ | \;\; | \\ H \;\; H \end{array}
\rightarrow
\begin{array}{c} H \;\; H \;\; H \;\; H \\ | \;\; | \;\; | \;\; | \\ R - C - C - C - C\bullet \\ | \;\; | \;\; | \;\; | \\ H \;\; H \;\; H \;\; H \end{array}
$$

The polymer chain is generated by repeating this process again and again until the growing chains collide or all of the free radicals have reacted.

### Termination

Free radicals can react to form a stable molecule:

$$
\begin{array}{c} [H] \;\; H \\ | \;\;\; | \\ R - C - C\bullet \\ | \;\;\; | \\ [H]_n \;\; H \end{array}
+ R\bullet \rightarrow
\begin{array}{c} [H] \\ | \\ R - C - R \\ | \\ [H]_{n+1} \end{array}
$$

Since n will vary from polymer chain to polymer chain, a wide range of long-chain molecules are produced. In most situations, there will also be some unreacted monomer and some *oligomers*, which consist of just a few repeating units.

# Condensation Polymerisation

*Condensation polymerisation* occurs when two molecules (not usually the same) react to form a larger molecule with the elimination of a smaller molecule (often, but not always, water).

In this case, monomer units with a carbon–carbon double-bond are not necessary, as shown in the following example of a silicone, which is an inorganic polymer formed by the condensation of silanols:

$$
\begin{array}{c} R \\ | \\ HO - Si - OH \\ | \\ R \end{array}
+
\begin{array}{c} R \\ | \\ HO - Si - OH \\ | \\ R \end{array}
\rightarrow
$$

$$
\begin{array}{c} R \;\;\;\; R \\ | \;\;\;\; | \\ HO - Si - O - Si - OH \\ | \;\;\;\; | \\ R \;\;\;\; R \end{array}
+ H_2O
$$

In this case, R is an organic group, such as a methyl ($CH_3$), and the by-product is water.

# Polymeric Structures

## *Molecular Weight*

The molecular weight of a polymer is equal to the number of repeating units (i.e. the *degree of polymerisation*) multiplied by the molecular weight of the repeating unit. In both addition and condensation polymerisation, the length of the chain is determined by purely random events, and not all of the chains will be of the same length, and in general, many different chain lengths will be present. Thus, the molecu-

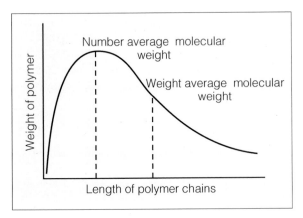

**37** The molecular weight distribution of a typical polymer.

lar weight can only be represented by an average value.

There are a number of ways in which the molecular weight can be determined for a polymer. Two main ones are the *number average molecular weight*, $M_n$, and the *weight average molecular weight*, $M_w$.

**Number Average Molecular Weight ($M_n$)**

$M_n$ is obtained by counting the number of molecules in a given weight of sample. The general expression would be given by:

$$M_n = \frac{\sum n_i M_i}{\sum n_i}$$

**Weight Average Molecular Weight ($M_w$)**

$M_w$ is obtained by measurement of the weight of the molecules in the total sample weight, given by the general expression:

$$M_w = \frac{\sum w_i M_i}{\sum w_i}.$$

The difference in the definitions for a distribution of molecular weights in a typical polymer is shown in **37**. $M_w$ is particularly sensitive to the presence of high molecular weight polymers, while $M_n$ is sensitive to the presence of low molecular weight polymers. For example, if equal weights of two polymers of $M_a$=10 000 and $M_b$=100 000 are mixed, $M_w$ is given by:

$$M_w = \frac{(w_a \times M_a + w_b \times M_b)}{(w_a + w_b)}$$

where $w_a$ and $w_b$ are the weights of $M_a$ and $M_b$ respectively.

In this case, $w_a$ and $w_b$ are equal to $1/2W$, and $M_a$=10 000 and $M_b$=100 000. Substituting these values in the above expression gives:

$$M_w = \frac{(1/2\,W \times 10\,000 + 1/2\,W \times 100\,000)}{W}$$
$$= 55\,000$$

The number average molecular weight is given by:

$$M_n = \frac{(n_a \times M_a + m_b \times M_b)}{(n_a + m_b)}$$

where $n_a$ and $m_b$ are the number of molecules of molecular weight $M_a$ and $M_b$ respectively. In this case, $n_a$=10 and $m_b$=1 such that:

$$M_n = (10 \times 10\,000 + 1 \times 100\,000) / 11$$
$$= 18\,200.$$

The molecular weight of a polymer is of great value in explaining the variations in the physical properties of different polymers. For example, the tensile strength and the elongation required to break the polymer increase steeply for some polymers in the molecular weight range of 50 000–200 000.

However, improving the physical properties by increasing the molecular weight is accompanied by a rapid increase in viscosity of the melt, and this raises the glass transition temperature, making it more difficult for the polymer to be processed.

## Chain Configurations

Polymer chains are held together by weak secondary (or van der Waal's) bonds, and by entanglement of the chains if they are sufficiently long. The higher the molecular weight, the more entanglements there will be, giving a stiffer and stronger polymer.

In a polymer such as polyethylene, which has a linear chain configuration, the weak bonds between the chains can easily be broken by increasing the temperature of the polymer. When this happens the chains can flow past one another so that the polymer softens and readily deforms.

H
Propyl
side
branch

**38** Branched polyethylene.

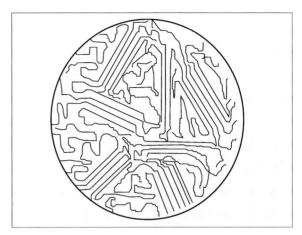

**39** Partial crystallinity in a polymer.

On cooling, the bonds are re-established, and the polymer becomes hard again, and retains the shape it was in at the higher temperature.

The temperature at which a plastic softens such that the molecules can begin to flow is defined as its *glass transition temperature*. They are similar to those for glasses, except that the temperatures involved are much lower in the case of plastics (see section I.IV).

A polymer that can be softened and subsequently shaped by heating it above its glass transition temperature is known as a *thermoplastic polymer*. Examples of such thermoplastic polymers are polystyrene, polymethyl methacrylate and polyethylene.

For many polymer systems, the chains are not as linear as polyethylene. In fact, polyethylene should be identical to polymethylene, but this is not so because the chains in polyethylene are branched, and hence non-linear (**38**). These branches give the polymer a three-dimensional network structure which prevents the chains from moving past each other easily, even when heated. Thus, the polymer will retain its properties up to reasonably high temperatures, until chemical breakdown of the polymer structure occurs.

Polymers which decompose on heating without showing a glass transition are known as *thermosetting polymers*.

## Crystallinity In Polymers

In a polymer the molecules usually twist and turn, coil up, and criss-cross in a random fashion. Sometimes, however, there will be zones where

the molecules are able to lie more or less parallel to each other, as shown in **39**. When this happens, the polymer exhibits a limited degree of crystallinity.

The relative proportions of crystalline and non-crystalline regions in a polymer will depend upon the chemical composition, the molecular configuration and the method of processing. These polymers are not wholly crystalline solids, but are composed of a large number of small crystalline regions in close proximity to one another, in an amorphous matrix.

Polyethylene is able to crystallise because of the regularity and simplicity of its polymer chain. As polymer molecules become more complex (whether due to branching or large side groups that restrict the motion of the chain), so it becomes more difficult for them to have crystalline regions.

## Cross-linking

When polymer chains are joined together by chemical bonds, the polymer is said to be *cross-linked*. As noted above, crosslinking has a profound effect on the properties of a polymer; it can make the difference between a thermoplastic polymer and a thermosetting polymer. More importantly, it can convert a liquid polymer into a solid polymer, a process used in the setting of many impression materials.

Silicone polymers have a glass transition temperature below room temperature, and therefore are liquids at, and above, this temperature. When these polymers are crosslinked, the chains are no longer able to slide past each other,

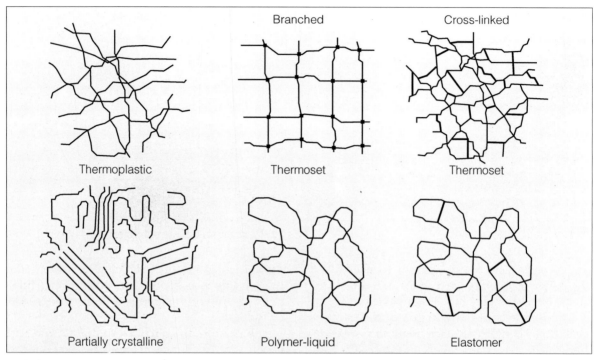

**40** Polymer chain configurations.

and a solid material is obtained. Extensive cross-linking in polymers results in hard, brittle materials.

If the polymer consists of particularly long and flexible molecular chains, there may be cross-linking at several points along their lengths.

The molecules can take up a highly coiled configuration when relaxed, and can stretch over long distances (by uncoiling) when stress is applied. When the stress is removed, the chains will again take up their coiled configuration, governed by the cross-links.

The amount of extension, and the stress that can be borne by such a polymer depends on the lengths of the chains, the degree of crosslinking, and the strength of the bonds.

Materials which show the ability to stretch large amounts, even to many times their original length, are known as *elastomers*. The characteristic features of an elastomer are that:

- The material is soft and has a low elastic modulus.
- Very high strains (>100%) are possible.
- The strains are reversible.

- The material is above its glass transition temperature.

The various polymer chain configurations for polymers are shown in **40**.

# Composition Of Real Polymers

Polymers are very rarely used in their pure form, for the same reasons that pure metals are rarely used in comparison to alloys. Instead, modifications are carried out in order to improve the properties of the polymers.

One such modification that has already been considered is the cross-linking of polymer chains, to form thermosetting polymers from thermoplastic polymers. As thermosetting polymers cannot be softened and reshaped, the shape of the object has to be created before cross-linking, and this places serious constraints on the means of processing. However, various other processing options are available, such as blending, and the uses of copolymers and composites.

## Blending

Blending is a process commonly used in the processing of thermoplastic polymers, and involves mixing two or more polymers prior to moulding. The properties of the blended polymer will usually lie somewhere between those of the constituent polymers.

As the polymers have to be miscible (i.e. mix freely with one another) they tend to be of a similar chemical composition. This places a limit on the changes in properties that are possible by the blending process.

## Copolymers

An alternative to blending is the mixing of two polymer producing systems during the polymerisation process; this is *copolymerisation*.

For example, if monomer A and monomer B are mixed prior to polymerisation they will *copolymerise* to form polymer chains consisting of both A and B monomer units. The sequence of the original monomers in the polymer may be random, producing a *random copolymer*, giving a sequence such as:

–A–A–A–A–B–B–A–B–A–B–B–B–A–A–B–B–A–B–

If the monomers self-polymerise more readily than they copolymerise, what will result is a *block copolymer*, where segments of each homopolymer are linked:

–A–A–A–B–B–B–B–A–A–A–B–B–B–

Such systems can produce polymers with properties that are quite different from the homopolymers. For example, one polymer may be quite rigid, while the other is very flexible. Producing a block copolymer would allow one to control the degree of flexibility of the final material by controlling the length of the blocks and the relative amounts of each polymer.

An example of a block copolymer is ABS (acrylonitrile butadiene styrene), which is formed from a mixture of three polymers. The acrylonitrile and styrene copolymerise to form a glassy block copolymer, while the butadiene forms spherical rubbery regions bonded to the rigid polymer matrix. Although this material has a lower stiffness and creep resistance than poly-styrene, it is much tougher, to the extent that it has been considered for the manufacture of car body parts.

## Plasticisers

If a low molecular weight substance is added to a polymer, it has the effect of lowering the glass transition temperature and the elastic modulus of the material. These plasticisers reduce the forces of attraction between the polymer chains, so the chains become more flexible, and begin to flow past one another at a lower temperature, which accounts for the reduction in $T_g$.

If enough plasticiser is added, a brittle polymer can be transformed into a soft, flexible and tough polymer.

Plasticisers are usually added to polymers to improve their flow (and hence their processability), and to reduce the brittleness of the product. An example is PVC, which is a very rigid polymer in its pure form, but can be formed into flexible tubing after the addition of plasticiser.

The basic requirement to be met by a plasticiser is that it must be compatible with the polymer, and have a permanent effect. Compatibility means that the plasticiser must be miscible in the polymer, and this implies the need for a similarity in the molecular forces active in the polymer and plasticiser.

For a plasticiser to be permanent and to not be easily leached out of the material, it must have a low vapour pressure and a low diffusion rate through the polymer.

A dental example of the use of a plasticiser, is when dibutyl phthalate is mixed with polymethyl or polyethyl methacrylate for the production of soft liners for dentures (see section III.II).

## Composites

A composite may be defined as a combination of materials in which the individual components retain their physical identity.

In two component composites, it is usual to refer to the *matrix* and the *filler*, the former being the component that binds the filler together. In polymer composites, the matrix may be a thermoplastic or a thermosetting polymer. The filler may be present simply to reduce the cost, or may be used to perform a specific role, such as to impart colour to an otherwise clear polymer. Their most crucial function however, is when they are used to improve the mechanical properties of the polymer. For instance, the inclusion of glass in a polymer increases the stiffness, and sometimes increases the strength.

The shape of the filler plays an important role in the way the properties are modified. Fillers may be *particulate*, *fibres* or *whiskers*, with fibres being the most effective. Significant improvements in toughness and creep resistance can be achieved by the judicious use of a filler. In dentistry, particulate fillers are most common, with two of their many important applications being in the use of impression materials and resin-based composite restorative materials.

# MECHANICAL PROPERTIES

## Introduction

When one stretches a steel wire or a rubber band the responses of the materials are quite different. The steel wire will hardly appear to change (although it will become longer), but this change is normally so small that it is difficult to perceive. On the other hand, the rubber band will stretch quite readily, and can virtually double in length. Obviously, different materials respond quite differently to the application of a load.

We could make a component and determine its response to an external loading. However, the data collected would be applicable only to that component, and would not allow us topredict the behaviour of a differently shaped component that was made from the same material.

How are we to compare the performances of materials in different applications? Obviously, we need some objective standard of comparison that is independent of the size and shape of the material. Once we have such a standard, it should be possible to compare the properties of different materials, and to predict the behaviour of objects made from them.

The basis for such an objective standard are the quantities called *stress* and *strain*. The description of the mechanical properties of materials is based on these, so we shall now consider them in some detail.

## Stress And Strain

The simplest approach to understanding stress and strain is to consider a rod of material that is held under tension by being subjected to a *tensile force*, or *load*. As shown in **41**, the rod will extend.

Naturally, one would expect the rod to fail (i.e. to snap or to deform irreversibly) under a high enough load. The load at which failure occurs is a measure of the strength of the rod, but it is particular to a rod of those specific dimensions and specific material. The load that the rod could bear without failing would be increased if the diameter of the rod was increased, and would decrease if the diameter was decreased.

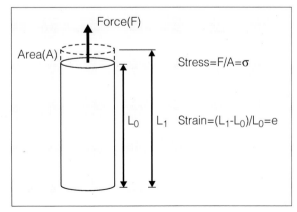

**41** Rod of material being pulled in a uniaxial direction.

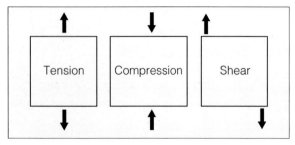

**42** Three principal types of stress.

The amount of extension of the rod at the time of failure depends upon the starting length of the rod, such that the longer the starting length, the greater the extension. Thus, force and extension do not represent the ideal means of defining the mechanical properties of a material.

The way to overcome these dependences on the dimensions of the rod is to introduce the parameters of stress, $\sigma$, and strain, e, for the material under test.

The definitions for these parameters are:

- *Stress* is the force per unit cross-sectional area, that is acting on a material.
- *Strain* is the fractional change in the dimensions caused by the force.

Thus, if a rod is subjected to a tensile force, F, along its length, the stress, $\sigma$, is given by

$$\sigma = \frac{F}{A},$$

where A is the cross-sectional area of the rod. When the force is applied, the rod's length changes from its original length $L_0$, to the extended length $L_1$. The strain that results, e, is given by

$$e = \frac{L_1 - L_0}{L_0}.$$

The units used to measure stress are Newtons per metre squared ($N.m^{-2}$), whereas the strain is dimensionless.

In practice, we can measure the load–extension curve for a material, and then convert this to a stress–strain curve. Once we have this information, it is possible to predict the load–extension curve for a rod of any cross-sectional area and length. We can also compare the response of different materials to the same tensile force.

Stress and strain are not properties in themselves, but allow the definition of a number of mechanical properties that could not be defined otherwise. In the example described above, the stress was generated by a load applied in an axial direction (i.e. along the rod), but in practice, a load could be applied in any direction, and in most situations there will be more than one load involved. These loads give rise to complex stress patterns in the structure.

The three principal types of stress are tensile stress, compressive stress and shear stress, and are shown schematically in **42**.

# Definitions Of Some Mechanical Properties

A typical stress–strain curve for a metal such as a brass alloy is shown in **43**. It can be used to identify several of a material's properties.

## *Elastic Limit And Plastic Flow*

An important feature of the mechanical behaviour of materials is the relationship between the stress and the strain. Immediately noticeable in **43** is that this brass alloy does not show a linear relationship between stress and strain along the full length of the curve.

The region where the stress–strain curve is linear is known as the *linear elastic region*, and represents the range where *elastic deformation* occurs. In this region, removal of the stress from the material results in the material returning to its original shape.

Where the curve begins to deviate from its linear path, the material will have exceeded its *elastic limit* and will begin to deform permanently; removal of the stress from the material does not result in the return of the material to its original shape. This is known as *plastic flow*, and is represented by the *plastic deformation region* on the graph.

## *Young's Modulus*

When a material is stressed, it is usually found that the stress is initially proportional to the strain, so their ratio is constant. In other words, the material deforms linearly and elastically. This can be represented by the expression:

$$\frac{\sigma}{e} = E,$$

which allows us to define an other property of the material, namely the *Young's modulus*, denoted by E. Young's modulus is the constant that relates the stress and the strain in the linear elastic region, and is a measure of the stiffness of the material.

Note that the stiffness of a rod is dependent upon its shape and dimensions, *and* upon the Young's modulus of the material from which it is constructed. Once we know the Young's modulus of a material, it is possible to determine the stiffness of any structure made from that material.

Since Young's modulus is obtained by dividing the stress by the strain, the units are the same as those of stress ($N.m^{-2}$). The value of Young's modulus is often very large for real materials. To make the values more manageable, it is usual to express the value of Young's modulus in Gigapascals (GPa) where one Pascal is $1\ N.m^{-2}$, and one Gigapascal is $10^9\ N.m^{-2}$.

The Young's modulus is often described as simply the *elastic modulus*, or the *modulus of elasticity*.

## Fracture Strength

It is now possible to define the *fracture strength* of the material, $\sigma_f$, since this is simply the stress required to break it.

## Yield Stress And Proof Stress

The stress at which plastic deformation begins is defined as the *yield stress*, $\sigma_y$. In practice, this point is often difficult to detect since there is a gradual transition rather than a rapid change in the slope of the stress–strain curve.

The quantity known as *proof stress* is used as a measure of the onset of yielding of the material, and is defined as the stress required to produce a certain amount of plastic strain, usually 0.2%.

## Ultimate Tensile Strength

In the tensile response depicted in **43**, there is a maximum stress that the specimen can with-

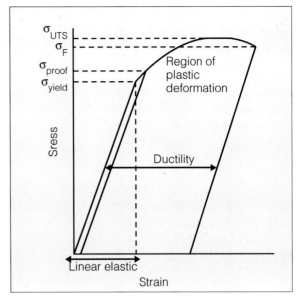

**43** Stress–strain curve for a ductile metal.

stand. This maximum stress is defined as the *ultimate tensile strength* of the material, $\sigma_{UTS}$, and is often different from the fracture strength, which, as noted above, is the stress at the point of fracture.

## Ductility

The amount of plastic strain produced in the specimen at fracture is called the *ductility* of the material.

Ductility is measured by drawing a line from the point of fracture, that is parallel to the elastic region of the stress–strain curve. Where this line meets the strain axis is the measure of the ductility of the material, and is frequently presented in terms of percentage elongation.

## Resilience And Toughness

When a wire is bent and then released, it will spring back to its original shape as long as the stress does not exceed the elastic limit.

This is because the energy stored in the wire is recoverable when the stress is released. The amount of energy which can be absorbed and subsequently released is an indication of the potential springiness of the material.

The *resilience* is the amount of energy a material can absorb without undergoing any permanent deformation. It is measured from the stress–strain curve as the area under the linear elastic portion of the curve, and is given by

$$R = \frac{1}{2} \frac{P^2}{E}$$

where R is the modulus of resilience, P is the proportional limit (another name for the yield stress) and E is the elastic modulus. The units are those of energy per unit volume, $J.m^{-3}$ ( 1 Joule = 1 Nm).

The total amount of energy that a material can absorb before it fractures is a measure of the *toughness* of the material, and is indicated by the total area under the stress–strain curve. It is also expressed in terms of $J.m^{-3}$.

# Mechanical Tests

## Tensile Test

The *tensile test* is a relatively simple test to understand and interpret and is possibly also the most useful. In this test, a sample of the material is stretched in a uniaxial direction in a tensile tester, as shown in **44**. The test is carried out at a constant strain rate (i.e. a constant rate of extension), and the load is measured from a load

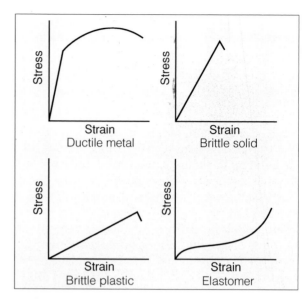

**45** Stress–strain curves for a range of materials. Note that the stress and strain scales are not meant to be comparable.

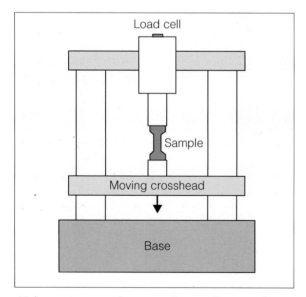

**44** An arrangement for measuring tensile strength.

cell. The elongation corresponding to the applied load is measured simultaneously, and can be done in a number of ways possibly involving measurement of the separation of the moving crosshead, or by attaching strain gauges to the material if the strains are very low. The stress and corresponding strain can then be calculated according to the definitions already described.

A stress–strain curve can be constructed, from which a number of properties can be determined. Some typical examples of stress–strain curves for a range of materials are shown in **45**.

An example of a ductile metal is mild steel, which shows a region of linear elastic behaviour, a well defined yield point and a considerable degree of ductility. In contrast, a hard brittle solid, such as plaster of Paris, shows only a linear elastic region and then fractures without any evidence of plastic deformation.

Many plastics, such as polymethyl methacrylate, are also brittle, although they are less stiff than plaster of Paris. The elastomer, of which silicone impression materials are examples, shows a very different behaviour when compared to the other materials. Firstly, it does not appear to have a linear elastic region, and the region of elastic recovery is very large. The percentage elongation is much higher than that observed with either steel or plaster of Paris, and

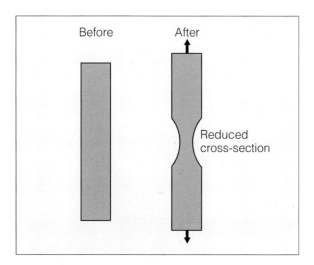

**46** Necking, exhibited by a ductile material.

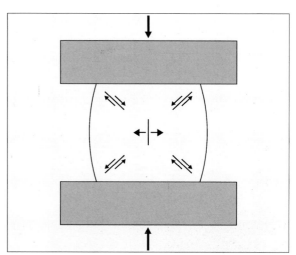

**47** An arrangement for measuring compression strength, showing where tensile and shear stresses develop.

it is elastic in nature, since the rubber will recover its original dimensions once the stress has been removed. The rubber also has a significantly lower tensile strength.

### Necking

During elastic deformation there is a slight increase in the volume of the material because the atoms which make up the solid are being pulled apart. However, no such change in volume occurs during plastic deformation. During such deformation an increase in the length of the material, must result in a decrease in the cross-sectional area. This tends to occur in a localised region of the material, as shown in **46**, and is known as *necking*. This phenomenon occurs most readily in highly ductile materials.

The results of tensile tests can be very useful when designing structures, because a knowledge of the elastic deformation characteristics of the material is required in order to predict the behaviour of the structure when it is placed under load.

The yield stress determines the maximum stress that the material can safely withstand, and, consequently, the maximum load the structure can withstand, although it is prudent to include some safety factor. The elastic modulus will allow the determination of the stiffness of the structure. For example, a combination of these properties would allow one to determine the resilience or springiness of a metal wire.

If fabrication techniques such as rolling, wire drawing or pressing are involved in the manufacture of a product, then it is necessary to know how much plastic deformation the material can withstand. If the material shows high ductility then it can be shaped, but if it shows no ductility then shaping by the application of loads will not be possible.

## Compression Test

For brittle materials in particular, the tensile test is difficult to carry out, and the results usually show a high degree of scatter. An alternative is a *compression test*, which is more easily performed on brittle materials and has results that show a lower degree of scatter. Another reason why such tests are done on brittle materials is that these materials are only used under conditions of compressive loading.

The configuration for a compression test is shown in **47**. As the sample is constrained by friction at points of contact with the platens of the tester, there is an increase in the cross-sectional area, with the material taking up a barrel shape. This 'barrelling' effect gives rise to a very complex stress pattern in the material (also shown in **47**) that cannot be analysed easily. This makes the interpretation of compression tests very difficult.

A compromise test is the measurement of *diametral tensile strength*, in which a disc of the material is subjected to a compressive load. The

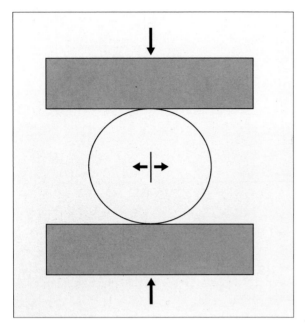

**48** An arrangement for measuring diametral tensile strength.

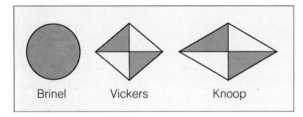

**49** Surface indenters from different hardness testers.

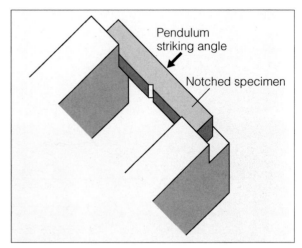

**50** Specimen arrangement for a Sharpy impact test. The pendulum has a hammer head which is released from a fixed height.

load applied to the disc results in a tensile stress in a direction perpendicular to the applied load, shown schematically in **48**. The tensile stress, $\sigma$, is calculated as follows:

$$\sigma = \frac{2P}{\pi DT}$$

where P is the load, D is the diameter of the disc and T is the thickness of the disc. It is a commonly used test for brittle dental materials, because it is simple and provides more reproducible results than a tensile test.

## Hardness Test

The *hardness test* measures the resistance of a material to an indenter or cutting tool. It provides an indication of the resistance of the material to scratching or abrasion. There is also a reasonable correlation between the hardness of a material and its ultimate tensile strength.

The test involves the use of an indenter, which can be in the shape of a ball (Brinell), a pyramid (Vickers or Knoop) or a cone (Rockwell), which of course must be harder than the material being tested. The indenter is pushed into the surface of the material for a given period of time, leaving behind an impression of the indenter (**49**).

The size of this impression will depend upon the hardness of the material. The sizes can be measured, and an empirical hardness number calculated. The choice of hardness tester depends to some extent on the nature of material being tested.

## Impact Test

The *impact test* is designed to test the resistance of a material to the sudden application of a load. A standard notched bar is subjected to an impulse load provided by a heavy pendulum. The arrangement for the test is shown in **50**.

The pendulum is released from a known height, and then strikes and breaks the sample, which is placed across parallel supports. Some of the energy of the pendulum is used up in breaking the sample. From a knowledge of the initial and final height of the pendulum after it has fractured the sample, the difference in energy can be calculated. This difference is a measure of the amount of energy that was absorbed by the

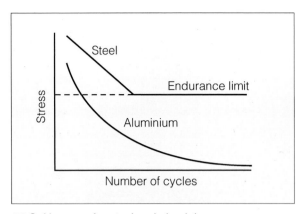

**51** S–N curves for steel and aluminium.

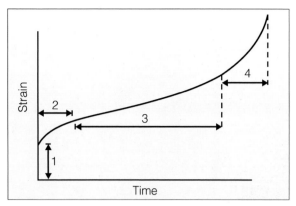

**52** Creep curve, showing the four stages of creep for long duration and high-temperature creep conditions.

sample, causing it to fracture. Although the test is empirical, it provides a useful means of comparing the impact resistance of a range of materials. The presence of the notch makes this a very severe test, and provides an indication of the sensitivity of a material to notches in its structure.

## Fatigue Test

In many practical situations, materials are subjected to fluctuating stresses rather than the static loads that are considered above. The gradual accumulation of minute amounts of plastic strain produced by each cycle of a fluctuating stress is known as *fatigue*.

Fatigue can lead to failure at stresses well below the yield stress of the material. The test for fatigue strength involves subjecting samples of the material to cyclic loading for a range of loads. The number of cycles required to cause failure is counted in each case.

The stress is plotted as a function of the logarithm of the corresponding number of cycles required to cause failure. This gives an S-N curve, as shown in **51**.

Two forms of behaviour can be observed. For some materials, as the number of cycles of loading is increased, the allowable stress decreases. In other materials however, there is what is known as an *endurance limit*, which corresponds to a level of stress to which the material can be subjected for an indefinite number of cycles without fracturing.

The fatigue strength is very dependent on the surface characteristics of the material. Improve-

ments in surface finish or surface compressive stresses, which may be induced mechanically or chemically, tend to raise the level of the S-N curve.

The testing environment will also have a profound effect on the S-N curve, with corrosive environments, particularly, lowering the fatigue strength.

## Creep Test

Under the influence of a constant stress, materials can deform permanently if the load is applied for a long time, even though the stress on the material may well be below its elastic limit. This time-dependent deformation of materials is known as *creep*, and will eventually lead to fracture of the material.

It is particularly important when a material is used at a temperature above about half of its melting temperature or softening point, e.g. some amalgam phases and many plastics. At temperatures 40–50% less than the absolute melting point, creep is negligible.

A typical creep curve is shown in **52**. Four stages of elongation can be identified:

- Initial elongation due to the application of the load.
- Transient or primary creep which tends to be a large effect.
- Steady state (secondary) creep.
- Tertiary creep.

We will not consider the mechanisms that give rise to creep.

47

# I.VIII

## PHYSICAL PROPERTIES

## Introduction

The uses to which dental materials are put are not conducive to mass production, as each patient is different from the last, and the material has to be specially moulded each time. As a consequence, most materials used by the dentist and the dental technician require some form of processing before they are hardened.

This processing often involves mixing the materials with others to produce a dough or liquid that can then be placed and shaped to suit the patient's needs. The successful use of dental materials therefore requires some understanding of the way in which materials flow when they are mixed, poured or moulded. The study of flow of materials is known as *rheology*.

When a patient drinks a cup of tea or eats an ice-cream, the temperature differences within the tooth can be quite pronounced. The pulp of the tooth would react severely if it were not protected from these temperatures that differ greatly from the norm of 37°C. When placing a filling, crown, bridge or denture, account must be taken of the need to protect the pulp from extremes of temperature. Therefore, the *thermal properties* of the dental materials need to be considered.

The restoration of the human dentition has moved more and more from the purely functional towards the aesthetic. Most patients now demand a level of restoration of their teeth where it is virtually impossible to detect that the dentist has intervened. Consequently, the *optical properties* of the materials that are selected and used by the dentist have become of great importance.

## Rheological Properties

Rheology is the study of the flow of materials. For liquids, flow is measured by the viscosity, whereas for solids one considers creep and *visco-elasticity*. Creep has already been described in the previous section and only the viscosity and the viscoelasticity will be considered here.

### Viscosity

When a substance flows under the influence of an external force (e.g. gravity), the molecules or atoms come into contact with different neighbours. Thus, bonds must be broken and remade, and this gives rise to a resistance to flow, known as *viscosity*.

For a liquid such as water, the forces binding the molecules together are very weak and easily overcome, so the water flows quite readily and has a low viscosity. For some fluids, the inter-molecular attractions are much stronger. This is usually associated with large molecules, such as

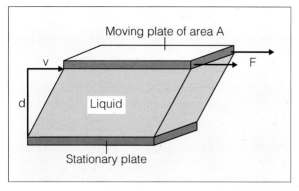

**53** Shearing of a liquid between two rigid plates that are separated by a distance, d. The upper plate is moving at a velocity, v, relative to the stationary plate and a force, F, is needed to overcome the resistance from the liquid.

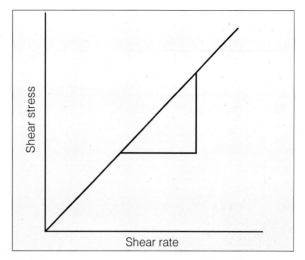

**54** Shear stress versus shear rate for a Newtonian liquid.

in the case of treacle. The molecules may even get tangled up in one another, giving rise to very high viscosities. This is what happens with high molecular weight polymers.

When we stir a liquid we are effectively applying a shear stress, and the degree of vigour with which we stir it can be quantified by the shear rate. Such a situation is shown in **53**. The shear stress and the shear rate are defined by:

$$\text{Shear stress} = \eta_s = \frac{F}{A}$$

$$\text{Shear rate} = \grave{e} = \frac{V}{d}$$

A number of methods are available for measuring the shear stress over a range of shear rates for a fluid, and the information collected can be plotted as a *shear stress–shear rate curve*. This relationship is linear for many fluids, and a typical curve for such a fluid is shown in **54**. The slope of the curve is equal to the viscosity, so that the exact scientific definition of viscosity, $\eta$, is given by:

$$\eta = \frac{\text{shear stress}}{\text{shear rate}}$$

The units of viscosity are Pascal seconds (Pa.s).

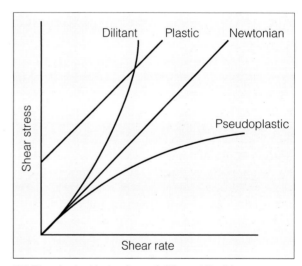

**55** Rheological behaviour of different liquids.

The viscose properties of substances that have a linear relationship between shear stress and shear rate are given entirely by this single value of viscosity, and are said to be 'Newtonian' in behaviour. However, not all materials behave in this simple fashion, and some of the different forms of behaviour are shown in **55**.

Liquids with *plastic* behaviour will not flow until an initial shear stress has been reached. The fluid will then flow in a Newtonian fashion.

*Dilatant* liquids show an increase in viscosity as the shear rate goes up. This means that the faster one tries to mix the fluid, the more difficult the liquid becomes to mix. It is not possible to

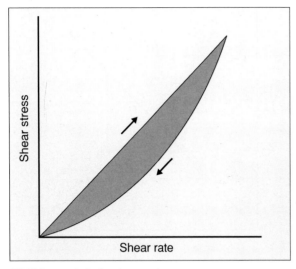

**56** Thixotropic behaviour.

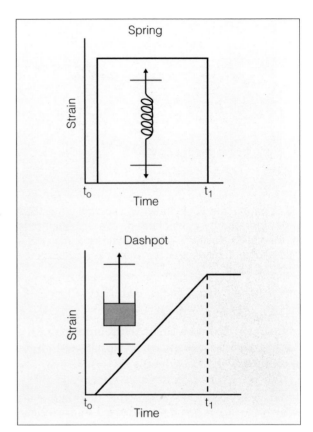

**57** Elastic and viscous response for a spring and dashpot model.

define the flow characteristics of such a liquid by a single viscosity.

For some liquids, an increase in shear rate does not lead to a corresponding increase in shear stress. This means that the liquid becomes easier to mix at higher shear rates than would be the case for a Newtonian or dilatant liquid. This behaviour is described as *pseudoplastic*, and leads to the feature of some liquids that is commonly known as *shear thinning*. A dental example of this type of behaviour is in silicone impression materials, where shear thinning makes the flow of the fluid from a syringe much easier than it would otherwise have been.

## Thixotropy

So far it has been assumed that the viscosity can be determined from a knowledge of the shear stress and shear rate at any one instant in time. For some substances, the viscosity will change at a particular shear rate, and if one plotted the shear stress against the shear rate for such a liquid, one would typically find the response shown in **56**.

In this case, the viscosity for an increasing shear rate is different from the viscosity for a decreasing shear rate, which is an example of *hysteresis*. In such cases, the viscosity of the fluid is dependent upon the previous deformations to which the fluid has been subjected.

This type of behaviour occurs when there is some molecular rearrangement caused by the mixing, and a lack of time for the molecules to return to their normal arrangement before mixing again. The effect of this is, that the longer the fluid is mixed at a given shear rate, the lower the shear stress and hence the viscosity will be. If the fluid were left for long enough, it would recover and the whole process could be repeated. This type of behaviour is defined as *thixotropic*, and a fluid that exhibits this is non-drip paint.

## Viscoelasticity

A wide range of materials show behaviour that is intermediate between that of a viscous liquid and an elastic solid. For an elastic solid, it has been assumed that the relationship between stress and strain is independent of any dynamic factors such as loading rate or strain rate. However, if given sufficient time to do so, some solids show a capacity to rearrange their molecules under the influence of an applied load, and this is reflected in a change in the strain. When the load is then released the material does not

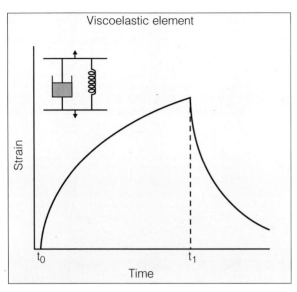

**58** Viscoelastic behaviour of a spring and dashpot in parallel.

immediately return to its original state. This means that the behaviour of the material is dependent upon such factors as the duration and the amount of load applied.

A simple and effective way of visualising this problem is through the use of models based on a spring and a dashpot, which combine to give a system rather like a shock absorber. The spring represents the elastic element, and the dashpot represents the viscous element. The variation of the strain with time for these models is shown in **57**. For the spring, the application of a load results in an immediate strain that is maintained for as long as the load is applied. Once the load is removed, the spring returns instantaneously to its original state. In contrast, upon the application of a load to the dashpot, there is a gradual increase in the strain, which continues to increase for as long as the load is applied. On removal of the load the strain is not relieved, and the dashpot remains in its new position.

When these two elements are placed in parallel, a simple viscoelastic model is created. The strain response for such a model is shown in **58**. In this model, the dashpot prevents the spring from responding elastically. Now, the dashpot gradually lets the spring approach its desired strained state. On removal of the load, the dashpot prevents the spring contracting to its unstrained state, which it can now only achieve after some time.

A dental example of a group of materials which show viscoelastic behaviour are the elastomeric impression materials. The strain–time curve for such a material, and the corresponding model based on the elastic, viscous and viscoelastic elements are shown in **59**.

In order to avoid excessive permanent deformation of these materials, they should not be loaded for any longer than necessary; this is why elastic impression materials must be removed from the mouth with a short sharp pull. The more rapid the material is loaded and unloaded the more elastically the material will respond.

# Thermal Properties

Material can either feel warm or cold to touch. This response of a material to a source of heat, in this case the finger tips, is dependent upon the ease with which heat is transferred through the material. A material which readily conducts heat is a *thermal conductor* and a material which resists the conduction of heat is a *thermal insulator*.

## Thermal Conductivity

One factor which determines the ease with which heat is transferred through a material is its thermal conductivity, where thermal conductivity (K) is defined as the rate of heat flow per unit temperature gradient; its units are cal. cm$^{-1}$.sec$^{-1}$.°C$^{-1}$.

## Specific Heat

For some materials, the initial 'cold feeling' can rapidly disappear as the material heats up due to the transfer of heat energy from the heat source to the material. How rapidly the temperature increases depends upon the specific heat of the material, which is defined as the heat energy required to raise the temperature of a unit volume by one degree Centigrade. Thus, its units are cal.gm$^{-1}$.°C$^{-1}$ and the symbol used is $C_p$.

## Thermal Diffusivity

The transfer of heat from a hot to a cold source is dependent on both the thermal conductivity and the specific heat, with the former regulating the rate at which the heat enters and passes through the material and the latter determining the rate at which the temperature will rise as heat enters

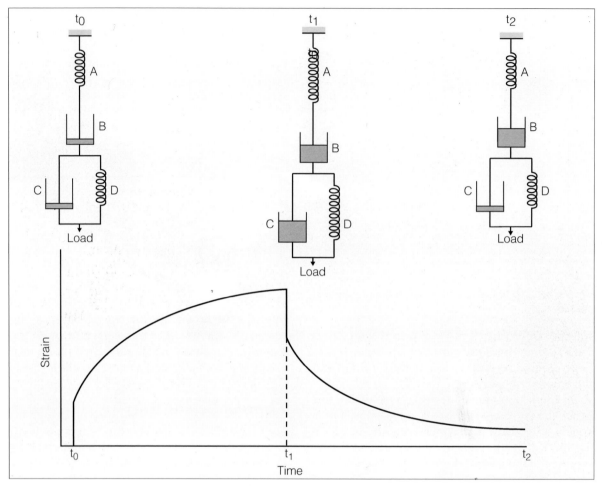

**59** Viscoelastic model corresponding closely to the rheological behaviour of a fully set elastomeric impression material. The load is applied at time $t_0$, and spring A extends instantaneously while spring D is prevented from doing so by the dashpot C. With time, dashpots C and B allow further strain to develop. At time $t_1$, the load is removed, and spring A contracts immediately. Spring D is prevented from doing so by dashpot C. Eventually, at time $t_2$, spring D has returned to its original length. Some permanent strain remains, since dashpot B will not return to its original state.

the material. This is presented by the thermal diffusivity, h, such that

$$h = \frac{K}{C_p \rho}$$

where $\rho$ is the density of the material. The thermal diffusivity gives a clear indication of the rate of rise of temperature at one point due to a heat source at another point, and may be considered the most relevant in dental applications.

Some typical values of the above properties for a range of materials are presented in *Table 5*. An interesting feature is the low diffusivity of water, showing it to be an excellent thermal insulator. For this reason, eskimos can be quite warm when sheltering in their igloos.

## Thermal Expansion

When a material is heated, the extra energy absorbed causes the atoms or molecules to vibrate with an increased amplitude. As a consequence,

**Table 5** Physical properties of dental materials.

|  | $\rho$ (gm.cm$^{-2}$) | $C_p$ (cal.gm$^{-1}$.°C$^{-1}$) | K (cal.cm$^{-1}$.sec$^{-1}$.°C$^{-1}$) | h (cm$^{-2}$.sec$^{-1}$) |
|---|---|---|---|---|
| Enamel | 2.9 | 0.18 | 0.0022 | 0.0042 |
| Dentine | 2.1 | 0.28 | 0.0015 | 0.0026 |
| Silver | 10.5 | 0.056 | 0.98 | 1.67 |
| Silica | 2.5 | 0.20 | 0.003 | 0.006 |
| Water | 1.0 | 1.00 | 0.0014 | 0.0014 |

the material expands. The most common way of measuring this expansion is by taking a length of material, heating it to a certain temperature and then measuring the resultant change in length. This change in length, when determined per unit length for a 1°C change in temperature, is called the linear coefficient of expansion, $\alpha$. This change is so small that it is more usual to express it in terms of parts per million per degree Centigrade (ppm/°C). Some typical values for $\alpha$ are given in *Table 6*.

In an ideal restorative material, the coefficient of expansion would be identical to that of the tooth tissues. If this is not the case, the thermal mismatch can give rise to marginal gap formation and the breakdown of adhesive bonds. Such effects will depend not only upon the coefficient of expansion but also on the thermal diffusivity of the material.

Some materials, such as silver, require only a small amount of heat energy to raise their temperature and readily expand or contract. In contrast, composite restorative materials have a low thermal diffusivity. This provides some protection against thermal stimuli, as more heat energy is required to cause a rise in temperature and the corresponding expansion. However, if sufficient heat *is* supplied, the material *will* show a significant expansion/contraction mismatch with tooth tissues.

Fracture of castings can occur due to hot tearing on cooling, when there is a big mismatch between the refractory material and the casting alloy. Dimensional correction of the cooling contraction of alloys is vitally important if crowns and bridges are to fit. Similarly, metal-bonded porcelain relies on a close match of the coefficient of expansion of the metal and the porcelain.

**Table 6** Coefficients of thermal expansion.

|  | $\alpha$ (ppm/°C) |
|---|---|
| Enamel | 12 |
| Dentine | 14 |
| Resin composite | 20–55 |
| Fissure sealant | 80 |
| Porcelain | 12 |
| Glass–ionomer cement | 8 |

# Optical Properties

The perception of colour is highly subjective as it is a physiological response to a physical stimulus. For example, the choice of colour of restorative material that is required to match a tooth tends to vary slightly from person to person, and presents a real problem for those who suffer from colour blindness. This happens because the eye is an ill-defined detector of light, having properties that vary from person to person. The *perception* of colour does not therefore lend itself to quantification, but this is not the case for the light itself.

Light is electromagnetic radiation that can be detected by the human eye. The spectrum of electromagnetic radiation from the ultraviolet to the infrared is shown in **60**. From this, it can be seen that visible electromagnetic radiation is in the range from 400–700 nanometers.

Light is focused on the retina and triggers nerve impulses that are transmitted to the brain. There are cone shaped cells in the retina that are responsible for providing sensitivity to different coloured light, and rod shaped cells that are sensitive only to the brightness (i.e. the amount of light) that is focussed on the retina. The

| X-ray | Ultra violet | Visible | | Infrared | RF |
|---|---|---|---|---|---|
| | Far | Violet | Red | Far | |
| | | Indigo | Orange | | |
| | | Blue | Yellow | | |
| | Near | Green | | Near | |
| 10 | 400 | Wavelength (nm) | 700 | 1 000 000 | |

**60** Spectrum of electromagnetic radiation.

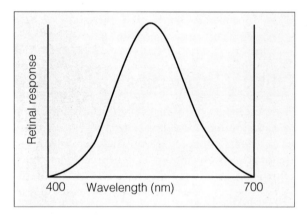

**61** The relative response of the retina to visible electromagnetic radiation.

response of the retina to light is indicated in **61**. It shows that the eye is most sensitive to light in the green–yellow range, and is least sensitive at the extremes of the visible spectrum, i.e. the reds and blues.

The cone shaped cells have a threshold intensity. Exposure to excessive light of a given wavelength can cause these cells to switch off, resulting in eye strain and a very different perception of colour.

The actual light that we see is not of a single wavelength, but is composed of a mixture of different wavelengths which combine to produce a distinctive colour. The wavelength and intensity spectrum of the light we see depends on the source of the light. The light spectra for daylight

and a tungsten filament lamp are quite different, as shown in **62**. This means that a surface's colour will appear different when it is viewed under light from different sources.

For a description of colour we can consider three aspects:

- *Hue* – This represents the dominant colour (i.e. wavelength) of the spectrum of light from the source. The possible colours are violet, indigo, blue, green, yellow, orange and red. The three primary colours, from which all other colours can be produced, are red, green and blue. This fact is used in TV sets to create a full colour picture from only three distinctly coloured sets of dots.
- *Chroma* – This is the *strength* of hue, in other words how vivid the colour is. On the TV set, this would be represented by the colour adjustment.
- *Value* – This is the brightness or darkness of the object, and ranges from black to white for diffusive or reflective objects, and from black to clear for translucent objects.

Whereas hue and chroma are properties of the object, the value will depend on the incident light, the surface finish of the object and the background if the material transmits light. With dental restorative materials, the latter dependence invariably has to be considered. For this reason, it is important that colour matching

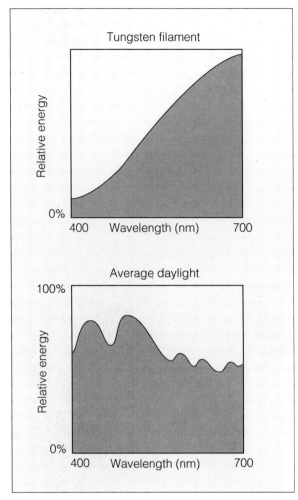

**62** Light spectra for a tungsten filament lamp and daylight.

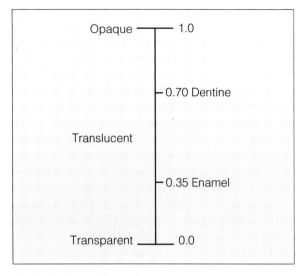

**63** A simple opacity scale.

should be carried out under a variety of light sources, with bright daylight being by far the best. The fact that objects can change colour under the influence of different light sources is known as *metamerism*.

Another important feature of light is that some objects are able to absorb light of a wavelength near ultraviolet range (300–400nm), and then release it as light of a longer wavelength (400–450nm). This is the property of *fluorescence*, and it occurs in natural tooth enamel. This is the reason why natural teeth look so white under a fluorescent light and why some crowns, bridges or fillings are more noticeable in such light, as they do not fluoresce, and look dark next to the fluorescing natural tooth.

Another important property of a material which affects the way it looks is its *opacity*. An opaque material is one that does not transmit light, but instead absorbs light or reflects or scatters from the surface.

The colour of the object will depend on which wavelengths of light are reflected and which are absorbed.

A translucent material allows some light to pass through it, absorbs some of the remainder, and scatters and reflects the rest from its surface. An object viewed through such a material would have a distorted appearance.

A transparent material allows the passage of light in such a way that little distortion takes place, meaning that an object can be seen quite clearly through it. Selective absorption of certain wavelengths may take place, and this forms the basis for optical filters.

For example, red glass is red because it allows light with the wavelength of red light to pass through it but absorbs all other wavelengths. Consequently, it would appear opaque if the light source did not contain light with the wavelength of red light, since all the other wavelengths are absorbed.

A simple scale for quantification of the degree of opacity is shown in **63**. Restorative materials can be compared easily with enamel and dentine on this scale, to find their relative degrees of opacity.

# I.IX

# CHEMICAL PROPERTIES

## Introduction

The oral environment is an aggressive environment. Materials may dissolve in the water that is present or release soluble components; they may erode due to the presence of acids; they may discolour or break down due to absorption of substances from the water; or they may tarnish and corrode.

All of these possibilities can adversely affect the chemical stability of the materials and limit their durability. The products released may have an adverse effect on the biological environment, both locally and systemically.

In general, it could be said that polymers tend to suffer from absorption and loss of soluble components, metals are prone to tarnish and corrosion, and ceramics may be subject to erosion.

## Water Sorption And Soluble Fraction

Polymers such as those used in resin composites, dentures and soft liners are susceptible particularly to water absorption and the loss of soluble components. In the case of resin composites, this is believed to be a contributory factor to the eventual discoloration of the restorations and the hydrolytic degradation of the resin–filler interface. Soft denture liners lose their flexibility due to the loss of water soluble plasticisers, have an increased propensity to creep, and may even fracture under the osmotic pressure that can build up.

Thus, it is desirable for both the water sorption and soluble fraction of polymers to be as small as possible. This ensures that the polymer retains its characteristic properties, and that no components are leached out which might adversely influence the biocompatibility of the material.

The simplest method of assessing the water sorption and soluble fraction of a polymer is to monitor the weight change of a sample when immersed in water. The detailed analysis of the amount of water sorption by polymeric materials is complicated by the concurrent loss of water soluble components such as residual monomers or plasticisers, as these two processes take place simultaneously, although at different rates. It is important in the characterisation of these factors that the two processes are separated.

Both processes are controlled by the rates of diffusion of water and the water soluble components through the material, such that the higher the rates of diffusion, the faster water will be absorbed and the faster the soluble fraction will be lost. It is important that any water that the sample has absorbed from the atmosphere has been removed prior to its immersion in water. To this end, samples must be stored in a dessicator until a constant weight is obtained.

The kinetics of a sorption and desorption cycle are shown in **64**. The peak in the weight of the sample in the first cycle is a consequence of the different rates of diffusio of water *into* the sample and diffusion of the soluble fraction *out of* the sample. Water is usually absorbed more rapidly than the soluble components are removed, such that there is an initial rapid weight gain until the sample is nearing saturation, at which point the loss in weight due to the soluble fraction begins to show, as its release is aided by its dissolution into the absorbed water. The amount of water sorption and the soluble fraction can be calculated from the following:

$$\text{Weight \% water sorption} = \frac{(W_1 - W_2)}{W_2 \times 100}$$

$$\text{Weight \% soluble fraction} = \frac{(W_0 - W_2)}{W_2 \times 100}$$

If the volume, V, at the end of the desorption cycle is calculated, and $W_2$ replaced by V, then the water sorption and soluble fraction can be expressed in terms of $\mu g/mm^3$, as recommended in the international standard (ISO/DIS 4049).

For most polymers, the amount of water sorption is approximately 30–50 $\mu g/mm^3$. For resin composites, the value will be lower, due to the presence of the glass fillers, but if this is taken into account, the amount of water sorption into the resin should be in the range given above for polymers. Higher values for water sorption have been recorded for some resin composites, which may be associated with the presence of porosity, free space formed due to removal of the soluble fraction, hydrolytic breakdown of the resin–filler interface, or dissolution of the glass filler.

# Tarnish And Corrosion

Tarnish is a surface discoloration due to the formation of hard and soft deposits, e.g. sulphides and chlorides. Tarnish does not cause a deterioration of the material itself, but can be

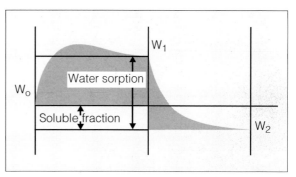

**64** A schematic representation of the kinetics of water sorption and the dissolution of the soluble fraction.

unsightly, and is easily removed from the surface by polishing the metal. In contrast, corrosion is a chemical reaction between the material and its environment and is therefore a potentially much more serious problem.

Ceramics, such as oxides, silicates and aluminates, are compounds of oxygen. They are chemically stable under most circumstances, whereas metals are not. Except for some *noble metals*, such as gold and platinum, metals are usually found in nature as compounds (principally oxides or sulphides), from which the metal is extracted. Corrosion is, to all intents and purposes, the reversal of the reactions employed in the extraction process. Frequently, the corrosionproduct of a metal is very similar to the compound from which the metal was originally extracted. For instance, iron is extracted from naturally occurring iron oxide, and rust is simply hydrated iron oxide. Generally, polymers are not stable either, as many will burn once ignited, showing that the polymer oxidises readily.

The corrosion process for metals is driven by a decrease in the free energy as the metal reacts with a liquid or a gas. All metals are prone to corrosive attack when the environment is aggressive enough. Corrosion is highly undesirable, as it weakens materials and may lead to fracture. Similarly, the corrosion products may react adversely with the biological environment. This latter factor is of major concern in the use of metals in dental applications.

## *Dry Corrosion*

Other than gold and a few other noble metals, all metals will form a surface oxide coating when the surface comes into contact with the oxygen in

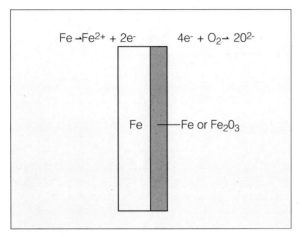

**65** Oxide formation on the surface of a metal.

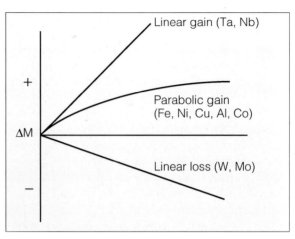

**66** Weight change due to surface oxidation.

the air (**65**). Sometimes this thin film of surface oxide can be seen, as is the case of titanium when it produces interference colours that are used to good effect in the production of jewellery.

Since the formation of the surface layer of oxide involves the addition of oxygen atoms to the surface, a material which oxidises will gain weight. This process can be monitored, and the three possible outcomes of such an experiment are shown in **66**. Which of these will actually happen depends upon the stability of oxide formed.

If the oxide is very stable then the corrosion process is self-limiting and there comes a point where the metal ions take so long to diffuse through the thickening oxide layer (whereupon they come into contact with oxygen and react with it), that the oxidation virtually stops. In this case there is an initial rapid weight gain that gradually tails off; this gives the parabolic weight gain curve.

Some other oxides are not very stable, and as they form on the metal surface, they tend to crack or to separate partially from the surface, exposing the underlying metal and allowing a new oxide coating to form. In this case there is a gradual build-up of the oxide, causing a continous gain in weight.

The third possibility, that of weight loss, is less common, and only occurs during the oxidation of certain metals at high temperatures. If the temperature is sufficiently high, the oxide evaporates as soon as it is formed, offering no barrier to further oxidation of the metal. Consequently, weight is lost as the oxide layer evaporates.

These forms of oxidation are described as *dry corrosion*. Most metals are stable under such processes due to the protective first layer of the oxide coating itself. Hence, surplus aircraft are stored in the desert, where it is hot, but more importantly dry, and cars are less susceptible to rust in hot, dry climates. In the presence of an aqueous environment, different conditions prevail and the material's response is much altered.

## Wet Corrosion

Wet corrosion can take place in neutral, acid or alkaline environments. When a metal is placed in an aqueous environment, metal ions and electrons are released into the water (**67**).

An oxidator, commonly oxygen dissolved in the water, withdraws electrons from the metal, in what is known as the *cathodic process*. This extraction of electrons produces a current called the *cathodic current*. This loss of electrons from the metal causes the metal to become positively charged, and positive ions are released into the water, producing an *anodic current*.

If the metal ions are removed from the surface evenly, the process is called *uniform* corrosion. Under suitable conditions, *localised* as opposed to *uniform* corrosion can take place, and this is generally far more dangerous. *Galvanic* and *crevice* corrosion are examples of such localised corrosion.

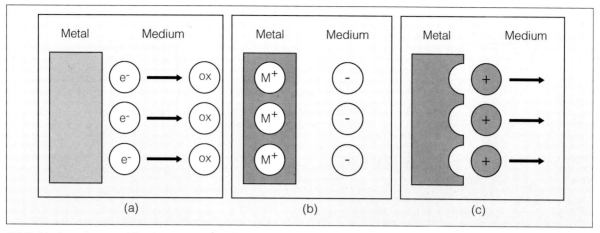

**67** Oxidation of a metal in an aqueous environment. The oxidator withdraws electrons from the metal in what is known as the cathodic process (a). This causes the metal to become positively charged and the medium negatively charged (b). Due to the positive charge of the metal, metal ions are released, in what is known as the anodic process (c).

### Galvanic Corrosion

Galvanic corrosion occurs when two dissimilar metals are combined, resulting in the corrosion of one of the metals being significantly increased.

A classic example of this is the corrosion of zinc in acid. When zinc is in contact with platinum, as shown in **68**, the platinum reacts very quickly with the hydrogen ions that are supplied by the acid, and releases electrons, producing hydrogen (this is an example of the cathodic process). This generates an electrical imbalance between the zinc and the platinum, such that electrons flow from the zinc to the platinum. This enhances the release of metal ions from the zinc (the anodic process), such that the zinc corrodes faster when it is in contact with the platinum.

To what degree dissimilar metals will be susceptible to this form of corrosion depends primarily on their relative rates of reaction. Platinum is a particularly effective oxidiser. Other noble metals will not have quite the same effect, as they are not quite so effective at oxidation.

A combination of metals behaving in this way is described as a *galvanic cell*, and can occur within alloys due to the presence of different phases with different rates of oxidation. An example is the galvanic cell set up between the $\gamma_1$ and $\gamma_2$ phases in dental amalgam, where the $\gamma_2$

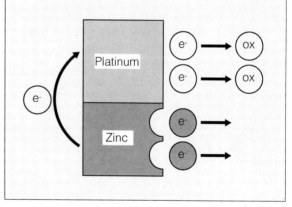

**68** Galvanic corrosion of zinc in contact with platinum. The noble metal (platinum) is more easily oxidised than the base metal (zinc) such that the anodic process takes place at the zinc surface and zinc ions are released into the aqueous environment.

phase corrodes significantly faster than the $\gamma_1$ phase.

### Crevice Corrosion

When there is a sharp crack or fluid filled space, as shown in **69**, this space is usually depleted of oxygen. The metal ions will still be released into the space and will form corrosion products, whereas the electrons are unable to react because of the lack of oxygen. Thus, the oxidation reaction must take place where there *is* oxygen,

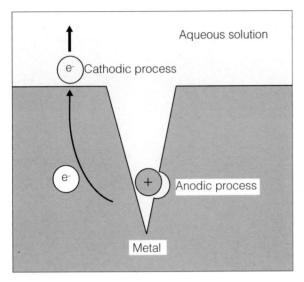

**69** In crevice corrosion the oxidation takes place at the surface (cathodic process) and metal ions are released from within the crevice (anodic process).

which will be at the main surface, such that the electrons will have to travel through the metal, making the base of the crevice anodic and the surface cathodic. Material is therefore lost from the base of the crevice. As the corrosion products are formed, they tend to build up in the crevice such that the supply of oxygen is further restricted. There is nothing to stop this reaction from continuing, which makes this form of corrosion highly insidious. The same process can happen when there is a break in the surface oxide coating, which is known as *pitting* corrosion.

The concentrated attack on one area of the metal is highly undesirable, as it causes the metal to weaken due to the formation and growth of cracks. The damage done is totally out of proportion to the amount of material destroyed by the corrosion process. Thus, localised corrosion is far more dangerous than uniform corrosion.

# I.X

## PRINCIPLES OF ADHESION

## Introduction

Since the acid-etch technique of bonding to enamel was introduced into dentistry, the use of adhesive procedures has developed to such an extent that it now constitutes a major part of the dental discipline. Many concepts which have served the profession well for many decades in providing good dental care have had to be revised in the light of these developments, and many new techniques and materials have been introduced.

Two examples of new, adhesive restorative procedures that spring to mind readily are resin-bonded bridges and porcelain veneers. These procedures have been possible because of our improved knowledge and understanding of the surface characteristics of enamel and dentine, and of the requirements that need to be satisfied in order to obtain good bonds to them.

These advances in themselves would not have been sufficient, but they laid a foundation for the development of the new materials and techniques that are used in enamel and dentine bonding today. A combination of factors has provided the dentist with a variety of procedures for restoring the dentition. Although these procedures have been available for only a relatively short time, their impact has already been quite considerable.

There are now many materials that we wish to bond to enamel and dentine and to each other. Consequently, numerous adhesives have been developed to cope with the diversity of the applications; such adhesives include composite resins, glass–ionomer cements and dentine bonding agents.

New methods of surface preparation, such as etching and silane coupling, have had to be investigated to find ways of using them in conjunction with materials such as the new glass-ceramics and a wide variety of alloys.

It is the variety of applications that has contributed to the growing complexity of adhesive restorative dentistry. In order to appreciate fully and understand the clinical application of adhesive techniques, it is important for the clinician to have a thorough knowledge of the principles of adhesion, the materials used, the dental adhesive systems and how these are applied in the clinical situation.

## What Is Adhesion?

*Adhesion* can be defined as the force that binds two dissimilar materials together when they are brought into intimate contact. That this is distinct from *cohesion*, which is the attraction between similar atoms or molecules within one substance.

61

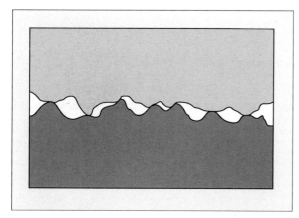

**70** Point to point contact of two solid surfaces at a microscopic level.

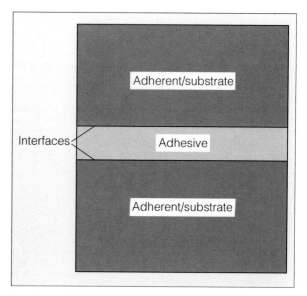

**71** Terminology for the description of an adhesive joint.

## Adhesion Between Solids

At an atomic level, surfaces are rough. This means that when they are brought into contact, the only places where intimate contact is achieved is at the tips of the *asperities* (**70**).

Very high pressures can be generated at these points, such that in the absence of any contaminants an effect called *local adhesion* or *cold welding* can result. If an attempt is then made to slide the one surface over the other, a resistance known as *friction* is experienced.

Friction is caused by the need of the local adhesions to be sheared, or broken. In general, the local adhesions are so strong that the shearing process does not take place at the interface but actually within the solids themselves; this explains the general phenomenon of frictional wear.

While frictional forces due to local adhesion can be quite high, adhesion *normal* (i.e. perpendicular) to the surface is usually undetectable. This has been attributed to the build up of elastic stresses in the normal direction, which are released when the load on the material is removed.

Only very soft metals, such as pure gold, can relieve these elastic stresses by flow and prevent rupture of the junction when a normal load is applied. A dental example of this is the use of cohesive gold.

## Adhesion Between A Solid And A Liquid

It is a matter of common observation that a drop of water will cling to the underside of a glass slide. This effect demonstrates the adherence of water to glass that arises by virtue of molecular attraction between the two substances. The attraction is due to secondary (van der Waals) bonds. Even a hard shake of the slide will not remove all of the water and merely drying the glass with a cloth will still leave a very thin residual layer of water. The only way of ensuring that all the water has been removed is by heating the glass in an oven.

This illustrates the good adhesion that may be obtained between a solid and a liquid. Such good adhesion is due to the liquid's ability to make intimate contact with the solid over a large surface area. This is in contrast to the poor adhesion (described above) that usually occurs between two solids, where the contact is at points only.

Thus, one of the fundamental requirements of adhesion is that the two substances to be bonded must be in close contact with each other.

The importance of this statement can not be overemphasised, as a strong bond can be created only in the case of intimate molecular contact. This may seem a simple requirement, but it is not particularly easy to achieve intimate contact at the microscopic level, as noted for solids above.

Given that the distance between the interacting molecules must be less than 0.0007 microns for adhesion to occur, one appreciates that adhesion is virtually impossible for two solid surfaces. This is a serious obstacle when there is a need for adhesion between two solids, and in order to overcome this, we use a third substance, usually in a fluid or semi-fluid state, to act as an intermediary.

The substance that binds the two materials is defined as the *adhesive*, and the surfaces of the materials are the *adherents* or *substrates*. The point at which the substrate meets the adhesive is described as the *interface* (**71**).

Naturally, what happens at the interface is crucially important to the success or failure of an adhesive bond. This applies equally to industrial and dental adhesives, so it is useful in the first instance to consider the general requirements of an adhesive and then to look more closely at the bonding mechanisms.

# Criteria For Adhesion

When reading the instruction leaflet of any adhesive, one of the first requirements is invariably that the surfaces to be bonded are both clean and dry. This is important for a variety of reasons. A clean, dry surface ensures that the adhesive has the best possible chance of creating a proper bond with the solid material; the presence on the surface of anything that could be considered as a contaminant will prevent the formation of a strong bond, since the contaminant itself is weakly bonded to the solid and will prevent the adhesion of the adhesive to the substrate.

The factors which govern the ability of the adhesive to make intimate contact with the substrate are:

- The *wettability* of the substrate by the adhesive.
- The *viscosity* of the adhesive.
- The *morphology* or *surface roughness* of the substrate.

## *Wettability*

In order for the adhesive to create a bond between two materials, it must make intimate contact with the surfaces of the substrates such that no air voids (which would weaken the bond) are formed. The ability of an adhesive to contact a substrate depends on the *wettability* of

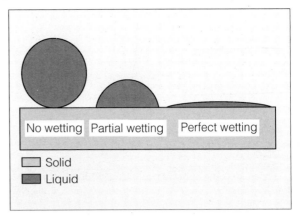

**72** The possible wetting characteristics for liquids on a solid surface.

the adhesive on that particular substrate. *Good wetting* is the ability to cover the substrate completely, so that the maximum benefit is obtained from whichever adhesive mechanism is activated.

The ability or inability of fluids to wet a surface is frequently encountered in everyday life. An example of a surface which is extremely difficult to wet with water is PTFE (polytetrafluoroethylene) as used in non-stick saucepans. Water placed on a PTFE surface forms globules that will not spread in an even layer across the surface. This is an example of poor wettability. This, and the other possible responses, are depicted in the **72**.

The interaction between the substrate and the adhesive is governed by a driving force that tends to spread the adhesive over the substrate, and resistance to spreading that depends upon the viscosity of the adhesive, the surface irregularities and the presence of contaminants. The driving force is provided by the surface energies of the adhesive and the substrate (see below)

## *Surface Energy*

In the bulk of a solid or a liquid, the molecules are subjected to attractive forces in all directions such that the molecule is in dynamic equilibrium with its surrounding molecules. At the surface however, this delicate balance is destroyed, resulting in a net attraction inwards, towards the large number of molecules in the mass of the material. It is this inward force which gives rise to the *surface energy* of a material. In liquids, the surface energy is known as the *surface tension*.

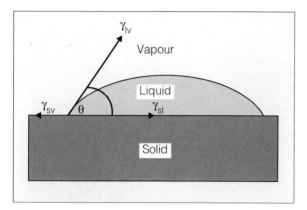

**73** The contact angle θ between a liquid and a solid, where $\gamma_{sv}$ is the surface tension between the solid and the vapour, $\gamma_{sl}$ is the surface tension between the solid and the liquid and $\gamma_{lv}$ is that between the liquid and the vapour.

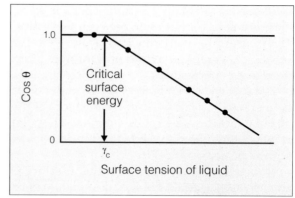

**74** Zisman plot for the determination of the critical surface energy, $\gamma_c$, of a solid.

One of the effects of surface tension is the tendency for liquids to take up a spherical shape in preference to any other. This arises because a sphere has the minimum surface area (and hence the minimum surface energy) for a given volume of liquid, allowing the total energy stored in the liquid to be a minimum.

Whereas the surface tension of a liquid is a real surface stress, in the case of a solid, work is done in stretching, and not in forming the surface. The measurement of the surface energy of a solid is not achieved as readily as it is with liquids. An approach that has now gained wide acceptance is one pioneered by Zisman, who introduced the concept of the *critical surface energy*.

## Contact Angle

When a solid and a liquid make contact, the angle between the liquid surface and the solid surface is known as the *contact angle*, and is dependent upon the surface tension of the liquid and the surface energy of the solid (**73**).

By measuring the contact angle between the solid and the liquid, a useful measure of the wettability of the liquid on a particular substrate can be obtained. For perfect wetting, which is the ideal situation for adhesion to occur, this angle should be zero degrees. In this case, the surface is completely covered with the adhesive and the maximum bond strength can be achieved. The driving force that gives rise to the tendency, or otherwise, of a fluid to spread on a solid surface

depends upon the surface tension of the liquid and the surface energy of the solid. At the point where the surface of the liquid meets the surface of the solid their surface tensions must balance, in order to be in equilibrium:

$$\gamma_{sv} = \gamma_{sl} + \gamma_{lv} \cos\theta.$$

This relationship can be rearranged to give the contact angle, θ, and in this form is known as the *Young equation*:

$$\cos\theta = \frac{(\gamma_{sv} - \gamma_{sl})}{\gamma_{lv}}$$

where $\gamma_{sl}$ is the surface energy at the solid–liquid interface, $\gamma_{sv}$ is the surface energy at the solid–vapour interface and $\gamma_{lv}$ is the surface energy at the liquid–vapour interface.

## Critical Surface Energy

If one measures the contact angle of a number of different liquids on the same substrate and plots the cosine of the contact angle against the known surface tension of the liquids, then a linear relationship results.

This relationship is shown in **74**; it shows the linear curve being extrapolated to the point where it crosses the line at which the cosine of the contact angle is equal to one. This is the situation under which the contact angle will be zero degrees, representing the condition of perfect wetting.

The value of the surface tension at which the cosine of the contact equals one is defined as the *critical surface energy* of the solid. This critical surface energy is equal to the surface tension of a liquid that will *just* spread on the surface of the solid; such a liquid may be real or hypothetical. Any liquid which has a surface tension less than the critical surface energy of the solid will wet the surface of the solid effectively.

Thus, a low surface energy liquid will readily spread over a high surface energy substrate, because the surface of the substrate is replaced by a surface with a lower surface energy.

PTFE has a very low surface energy, making it difficult to find liquids with lower surface tensions that could wet it successfully. Another material with a similarly low surface energy is silicone rubber. Again, it is extremely difficult to get anything to adhere to this material.

On the other hand, silicone polymers in their liquid form tend to adapt well to most surfaces due to their low surface energies. These polymers are used to great effect in impression materials.

Examples of the surface energy of a number of substances, expressed in units of J.m$^{-2}$ (N.m$^{-1}$) for convenience, are provided in *Table 7*. In the case of perfluorolauric acid, only condensed inert gases can spread on this surface.

## Viscosity

For an adhesive to be effective, it must be able not only to make intimate contact with the substrate, but also to spread easily on it, yet not so easily that it is impossible to control. The driving force for the spreading of the liquid is provided by its wettability on the solid surface, and is resisted by the liquid's viscosity. Too high a viscosity is undesirable, as it prevents the fluid from flowing readily over the surface of the solid.

In general, contact angles are directly proportional to the viscosity of the adhesive, but this can be a misleading statement if the adhesive is a solvent containing additives.

The use of low surface tension solvents with highly viscous solutes will give misleadingly low contact angles. Although, a low contact angle is obtained, the resistance to flow offered by the high viscosity of the solute will continue to resist the spreading.

**Table 7** Typical surface energies

| | Surface Energy (×10$^{-3}$ J.m$^{-2}$) |
|---|---|
| Perfluorolauric acid | 6 |
| Methyl chloride | 16 |
| Polytetrafluoroethylene (PTFE) | 18 |
| Polytrifluoroethylene | 22 |
| Ethyl alcohol | 24 |
| Polyvinyl chloride (PVC) | 39 |
| Water | 73 |
| Plate glass | 20 |
| Steel | 230 |
| Iron oxide | 350 |
| Alumina | 560 |
| Mercury | 488 |

Similarly, a highly filled adhesive, such as a composite resin, can be difficult to spread, which may lead one to think it has a high surface tension and poor wettability. However, the substrate only experiences contact with the low viscosity resin that may readily wet the surface if it has the correct surface tension. Spreading of the composite resin is merely resisted by its own stiffness and not by any reluctance on the part of the resin to wet the underlying surface.

## Surface Roughness

The measurement of contact angles assumes that the surface of the substrate is perfectly smooth. In reality, the surface may be quite rough at a microscopic level. This roughness has the advantage of increasing the potential area for bonding, but can also give rise to the entrapment of air. Such entrapment will significantly reduce the effective bonding area and result in a weak bond. Cracks and crevices constitute surface irregularities and the adhesive must be able to flow into these.

Adhesives with a high viscosity are particularly prone to causing entrapment of air, because their stiffness may be such that they bridge the small cracks and crevices in the surface, rather than flowing into them.

In the absence of air, capillary action ensures that the adhesive penetrates the cracks and crevices. For this penetration to occur readily, a

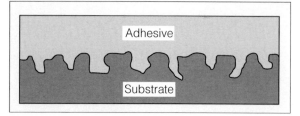

**75** Microscopic mechanical interlocking between an adhesive and the substrate.

high surface tension adhesive is desirable, as this means that the capillary attraction is also high. This effect is demonstrated by the fact that the higher the surface tension of a liquid, the higher the liquid will climb up a capillary placed in it.

The driving force that causes capillary action must work against the pressure of the air that is trapped by the adhesive, and must also overcome the viscous resistance forces. However, the surface tension of the liquid must also be sufficiently low to wet the substrate perfectly. Hence, the ideal adhesive would have a surface tension just below the surface energy of the solid. If this condition is satisfied, then the surface irregularities can be advantageous in improving the bond strength of the adhesive.

An irregular surface has a higher surface area than a smooth surface, so more chemical bonds can be created. If the irregularities are of a certain morphology, such that undercuts are present at the microscopic level, the bond can be enhanced by the process of micromechanical interlocking.

# Mechanisms Of Adhesion

First, let us assume that the initial criterion for adhesion is met, in that intimate contact at the molecular level between the adhesive and the substrate is achieved. Let us now look at what happens when the materials are in contact, and see how they may interact. The way in which an adhesive bond is created can be either mechanical, physical or chemical, and is more usually a combination of all of these.

## Mechanical Adhesion

The simplest method of adhesion is that of the mechanical interlocking of components. This form of adhesion can result from the presence of surface irregularities, such as pits and fissures, that give rise to microscopic undercuts.

A primary condition for this form of adhesion is that the adhesive can penetrate readily into the pits before it begins to set. This condition is determined by the wettability of the adhesive on the substrate, which in turn is governed by the relative surface energies and the resultant contact angle; the ideal situation being that of perfect wetting. To improve the level of contact, any air or vapour in the pits must be able to escape in front of the advancing liquid. If the adhesive is able to penetrate these spaces and subsequently to set solid, it remains locked in by the undercuts (**75**). The degree of penetration will depend upon both the pressure used in the application of the adhesive, and upon the properties of the adhesive itself.

If the adhesive is to disengage from the substrate, then it must fracture in the process of debonding as it can not withdraw from the undercut. This is not unlike the concept of retention, used in the placement of restorations, except that it occurs at a microscopic level. However, one important difference is that good wettability is not a prerequisite for macro-retention, whereas it is of paramount importance for micromechanical interlocking.

The general view is that undercuts frequently provide important mechanical characteristics, but that they are not usually sufficient to act as the mechanism of adhesion in themselves. There are a number of additional adhesive mechanisms that are due to what can be described as physical and chemical causes. The term *true adhesion*, or *specific adhesion*, is commonly used to distinguish physical and chemical adhesion from mechanical adhesion. However, these terms should be discouraged as these are inappropriate.

True adhesion implies that there is also false adhesion, but a material is either adhesive or not. Physical and chemical adhesion are distinguished from mechanical adhesion by the virtue that they involve a molecular attraction between the adhesive and the substrate, whereas mechanical adhesion does not require such interaction at the interface.

## Physical Adhesion

When two surfaces are in close proximity, secondary forces of attraction arise through dipole–

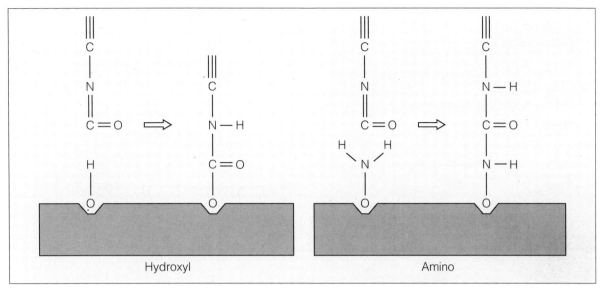

**76** Covalent bond formation between an isocyanate and a hydroxyl and an amino group on the surface of the substrate.

dipole interactions between polar molecules (see section I.III). The attractive forces that are generated can be quite small, even if the molecules have a substantial permanent dipole moment or have a large polarisability.

The magnitude of the interaction energy is dependent upon the relative alignment of the dipoles in the two surfaces, but is usually less than 0.2 eV. This is considerably less than primary bonds, such as ionic or covalent bonds, which are typically 2.0–6.0 eV.

This type of bonding is rapid (because no activation energy is needed) and reversible (because the molecules remain chemically intact on the surface). This weak physical *adsorption* is easily overcome by thermal energy, and is not suitable if a permanent bond is desired. Even so, the hydrogen bond in particular, can be an important precursor to the formation of a strong chemical bond.

It follows that non-polar liquids will not readily bond to polar solids and *vice versa*, because there is no interaction between the two substances at the molecular level, even if there is good adaption. Non-polar liquid silicone polymers exhibit such behaviour, and will not form bonds to solids other than themselves; this bonding is only possible because the chemical reaction of cross-linking provides sites for bonding between the solid and the liquid.

## Chemical Adhesion

If a molecule dissociates after adsorption onto the surface and the constituent components then bond themselves separately by covalent or ionic forces, a strong adhesive bond will result. This form of adhesion is known as *chemisorption*, and can be either covalent or ionic in nature.

The sharing of electrons between the two atoms in the chemical bond distinguishes it from the physical interaction. Adhesives must be strongly chemically attracted to the surface of application in order for strong bonds to form, and require the presence of reactive groups on both surfaces. This is particularly so for the formation of covalent bonds, such as occurs in the bonding of reactive isocyanates to polymeric surfaces containing hydroxyl and amino groups (**76**).

In contrast, a metallic bond is readily created between a solid metal and a liquid metal, and this forms the basis for soldering or brazing. The metallic bond is provided by free electrons and is chemically unspecific. However, the bond will only be possible if the metal surfaces are scrupulously clean.

In practice this means that fluxes need to be used to remove oxide films which would otherwise prevent the metal atoms from meeting.

The mechanical breaking of these chemical bonds becomes the only way of separating the

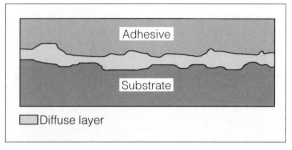

**77** Diffuse interpenetrating layer arising from molecular entanglement between the adhesive and the substrate.

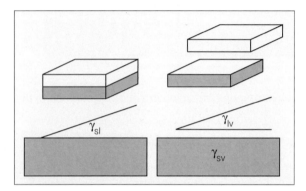

**78** Separation of a liquid from a solid surface, resulting in the creation of two surfaces.

adhesive and the substrate, and there is no reason why these bonds should be broken in preference to any other valence bond. This places a restriction on the strength that can be achieved. If the bond strength exceeds the tensile strength of the adhesive or the substrate, then a cohesive failure of the adhesive or substrate will occur before the bond fails.

### Adhesion Through Molecular Entanglement

So far it has been assumed that there is a distinct interface between the adhesive and the substrate. In effect, the adhesive is adsorbed onto the surface of the substrate and can be considered as being *surface-active*, collecting on the surface but not dissolving in the medium below. In some instances, the adhesive, or a component of the adhesive, is able to penetrate the surface of the substrate and absorb *into* it rather than *onto* it. It should be stressed that the absorption of molecules is a **result** of good wetting and not the cause.

If the absorbing component is a long chain molecule, or forms a long chain molecule within the penetrated layer, the resultant entanglement between the adhesive and the substrate is capable of producing very high bond strengths (**77**).

Thus, adhesives must be strongly chemically attracted to the surfaces of application in order to form a strong bond.

# The Strength Of The Adhesive Bond

A reasonably strong bond can result from the cumulative action of a number of bonding mechanisms that act in concert, such as a large area of intimate contact providing numerous sites for the creation of weak secondary bonds, and the presence of surface undercuts at the microscopic level.

### The Theoretical Strength

It is possible to determine roughly the theoretical strength of an adhesive joint between a liquid and a solid.

If we assume that we have unit surface area of the solid in contact with the liquid, the energy required to separate these materials will be the difference between the energy of the surfaces when joined and the energies of the individual surfaces when separated (**78**).

Thus, the work of adhesion per unit surface area can be defined as:

$$W_a = \gamma_{sv} + \gamma_{lv} - \gamma_{sl}.$$

This is known as the *Dupré equation*, which states that the work of adhesion is the sum of the surface free energy of the solid and the liquid, less the interfacial energy between the solid and the liquid.

From the Young equation,

$$\gamma_{sv} - \gamma_{sl} = \gamma_{lv} \cos \theta.$$

Thus, the work of adhesion can be rewritten as:

$$W_a = \gamma_{lv} (1 + \cos \theta).$$

This adhesion will be a maximum when we have perfect wetting, in which case cos θ = 1, so

$$W_a = 2\,\gamma_{lv}.$$

For a hydrocarbon liquid, the surface tension is approximately 30 mJm$^{-2}$, and if it is assumed that the attractive force falls to zero at a distance of $3\times10^{-10}$ metres, then the force required to pull the liquid away the solid surface is given by the work of adhesion divided by the distance, giving about 200 MPa. This value is in fact far in excess of anything found in the real situation. For example, two slides held together by an interposing liquid are difficult to separate by pulling apart but separation is readily achieved by shearing the two slides apart, as the liquid has no resistance to such a shearing action other than its viscosity.

Thus, it is not enough for the fluid adhesive to wet the surface of the substrate and provide a chemical bond. It must also be able to resist tensile and shearing forces, which would cause failure within the adhesive. Increasing the viscosity would make shearing more difficult, and this is the basis on which adhesives such as sellotape work.

When two plates that are held together by an interposing viscous substance are separated (**79**), the relationship between the force required to do so and the viscosity of the liquid is given by

$$F = \frac{3}{2}\,\frac{\pi\eta R^4}{h^3}\,\frac{\delta h}{\delta t}$$

where is η the viscosity, R is the radius of the plates, and h the thickness of the adhesive.

We will not concern ourselves with how this expression is derived, but it is based on the need for additional fluid to enter the space between the two plates as they are separated. The expression shows that the force is dependent upon the viscosity and the thickness of the adhesive layer. The higher the viscosity of the adhesive and the thinner the adhesive layer then the more force is required to separate the two plates. This expression also shows that the force depends upon the rate of separation.

High rates of separation are resisted more strongly than low rates. The adhesive bond is not resistant to long-term low loads, as it would

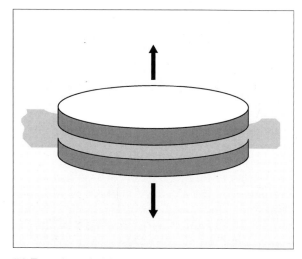

**79** Two plates held together by a viscous liquid.

eventually fail by viscous flow in this manner. The best resistance to shear would therefore be offered by a liquid which turns into a solid, as this greatly increases its shear strength.

## Real Bond Strengths

The actual strengths of adhesive joints are found to be at least an order of magnitude smaller than those predicted from theoretical strength calculations. Another common observation is that bond failure does not often take place at the interface between the substrate and the adhesive but actually somewhere *within* the adhesive, which is essentially a cohesive failure.

Where the failure is genuinely adhesive in nature, it is most probably due to the inability of the adhesive to adapt to the substrate, such that no interaction at the molecular level is possible. Alternatively, contamination or the entrapment of air or other gasses at the interface can prevent a good contact from being established. In this case again, the failure will be at the interface, occurring due to the nucleation and growth of cavities at weak spots along the joint. This highlights the importance of contaminant-free surfaces for bonding.

In practice, the strengths of many adhesive bonds are governed by the presence of stress concentrations in the adhesive or at the interface, rather than the local forces of attraction at the interface. This is especially the case when the bonded structure is subjected to environmental attack or highly stressed loading conditions. In general, adhesives tend to have poorer mechanical properties (i.e. tensile strength and shear strength) than the substrates being bonded, such that surface and internal defects can play a major role in determining the bond strength of the adhesive joint.

For example, if the exposed surface of the adhesive contains numerous defects, then the probability of finding a defect of a critical size is increased as the exposed surface area of the adhesive is increased. For this reason, it is important that the thickness of the adhesive layer is kept to a minimum. The adhesive must be able to adopt a very thin film thickness, which imposes limits on the addition of fillers which might be incorporated to improve the strength.

There is another reason why the minimal application of adhesives is desirable, and that is because of the shrinkage associated with the setting process. When an adhesive shrinks on setting, the contraction may be away from the surface of the substrate such that debonding of the adhesive occurs immediately after placement. Even if the bond holds out during the initial contraction, the stresses generated may be sufficient eventually to cause breakdown of the bond. The thinner the layer of adhesive, the smaller the shrinkage will be.

# Adhesion Promoters

There are many instances in which two materials need to be bonded to each other, but will not do so under normal circumstances because they have no particular affinity for each other and consequently will not wet each other.

A dental example of this would be the desire to obtain a strong and durable bond between the glass filler particles used in a composite resin and the resin itself. To allow these two materials to bond by means other than the physical adsorption of one onto the other (which would be inadequate in itself), it is necessary to modify one or other of the two surfaces to achieve a bond. Sometimes, an intermediary substance can be used that is able to bond to both of the materials in question, and such a material is known

as a *coupling agent*. Alternatively, it is possible to modify the characteristics of the surface of one of the two materials so that a bond can be created. These materials are known as *primers*.

## Coupling Agents

The surface of glass, being ionic in nature, readily adsorbs water, forming a well-bonded surface layer which may be many molecules thick. The formation of this water layer can not be avoided during the commercial processing of glass.

As a consequence of this, when glass is mixed with a resin to produce a composite, be it a fibre composite or a particulate composite, the resin will not wet the surface of the glass and the two are poorly bonded. This has the effect of producing a very weak composite because the glass is not able to take on a load-bearing role and acts merely as a space filler. Some method needs to be devised to dispose of the adsorbed water. One such approach is the use of *coupling agents*. An appropriate coupling agent, applied to the glass, will displace the water on the surface if the bond created between it and the glass is more stable than that between the water and the glass.

The function of the coupling agent is to displace the adsorbed water and provide a strong chemical link between the oxide groups on the glass surface and the polymer molecules of the resin. Silane coupling agents are extensively used for this purpose and have the general formula

$$R - Si - X_3,$$

where R represents an organo-functional group and the X units are hydrolysable groups bonded to the silane. The latter are only present as an intermediate, since they are hydrolysed to form a silanol as follows:

$$R - Si - X_3 + 3 H_2O \rightarrow R - Si (OH)_3 + 3HX$$

These trihydroxy-silanols are able to compete with the water on the surface of the glass by forming hydrogen bonds with the hydroxyl groups on the glass surface.

When the silane coated glass is now dried, the water is removed and a condensation reaction occurs between the silanol and the surface. The two stages involved are shown in **80**. Once this bond is formed, it is no longer susceptible to hydrolysis.

When the resin is now placed in contact with the silane-treated glass, the organo-functional group, R, reacts with the resin, and forms a strong bond to it. For this process to succeed, it is important that the organo-functional group is so chosen so as to be compatible with the particular resin system employed.

This approach produces a strong, water resistant bond. Without the coupling agent, the bond would deteriorate rapidly as water diffuses through the resin and re-adsorbs onto the glass surface, displacing the resin.

The bond, as depicted in **80**, will be very rigid, as the organo-functional groups are very short. Strains generated by shrinkage during setting, or possibly by differential thermal shrinkage, could be sufficient to cause the bond to fail. This problem can be overcome by making sure that the organo-functional groups consist of reasonably long molecules, providing the necessary degree of flexibility. In a sense, the interface created by the use of coupling agents should be treated as two interfaces, namely the glass–silanol interface and the resin–organo-functional group interface.

Two commonly used silane coupling agents are γ-aminopropyltriethoxysilane, and γ-mercaptopropyltrimethoxysilane.

## Primers

Primers, like the coupling agents, are another group of substances which seek to make the surface of the substrate more amenable to accepting a bond. Primers are usually applied in conjunction with an adhesive.

A typical example of a primer is one that is used to seal the surface of wood prior to applying the adhesive. If a primer was not applied, the adhesive would be soaked up by the porosity of

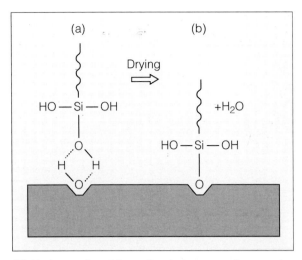

**80** Hydrogen bond formation between a silane and a surface hydroxyl group (a), which, after drying, forms into a covalent bond with the release of water (b).

the wood, such that none remained at the interface.

There are many dental examples of primers, such as phosphoric acid which is used for preparing the enamel surface, and the wide variety of dentine conditioners which are used in conjunction with dentine bonding agents. Unfortunately, in the dental literature, the distinction between primers and coupling agents is lost, and the two terms are used interchangeably.

# Summary

Adhesion is not a simple phenomenon, nor is it comprehensible with a single model. The formation of an adhesive bond depends on a multitude of factors and rarely involves a single adhesive mechanism.

# II
# CLINICAL DENTAL MATERIALS

A wide variety of materials are used in the dental surgery by both the dentist and the dental surgery assistant. It is important that the manner in which these materials are to be handled and for which clinical applications they are appropriate are well understood.

One of the biggest causes of failure of restorations is the misuse and abuse of dental materials. This problem can be minimised by a thorough appreciation of the physical and mechanical properties of the materials available.

# DENTAL AMALGAMS

## Introduction

Dental amalgam had a fairly inauspicious beginning, early in the 19th century, when it was used as a restorative material, being made by mixing Spanish or Mexican silver coins with mercury. Dental amalgams have come a long way since then, and are still a part of the everyday dental practice.

The development of dental amalgams is due, in no small way, to one of the most famous ever dentists, G.V.Black, who recognised the need to determine the properties of dental amalgams with some accuracy, if their performance was ever going to be predictable. At the beginning of the 20th century, because of his research work, amalgams could be produced with reasonably predictable handling characteristics.

Over the years, our understanding of these materials has advanced considerably, but up until the late 1960s, there was little change in this field and the composition was very much as it had been for the last 50 years.

During the last 20 years, it seems as though the developers of dental amalgams have tried to make up for this lack of activity, with new formulations appearing at frequent intervals. There has been an onslaught on the traditional applications of this material by new materials, such as the resin composites and the glass–ionomer cements. While this has led to some exciting new developments in dental amalgams, it has made the dentist's job more difficult, as the selection of the best available product at the best possible price becomes more and more complicated.

In this section, the development of the amalgams from the late 1960s to their current status is charted, high-lighting the important advances made.

## The Structure Of Traditional Dental Amalgams

### Composition

An amalgam is formed when mercury is mixed with another metal or metals. Mercury is liquid at room temperature (solidifying at -39 °C), and it reacts readily with metals such as silver, tin and copper, to produce solid materials. When the dentist selects a certain dental amalgam, it is effectively a selection of the alloy with which the mercury will be mixed and react.

Strictly speaking, the term *dental amalgam* can not be used until one is referring to the material produced as a consequence of the reaction between the mercury and the alloy. This alloy

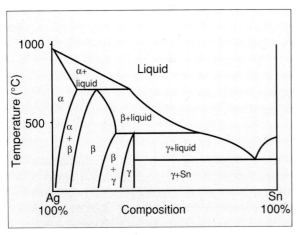

**81** Phase diagram for the Ag–Sn system.

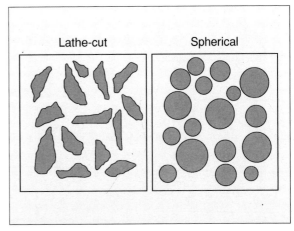

**82** Schematic representation of the lathe-cut and spherical shapes of alloy particles used in amalgams.

can vary either in composition or in form, and the dental amalgam manufacturers use this variability to produce a wide range of products.

## The Alloy

The alloy used in the traditional dental amalgams consists of a mixture of silver, tin, copper, zinc and sometimes mercury. A typical composition may be as shown in *Table 8*.

Silver is the main constituent, present in combination with tin as the inter-metallic compound $Ag_3Sn$, known commonly as the $\gamma$ *phase*. The phase diagram for the Ag–Sn system is shown in **81**, and shows that the $Ag_3Sn$ phase is the third pure phase in the system, hence the Greek symbol $\gamma$.

This $\gamma$ phase reacts readily with mercury to form the dental amalgam. Copper is present to increase the strength and hardness of the amalgam, and a more pronounced effect is produced when the copper content is increased beyond 6%, but this will be dealt with later. The zinc is present as a result of the initial production of the alloy, and is not considered to serve any useful purpose in the amalgamation process. Mercury is sometimes added to provide a more rapid reaction, in what is referred to as *pre-amalgamation*.

The alloy is used in the form of a powder, and the size and shape of the particles in this powder are critical to the handling characteristics and the final properties of the restoration. The alloy powder is available as either *lathe-cut* particles or spherical particles, as shown in **82**.

| Table 8 Constituents of a typical dental amalgam. | |
|---|---|
| Constituent | % of total |
| Ag | 67–74 |
| Sn | 25–28 |
| Cu | 0–6 |
| Zn | 0–2 |
| Hg | 0–3 |

### Lathe-Cut

The lathe-cut particles are produced by machining a solid ingot of the alloy on a lathe. The chippings that are produced are graded, and only those in the right size range are used in the powder to be amalgamated with mercury.

The alloy is available as coarse, medium or fine grained powder, and each will handle slightly differently. The individual chippings will have become highly stressed during the machining, and this makes their surfaces very reactive to mercury. A consequence of this is that the setting reaction is far too rapid unless heat treatment (which relieves the internal stresses) is applied. The heat treatment is usually carried out by placing the powder in boiling water.

### Spherical Particles

The production of the spherical particles is by a quite different route. The various ingredients of the alloy are melted together and then sprayed into an inert atmosphere, where the droplets solidify as small, spherical pellets of various

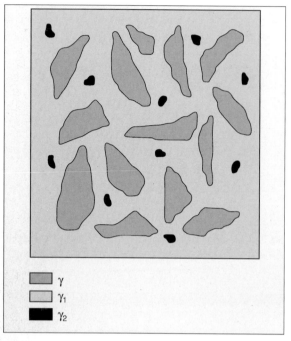

**83** Schematic representation of the microstructure of a lathe-cut alloy-based amalgam.

which are solid at room temperature. The reaction is as follows:

$$Ag_3Sn + Hg \rightarrow Ag_3Sn + Ag_2Hg_3 + Sn_7Hg$$
$$\gamma + mercury \rightarrow \gamma + \gamma_1 + \gamma_2$$

| powder | liquid | unreacted alloy | amalgam matrix |

As can be seen from the reaction, not all of the alloy dissolves in the mercury. On the contrary, a considerable amount remains, so that the final structure is one of a core of $\gamma$ held together by a matrix of predominantly $\gamma_1$ which is interspersed with $\gamma_2$. The structure of the set material is shown in **83**.

The copper in the lathe-cut alloy is present in the form of discrete areas of $Cu_3Sn$, and remains mainly within the original alloy in its unreacted form.

In the case of the spherical particles, the copper is uniformly distributed, and the alloy could be more accurately regarded as a ternary alloy of silver, tin and copper. Hence, in the final structure of the spherical alloy amalgam, the copper is not present as a discrete phase, but is widely distributed throughout the material. Although some voids will inevitably be present, in a well condensed amalgam there will be very little porosity.

# Properties Of Traditional Amalgams

It is not the intention here to cover all aspects of the properties of dental amalgams, and only those properties of some importance to the clinical use and development of the new alloys will be considered.

## *Strength*

The strength of an amalgam is extremely important, since the restoration has to be able to withstand the considerable loads generated during mastication, and any lack of strength is likely to lead to marginal ditching of the restoration or even gross fracture.

Although most attention has been paid to the final compressive strength of the set material, it is perhaps more important to consider the tensile

sizes. This method of manufacture has the advantages that no further machining processes are required, and that the composition of the alloy can be readily altered. What is important to the manufacturer is that the yield of particles of the correct size is as high as possible, since this minimises the cost of production. The particles which are rejected because they are either too big or too small are simply recycled.

### The Mercury

The mercury used in the preparation of an amalgam needs to be very pure, otherwise a surface layer of contaminants is formed which interferes with the setting reaction. For this reason, the mercury is triple distilled. The purity can easily be checked by visual examination. If a dull surface is observed, as opposed to the usually highly reflective surface, the mercury is contaminated.

## *The Setting Reaction*

The setting reaction between the Ag–Sn alloy and the mercury is initiated by a vigorous mixing of the two ingredients. This mixing causes the outer layer of the alloy particles to dissolve into the mercury, forming two new phases strength and the rate at which the final strength is acquired.

As might be imagined, the final strength of the amalgam will be a function of the properties of the individual phases. It is not easy to determine the properties of the three main phases of an amalgam, but micro-hardness measurements suggest that the $\gamma$ phase and the $\gamma_1$ phase have a similar hardness while the $\gamma_2$ phase is considerably softer. The tensile strength of the $\gamma_2$ phase has also been measured to be only a fraction of that of the original $\gamma$ phase, with the $\gamma_1$ phase falling in between (see *Table 9*).

This means that the weak link within the amalgam structure is the $\gamma_2$ phase, and if its proportion in the final composition could be minimised, a stronger amalgam would result. The amount of $\gamma_1$ and $\gamma_2$ formed is strongly dependent upon the amount of mercury in the final composition. The higher the mercury content, the weaker the material will be, because larger amounts of the weaker phases will be produced.

The final mercury content of the amalgam is dependent upon the quality of the condensation technique more than anything else, with a properly condensed amalgam having a mercury content of just less than 50%. Besides the condensation technique, the size and shape of the alloy particles will also affect the final mercury content. The initial ratio of alloy to mercury is lower in amalgam made with spherical alloy particles than with lathe-cut alloy particles, because the material is more easily condensed. With spherical alloy particles, a final mercury content of about 45% is readily achievable.

The particle size is important, too. Given an amount of alloy that is to be amalgamated with mercury, choosing smaller alloy particles results in more of the alloy surface being exposed to the mercury. This means that more of the alloy will dissolve in the mercury, producing more of the mercury containing phases. Consequently, too small a particle size is contraindicated.

Whatever the form of the alloy used, the conscientious removal of excess mercury during the placement of a restoration is vitally important.

## Flow And Creep

It has been postulated that the excessive flow of an amalgam, resulting from repeated occlusal loading, can cause flattening of contact points,

| Table 9 Tensile strengths of phases of amalgam. | |
|---|---|
| Phase | Tensile Strength (MPa) |
| $\gamma$ | 170 |
| $\gamma_1$ | 30 |
| $\gamma_2$ | 20 |
| amalgam | 60 |

overhanging margins, and protrusion of the restoration from the tooth surface at the margin. The latter has been implicated as a major source of marginal breakdown. While flow is measured for amalgams, the measurement is usually carried out over a short time period very soon after mixing.

A more appropriate measurement would be that of creep. This is the flow caused by loads acting over long periods. Creep is dependent upon both the yield strength of the material and the temperature of the environment, and only becomes a serious problem when the environmental temperature is greater than half of the materials melting temperature.

Since the amalgam phases have very low melting temperatures (about 80°C) and the restorations are subjected to repeated loadings, there is the possibility of creep occurring. The phases most prone to creep will be the mercury-based $\gamma_1$ and $\gamma_2$ phases. Consequently, the lower the proportion of these phases present (as may be achieved by proper condensation), the less susceptible the amalgam will be to creep.

## Corrosion

It is well recognised that amalgams corrode in the oral environment. Indeed, corrosion is often cited as an advantage, in that the corrosion products help to produce a good marginal seal. Crevice corrosion, caused by the formation of an oxidation cell in the marginal gap is the culprit.

The $\gamma_2$ phase is considerably more electronegative than the $\gamma$ and $\gamma_1$ phases. This means that in the presence of of an electrolytic solution, the $\gamma_2$ phase will act as the anode of the oxidation cell and will gradually dissolve. The reaction is as follows:

| tin–mercury | + | oral | $\rightarrow$ | tin | + | free |
|---|---|---|---|---|---|---|
| phase | | fluids | | salts | | mercury |
| $Sn_7Hg$ | | + oxygen | $\rightarrow$ | oxides & | + | Hg |
| | | | | chlorides | | |

Normally, the formation of oxides would help to slow down the corrosion process by forming a protective surface coating. However, in the gap between the amalgam and the tooth tissues a surface oxide is not formed, as the reaction products from the corrosion process precipitate out. The process is also very insidious, since the production of free mercury allows further reaction with $\gamma$, and the formation of more $\gamma_1$ and $\gamma_2$. This process will severely weaken the amalgam structure, and is often cited as a cause of marginal breakdown.

# High Copper Content Dental Amalgams

From the above discussion of the properties of the traditional dental amalgams, it can be deduced that an improvement in their performance may be possible if their strength could be increased. This strengthening is possible by reducing the amount of $\gamma_1$ and $\gamma_2$, or better still if the weak and corrosion susceptible $\gamma_2$ phase could be eliminated from the structure entirely, with the added benefit that creep could be reduced.

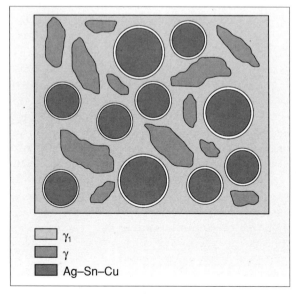

**84** Schematic representation of the microstructure of a dispersed-phase amalgam. The halo around the spherical particles is a Cu–Sn phase.

## Dispersed Phase Amalgams

In the early 1960's, attempts were made to increase the strength of dental amalgams by increasing the copper content of the alloy.

The idea was that the copper would act as a dispersion strengthening agent. A spherical alloy (basically silver and copper) with a high copper content was added to the conventional lathe-cut alloy. The choice of the spherical particles was made essentially because it was easier to alter the composition of spherical particles than lathe-cut particles on an experimental basis. The potential advantages, in terms of easier condensation, were also recognised at that time.

As it turned out, the increase in the copper content of the alloy resulted in a modification of the setting reaction, which proved to be highly beneficial.

The first reaction is the same as for the traditional alloys, but this is followed by the second reaction:

$$\gamma_2 + Ag\text{--}Cu \rightarrow Cu_6Sn_5 + \gamma_1.$$

Thus, the final amalgam contains little or no $\gamma_2$. The structure of this amalgam is shown in **84**.

Initially, it was thought that all of the $\gamma_2$ was eliminated by this reaction, but it has since been recognised that some $\gamma_2$ will remain, although it is only a small, and probably insignificant amount.

The modification in the setting reaction has resulted in a number of interesting and important changes in the properties of the amalgam, namely:

- A higher compressive strength.
- A more rapid set to full strength.
- A reduction in creep.
- A reduced susceptibility to corrosion.

## Other High Copper Content Formulations

With these sorts of improvements, it was not long before the idea of the *all-spherical high-copper amalgams* came into being. These combine all of the advantages of easier condensation with those mentioned above, and a number of such products are now available.

The powder in these cases is a ternary spherical alloy of silver, tin and copper and has a setting reaction as follows:

$$Ag-Sn-Cu + Hg \rightarrow Ag-Sn-Cu + \gamma_1 + Cu_6Sn_5.$$

The reluctance of many dentists to convert from a lathe-cut alloy to a spherical alloy, has led to the introduction of *high-copper content all-lathe-cut alloy* formulations. The composition of these alloys is essentially the same as for the all of the spherical alloys, except that there are wide differences in the total copper content, which can vary from 12–30%. As yet, it is not known what the optimum percentage of copper is.

For those dentists who prefer the dispersed-phase type of alloy, there are now a number available which have a mixture of spherical and lathe-cut particles, where both particle types have the same composition of ternary Ag–Sn–Cu alloy.

# Selection And Use Of Dental Amalgams

In the selection of the appropriate dental amalgam, there are two major factors which need to be considered:

- Variables under the control of the manufacturer.
- Variables under the control of the operator.

Each of these will have a profound effect on the properties of the dental amalgams, such as their handling characteristics and their clinical performance.

The clinical performance of an amalgam restoration is as much dependent upon the correct choice of the alloy as it is on the use of a good operative procedure. The need for a good procedure involves all of the stages of amalgam placement, from the proportioning stage to the final polishing.

## *Manufacturer's Variables*

The variables under the control of the manufacturer are the composition and the particle size and shape of the alloy.

### Composition

The most obvious differences in composition relate to the copper content of the alloy and the first question that might be asked is *'Should I use a traditional or a copper enriched amalgam alloy?'*.

The evidence obtained from controlled clinical trials indicates very strongly that the performance of the high-copper amalgams is superior to that of the traditional amalgams. The rate of marginal breakdown is most certainly lower than that of the traditional low copper content alloy systems, although this by itself does not necessarily mean that the longevity of these two systems will be very different.

It should be remembered that the traditional amalgams have provided excellent service for many years, and that a lifetime in excess of 10 years is by no means uncommon for these restorations, showing the potential of this amalgam. More often than not, the premature failure of an amalgam restoration is related to inadequate operative technique. Nevertheless, in the hands of experienced operators, and under highly controlled conditions, high-copper amalgams appear to perform better.

Why the high-copper amalgams should give better clinical performance is not as yet clear. The resistance to creep has improved significantly, as has the resistance to corrosion. Both of these have been implicated as causes in the reduction in marginal breakdown, but it is not clear whether the reduced corrosion or the reduced creep is responsible for the improved properties. Perhaps it is as well to be pragmatic and just accept that there is an improvement in performance, whatever the cause.

A feature of the high-copper amalgams is their increased compressive strength, when compared to the traditional alloys. Just one hour after placement, the high copper content amalgams can be twice as strong as the traditional amalgams, and this must contribute to a reduced incidence of gross fractures. It should be noted, though, that the final compressive strength may not be that different.

Another feature of the high-copper amalgams is that they do not contain any zinc. Since zinc is understood to be the source of delayed expansion when an amalgam becomes contaminated with saliva this is an additional advantage.

One disadvantage that has been noted with some of the high-copper amalgams is that their surfaces are more prone to tarnish.

## Particle Size And Shape

The particles' size and shape need to be considered seriously because they determine not only the handling characteristics of the alloy, but also affect the final composition.

There is a tendency to opt for the very fine particle size alloys, because they are easily carved to give a very nice surface finish. However, the small particle size of the powder means that more mercury will react with the alloy, giving a higher final mercury content and hence higher proportions of $\gamma_1$ and $\gamma_2$. In addition, the early compressive strength of these amalgams is much lower than those of amalgams made with either the fine or medium sized alloy particles.

Some studies have shown that the use of a very fine alloy powder gives rise to a higher rate of marginal breakdown, and that its use is contraindicated.

The coarse grained alloys are difficult to carve because particles are easily dislodged from the surface during the initial set. Medium or fine particles appear to be the best compromise in this respect.

The concern over particle shape is a choice between lathe-cut and spherical alloy, or perhaps a mixture of the two. This is very much a matter of personal preference, but it is said that the spherical-alloy systems condense more readily than the lathe-cut alloy compositions. In the end, this is something that only the dentist can decide, by being prepared to try different types of amalgams.

To date, the clinical performance of the new high-copper amalgam alloys has been compared with that of the traditional alloys, using maintenance of marginal integrity as the yardstick of performance. It may be that the longevity of amalgam restorations is not a function of the rate of marginal breakdown, in which case it would be impossible to state categorically which of the amalgam alloys will provide the best result. Nevertheless, given all of the advantages in physical and mechanical properties of the high-copper amalgams over the traditional alloys, the balance must swing in favour of the high-copper amalgams.

## Operator Variables

The variables that are under the control of the dentist and which may affect the final quality of the restoration are:

- Proportioning of the alloy and mercury.
- Trituration.
- Condensation.
- Carving and polishing.

### Proportioning

Proportioning is most commonly carried out using volumetric dispensers or pre-proportioned capsules.

The advantages of the latter are that the dentist does not have to worry about getting the right ratio of alloy to mercury (as this is pre-fixed by the manufacturer), and that there is less danger of mercury spillage during the handling stages of amalgam placement. Unfortunately, the capsules are more expensive than buying the alloy powder in bulk.

Thus, the volumetric dispenser is a more attractive proposition to some dentists, but it does limit the choice of the alloy to the fine-grained variety, since the medium or coarse-grained alloys tend to produce erratic mixes.

On the other hand, the volumetric dispenser allows more freedom in the alloy to mercury ratio, a feature which could appeal particularly to those dentists who like to start from a fairly wet mix.

The high initial mercury content should present no problem as long as a good condensation technique is employed. It is important that a sufficiently plastic mix is obtained to allow proper amalgamation and handling; a dry mix should be avoided at all costs. Generally, a 1:1 ratio of alloy to mercury will suffice for the lathe-cut alloys, but for the spherical alloys a higher ratio of alloy to mercury is allowed because of the lower total surface area of the spherical particles.

The lower mercury content in this case does not mean that this reduces the need for the removal of excess mercury. It is important that the final mercury content is as low as possible, and a good condensation technique is still required.

## Trituration

Trituration is one of the most important of the operator variables. Adequate trituration is essential to ensure a plastic mix and thorough amalgamation. The trituration time that is needed is depenndent upon both the type of alloy being used and the dispensing and mixing system.

The spherical alloys tend to mix more readily and in general require a shorter trituration time. This is because the particles are more easily wetted than the lathe-cut particles.

The exact trituration time depends on the mixing system. For a system running at a speed of 4000 rpm and a throw of some 50 mm, amalgamation times can be as short as five seconds. For a slower system, with a speed of 2600 rpm, the trituration time can be 20 seconds or more.

The general recommendation is that it is better to err on the side of over-trituration than under-trituration. If it is found that the amalgam sets too rapidly, then the trituration time must be *increased*, and not decreased as is often thought; the extra trituration will provide a more plastic mix with a longer working time.

Trituration times also affect the dimensional changes that occur when amalgams set. Ideally, the material should expand slightly on setting, as this aids marginal adaptation and will reduce the potential for marginal leakage.

Prior to the introduction of capsules and amalgamators, the traditional amalgams contained large alloy particles which were hand triturated; these formulations showed a slight expansion once fully set. The dimensional change with time is shown in **85**.

There is an initial contraction as the mercury diffuses into the alloy. This is followed by an expansion as the $\gamma_1$ phase forms, due to the $\gamma_1$ crystals impinging on one another and producing an outward pressure which opposes the contraction. This occurs only if sufficient mercury is present to produce a plastic mix.

The introduction of high speed mechanical amalgamators, low mercury:alloy ratios, small alloy particle sizes and high condensation pressures reduce the amount of mercury in the mix, and favours a contraction of the amalgam, such that modern amalgams show a net contraction once set.

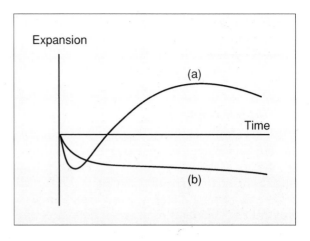

**85** Dimensional change for a traditional hand-mixed amalgam (a) and a modern mechanically mixed amalgam (b).

## Condensation

The most important demands on the condensation technique are that as much excess mercury is removed as is possible, and that the final restoration will be non-porous.

For the lathe-cut alloys, a final mercury content of 45% can be achieved. Although reductions below 50% mercury have little effect on the compressive strength after 24 hours, a much higher early compressive strength is achieved. A high early strength reduces the likelihood of gross amalgam fracture during the first few hours after placement. This applies equally well to the spherical alloy systems, except that in these cases the final mercury content should be approximately 40%.

The important components in condensation are the use of maximum force, the use of suitably sized condensers in relation to cavity size, the use of multiple and rapid thrusts and the placement of small increments.

Although condensation pressures of 30–40 N are generally recommended, this does not mean that lower condensation pressures will result in a poorer result, as low condensation pressures can be compensated for by the placement of small increments.

The placement of large increments will not only lead to the formation of large amounts of $\gamma_1$ and $\gamma_2$ but will also produce a high level of porosity.

The condensation of the spherical alloy amalgams requires a different approach from the lathe-cut systems. As the mix flows more readily under even light pressures, small loads need to be applied by larger condensers, if possible.

### Carving And Polishing

The carvability of an amalgam is a function of the size and shape of the alloy particles. In general, the spherical alloys produce a better initial surface finish than the lathe-cut alloys.

The need for polishing of an amalgam at a second visit is a matter of some debate. Some would argue that polishing is necessary for no other reason than that it improves the aesthetics, while others would point to the high level of residual mercury in the surface layer, and feel that this needs to be removed.

It may be true that a thin surface layer will have a preponderance of the $\gamma_1$ and $\gamma_2$ phases, but this layer is likely to be so thin that it would soon be worn away. Similarly, a controversy exists concerning the need, or not, for burnishing. It used to be said that the burnishing of amalgams will give rise to a mercury-rich surface layer, which increased the possibility of corrosion or fracture. However, more recent studies would indicate that the overall effect of burnishing is to increase surface hardness, reduce porosity and decrease corrosion, while also improving the marginal adaptation of the amalgam.

An as-carved surface finish for an amalgam is decidedly rough, and some form of additional finishing is necessary. The option is either to recall the patient the next day in order to polish the restoration, or alternatively to burnish the restoration at the time of placement. Burnishing may be an effective substitute for conventional polishing of lathe-cut amalgams, and so long as either is used, a better marginal integrity is attained.

# Limitations Of Dental Amalgams

The use of dental amalgams has been the subject of considerable discussion since the introduction of the new resin composites and glass–ionomer cements. Some have even suggested that the use

of amalgams should be discontinued. Given that amalgams have given stirling service for some 100 years, this would seem a rather extreme viewpoint. Nevertheless, dental amalgams have a number of shortcomings.

## *Poor Aesthetics*

Being metallic restorations, amalgams are not the most visually attractive of options, although if thay are polished more regularly than is the current practice they *can* look quite presentable.

The polished finish is lost with time, due to tarnishing. Although there is an increasing demand from patients for more aesthetic restorations, in the case of posterior restorations, the durability is the most important consideration.

## *Mercury Toxicity*

It can not be denied that mercury is a highly toxic substance; its use demands the greatest of care. The main sources of mercury exposure arise from:

- Accidental spills.
- Poor mercury hygiene.
- Direct contact with mercury.
- Amalgamators.
- Removing old restorations.

The most serious potential hazard is from mercury vapour, and the most significant source of this vapour is spillage of mercury in the surgery. The use of amalgam capsules should minimise this risk.

It is the dental surgery staff who are most at risk from mercury contamination, since the material is dealt with on a daily basis. If any spillage should occur, it is in the interests of everybody, particularly the dental staff, that it is dealt with it immediately and thoroughly. Any mercury left lying around will gradually vaporise and thence be inhaled.

Appropriate mercury hygiene procedures must be used, and these include:

- The use of no-touch technique.
- The use of mechanical amalgamators with good seals.
- The storage of mercury and old amalgams under water in unbreakable, tightly sealed containers.

- The cleaning up of spilled mercury immediately.

Patients are considerably less at risk from mercury than the dental staff are. Certainly there is some ingestion of mercury on placing a freshly mixed amalgam. After this, there are the wear and breakdown products, but, in most cases, the amounts are so small as to be insignificant. However, there have been a number of occasions when patients have reacted very badly to the presence of amalgams in their mouth, due to a hypersensitivity to mercury. Rare as these allergic reactions are, the symptoms can be quite severe, and the dentist should be aware of such a possibility.

## *High Thermal Conductivity*

As one would expect from a metallic material, the thermal conductivity of dental amalgams is very high. Problems presented by this, such as pulpal sensitivity due to the hydrodynamic effect of pumping fluid through the marginal gap and up and down the dentinal tubules, are readily dealt with by suitable cavity preparation techniques, involving the use of varnishes or liners (see section II.IV).

## *Galvanic Effects*

When two metallic restorations consisting of metals with different degrees of electronegativity are placed in close proximity to one another in an electrically conducting medium (in the dental case this medium is saliva), it is possible that a galvanic cell will be set up.

The resultant currents can cause patients discomfort or leave a strong metallic taste in the mouth, and can accelerate the corrosive breakdown of the more electronegative metal. Consequently, although the problem rarely arises, the use of different metals in the mouth is not recommended.

## *Lack Of Adhesion*

The need for the use of retentive cavity designs with dental amalgams imposes a severe constraint. Often, large amounts of perfectly sound enamel or dentine are removed, under the banner of 'extension for prevention'. This principle is questionable, as amalgam can never be a substitute for healthy tooth tissues.

New ideas in cavity preparation, aimed at minimising the loss of healthy tooth tissue have been developed, but these can never be as conservative as the approach of using adhesive restorative materials.

## *Limited Life Span Of Dental Amalgam Restorations*

Hundreds of thousands of amalgams are placed each year, and, on average, half of these are replacements of existing restorations. The longevity of amalgam restorations has been the subject of a number of clinical studies, with some suggesting that half need replacement within 4–5 years.

On average, the survival time of amalgam restorations is inversely proportional to their size. To compound this problem, every time an amalgam restoration **is** replaced the cavity outline is increased by at least 0.5 mm, leading to a larger restoration. In general then, the smaller the restoration, the longer it will survive.

Of all the disadvantages mentioned above, the lack of longevity and the destructive nature of the procedure are matters of the greatest concern. Ways of making restorations last longer will be considered in the next section.

# Improving The Longevity Of Amalgam Restorations

Several workers over the last decade have cast a critical eye over established amalgam techniques. They have made recommendations that, if adopted, should result in an increased life span of both new and replacement restorations. Before considering these recommendations, however, it is necessary to consider the various causes of amalgam failure.

Some of the problems are unavoidable, being related to inadequacies in the properties of the amalgams, but others *can* be avoided by considering the amalgams' limitations and by adopting appropriate techniques.

## *Causes Of Failure Of Amalgam Restorations*

The failure of an amalgam restoration may manifest itself as secondary caries, gross fracture

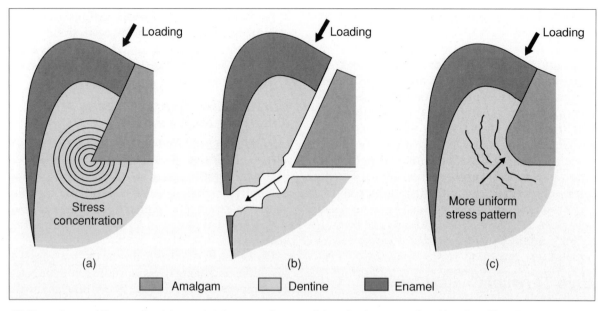

**86** Sharp internal line angles (a) may lead to cusp fracture (b) under heavy occlusal loading. Tensile stresses are concentrated at the line angle which can be considerably reduced by creating rounded line angles (c).

of the amalgam, gross fracture of the tooth, or marginal breakdown. The latter may arise from either the fracture of the amalgam margins or the enamel margins. Of these, the most common reason for replacing an amalgam restoration (accounting for some 70% or replacements) is secondary caries.

The causes of such failures can be grouped under three main headings:

- Faults in cavity design.
- Poor clinical technique.
- Limitations of the materials.

There are many aspects to each of these causes, and they will be considered in turn.

## Faults In Cavity Design

### Weakened Tooth Structure

The more tooth tissue that is removed, the weaker the tooth becomes. A dental amalgam acts as an effective space filler, but since it has no adhesive qualities, it does not help in strengthening the underlying tooth structure. Thus, techniques involving the minimal removal of tooth tissue should always be employed.

By cutting enamel along the plane parallel to the prism direction, it is possible to keep outline form to a minimum. This practice also ensures that cavo-surface angles will be close to 90°, which is optimal for the amalgam, with acute cavo–surface angles encouraging marginal breakdown of the amalgam.

There are now a number of adhesives available that allow bonding of the amalgam to the tooth tissues. The bond will provide additional support to both the restoration and the cusps, which should help to strengthen the restored tooth crown.

As the durability of the bond is as yet unknown, the design of the cavity should still be such as to avoid potential sites for fracture. With severely weakened cusps, alternative techniques such as gold onlays or resin-bonded ceramics might have to be considered.

### Sharp Internal Line Angles

The presence of sharp internal line angles concentrates stress at these sites, which increases the risk of fracture of both the tooth and the filling, as shown in **86**. Such sharp angles are avoidable, and rounded internal surfaces should be the aim. For example, proximal boxes should be pear-

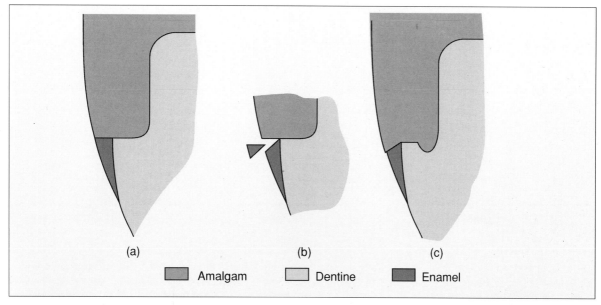

**87** If the gingival floor of the proximal box is finished (a), then unsupported enamel will break away (b) and lead to recurrent caries. Bevelling the enamel (c) prevents this occurring but it is necessary to place a groove in the gingival floor of the dentine to resist the displacement of the restoration proximally.

shaped, to conform to the extent of the underlying lesion, and should not be cut with sharp line angles in their corners.

### Non-Retentive Proximal Boxes

A frequently observed failure of MO, DO or MOD restorations is the fracture of the proximal boxes from the occlusal section of the filling.

To some extent, this is due to the low tensile strength of the amalgam restoration, as an occlusal load can force the amalgam to splay outwards. However, sharp internal line angles aggravate the situation, which ultimately leads to the fracture and loss of the box.

This risk of this happening can be reduced by cutting retention grooves in the lateral walls and gingival floor of the boxes. This technique ensures that the box is self-retentive and opposes the splaying action from an occlusal load by resisting the displacement of the restoration in a proximal direction. An added advantage is that an occlusal lock is not required for retention of the restoration. Thus, the additional preparation of occlusal fissures is not required when a primary lesion is confined to the proximal surface only; this type of preparation is generally described as a 'wedge' preparation.

### Incorrect Cavo-Surface Angles

The primary cause of marginal breakdown of a restored tooth is the presence of an incorrect cavo-surface angle, leading to marginal fracture of the enamel or the amalgam.

The principle of providing flat walls and floors to a cavity can give rise to undermined enamel, as shown in **87** for a box in a proximal restoration. The unsupported enamel will break free and leave a gap which can lead to recurrent caries.

Marginal breakdown of the amalgam occurs more readily when the amalgam has an acute margin angle. Amalgam is extremely brittle and has a very low tensile strength, (60–70 MPa), so any resultant thin wedges will fracture very easily as they bend under the application of an external load. This contrasts with gold alloy inlays which do not show symptoms of marginal breakdown of the alloy because this material is tough and ductile. Consequently, marginal breakdown is less likely to occur with margin angles greater than 70° as this avoids thin wedges of the amalgam.

The practice of cutting perpendicular cavity walls on the occlusal aspect of the cavity, is conducive to producing an acute margin angle

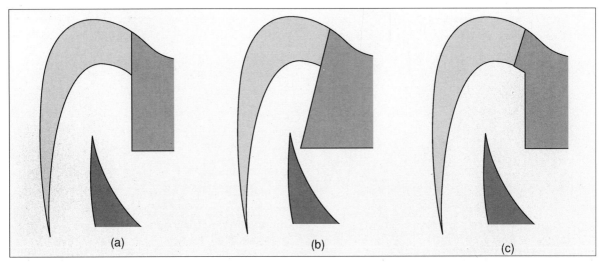

**88** An obtuse cavo-surface angle (a) produces an acute margin angle in the restoration that will lead to marginal fracture and should be corrected. In (b), the cavo-surface angle is now closer to the ideal but may give rise to a pulpal exposure. An acceptable method is shown in (c), where adjustment is confined to the enamel without increasing the outline form.

for the amalgam (**88a**). Changing the angle for the whole of the cavity wall is not possible, as this may cause the cavity outline to come close to or to perforate the pulp horn (**88b**). An acceptable method of overcoming this problem is to confine the sharp angulation to the enamel only, as depicted in **88c**.

For occlusal cavities of minimal width, it is not necessary to prepare 90° cavo-surface angles in the enamel, because the amalgam may be carved flat without interference with the opposing dentition. The amalgam margin angle will then be obtuse, which will give the margin added strength due to the support of the underlying bulk of the restorative material.

Great care should be employed in the preparation of cavity margins, so as to avoid undermined enamel or acute margin angles in the amalgam.

### Shallow Preparations

Dental amalgams have a very low tensile strength. When placed in thin sections they are subjected to bending forces and will break. Shallow preparations are only acceptable in very small restorations, where the surface area is small compared to the depth. For large MOD restorations, there must be sufficient depth to the cavity on the occlusal floor to provide enough bulk to resist the bending forces. This may re-

quire the removal of large amounts of sound tooth tissue.

## Poor Clinical Technique

### Residual Caries

It is of paramount importance that any residual caries is removed. If not, the caries will spread and undermine the cusp, eventually causing it to fracture. The leakage of bacterial toxins will also cause pulpal inflammation.

### Poor Matrix Techniques

A poorly adapted matrix band can be the cause of proximal overhangs, or of poor contact points with the adjacent teeth. Overhangs are particularly prone to plaque accumulation, and may initiate secondary caries. If the overhang is subgingival, it may cause soft tissue irritation and can eventually lead to bone loss and pocketing.

Overtightening of the matrix band can cause the fracture of tooth cusps that have been weakened by the removal of large amounts of tooth tissue.

### Contamination

Contamination of the cavity with blood or saliva will result in poor adaptation of the restoration to the cavity margins. In the case of zinc containing alloys, the entrapment of saliva in the material as it is being placed can result in a phenomenon known as delayed expansion. The water reacts with the zinc as follows:

$$H_2O + Zn \rightarrow ZnO + H_2$$

Bubbles of hydrogen gas are formed within the amalgam. The pressure rises over time, as more and more hydrogen is produced and stored in the bubbles. Eventually, the pressure is so great that the bubbles expand, causing an expansion of the restoration. This expansion occurs during the early stages of slow setting amalgams, as they are unable to resist this pressure until they are fully set. The expansion can give rise to a downward pressure on the pulp, or cause the restoration to sit proud of the surface. The former will cause pulpal pain and the latter will lead to marginal breakdown. In badly broken-down teeth, the expansion could also cause cuspal fracture.

This hazard can be minimised by using proper isolation and the selection of a zinc-free amalgam with a rapid set.

### Poor Condensation

As already noted, poor condensation results in porosity of the amalgam and the presence of excess mercury, both of which reduce the strength of the amalgam. Marginal adaptation will also be poor, increasing the potential for marginal leakage, secondary caries and corrosion. For good condensation, it is important that the amalgam is well mixed, and that the appropriate trituration time is selected. Under-trituration, in particular, should be avoided, as this will result in a dry amalgam mix which will not condense properly.

### Over- And Under-Filling And Over-Carving

If a cavity is over-filled and is not then carved back sufficiently to provide a smooth transition from the tooth surface to the restoration surface, a ledge will result. This ledge will eventually fracture, and give the appearance of marginal breakdown of the restoration. This would encourage the dentist to replace the restoration, when, perhaps, all that is needed is to trim it back so that it is flush with the tooth surface. Such unnecessary treatment can be avoided by ensuring that the surface has been properly carved in the first place. Equally, underfilling or over-carving can result in an acute amalgam margin angle that will give rise to marginal breakdown.

## *Limitations Of The Materials*

The problems associated with amalgam as a filling material have already been covered in detail, both in terms of the limitations imposed by their mechanical and physical properties and their handling.

Most short-term failures are avoidable if the above factors are addressed and if careful attention is paid to the detail of cavity preparation and the handling of the materials.

In the longer term, amalgams will eventually fail. When such failures are specifically material-related, they are usually associated with creep or corrosion that has caused marginal breakdown. Ideally, the amalgam alloy used should show little or no creep, and should have a high corrosion resistance; a high copper content amalgam is the preferred choice.

## Summary

Dental amalgams will continue to be the restorative material of choice for many clinical situations. By paying careful attention to material selection and handling, and by having an appreciation of their limitations, amalgams should provide the patient with restorations that will give satisfactory function for many years.

## Further Reading

Brown D. (1984) The development of improved amalgams. Brit. Dent. J. **157**, 427

Brown D. (1988) Dental amalgams. Brit. Dent. J. **164**, 253

Cruickshank-Boyd D. W. and Patel S. (1980) High copper content amalgams. Dental Update June, 237

Elderton R. J. (1984) New approaches to cavity design. Brit. Dent. J. **157**, 421

Elderton R. J. (1984) Cavo-surface angles, amalgam margin angles and occlusal cavity preparation. Br. Dent. J. **156**, 319

Eley B.M. and Cox S. W. (1988) Mercury poisoning from dental amalgam – an evaluation of the evidence. J. Dent. **16**, 90

Grajower R. and Novickas D. (1988) The amalgam margin angle, marginal breakdown and adjacent caries in occlusal enamel, a pilot study on extracted teeth. J. Oral Rehab. **15**, 257

Hamilton C.J. *et al.* (1983) Marginal fracture not a predictor of longevity. J. Prosthet. Dent. **50**, 200

Letz H. and Vrijhoef M. A. (1984) Long-term influences on marginal fracture of amalgam restorations. J. Oral Rehab. **11**, 95

Mjor I. A. (1985) Frequency of secondary caries at various anatomical locations. Oper. Dent. **10**, 88

Papadogiannis Y., Boyer D. B. and Lakes R. S. (1987) Creep of amalgam at low stresses. J. Dent. Res. **66**, 1569

Sarkar N. K. (1978) Creep, corrosion and marginal fracture of amalgam fillings. J. Oral Rehab. **5**, 413

Staninec M. and Hold M. (1988) Bonding of amalgam to tooth structure: tensile adhesion and microleakage tests. J. Prosthet. Dent. **59**, 397

# II.II

# COMPOSITES

## Introduction

A composite, as the name implies, consists of a mixture of two or more materials. Each of these materials contributes to the overall properties of the composite, and are present in their discrete form. The resin-based composite restorative materials ('composites' in brief) that are used in dentistry have three major components:

- An organic resin matrix.
- An inorganic filler.
- A coupling agent.

The resin forms the matrix of the composite material, binding the individual filler particles together through the coupling agent (**89**).

## Composition And Structure

### The Resin Matrix

The resin is the chemically active component of the composite. It is initially a fluid monomer, but is converted into a rigid polymer by a radical addition reaction. It is this ability to convert from a plastic mass into a rigid solid that allows this material to be used for the restoration of dentition.

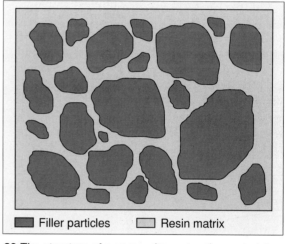

| ■ Filler particles | □ Resin matrix |

**89** The structure of a composite restorative material.

The most commonly used monomer for both anterior and posterior resins is Bis-GMA, which is derived from the reaction of bisphenol-A and glycidylmethacrylate. It has a higher molecular weight than methyl methacrylate, which helps to reduce the polymerisation shrinkage (**90**). There are now also a number of composites that use an urethane dimethacryate resin rather than Bis-GMA.

Bis-GMA and urethane dimethacrylate monomers are highly viscous fluids because of their high molecular weights; the addition of even a small amount of filler would produce a compos-

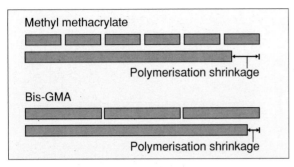

**90** Polymerisation shrinkage of a small and large monomer-based system.

ite with a stiffness that is excessive for clinical use. To overcome this problem, low viscosity monomers known as *viscosity controllers* are added, such as methyl methacrylate (MMA), ethylene glycol dimethacrylate (EDMA) and triethylene glycol dimethacrylate (TEGDMA); the latter of these is most commonly used. The chemical structures of some of these monomers are presented in *Table 10*.

To ensure an adequately long shelf life for the composite, it is essential that premature polymerisation is prevented. To this end an *inhibitor*, such as hydroquinone, is included, usually in amounts of 0.1%, or less.

The resin matrix also contains the activator/ initiator systems for achieving the cure. These components depend upon the type of reaction employed, which may be either chemical curing or visible-light activated curing.

### The Filler

A wide variety of fillers have been employed in composites to improve the properties.

This practice began in the late 1950's, when fillers such as quartz were introduced into methyl methacrylate-based filling materials. This offered three potential advantages. Firstly, the methyl methacrylate was subject to a high polymerisation shrinkage, even when used as a powder–liquid system. The shrinkage was much reduced, but never totally eliminated (because the filler does not take part in the polymerisation process), by producing a paste with a high filler loading. Secondly, methyl methacrylate has a high coefficient of thermal expansion. This coefficient was reduced by the addition of ceramic fillers, which have a coefficient of expansion similar to that of tooth tissues. Thirdly, the fillers

increased properties such as hardness and compressive strength.

The developments in filler technology lie at the root of many of the improvements that have led to the composites that are used today.

### Coupling Agent

In order for a composite to have acceptable mechanical properties, it is of the utmost importance that the filler and the resin are strongly bonded to each other. If there is a breakdown of this interface, the stresses developed under load will not be effectively distributed throughout the material; the interface will act as a primary source for fracture and the subsequent disintegration of the composite.

The bond is achieved by the use of coupling agents that are incorporated into the resin. These coupling agents are silanes of one form or another (see section I.X).

# Developments In Composites

A look at the changes in composites over the last ten years readily identifies two important new areas of development:

- New polymerisation techniques.
- New filler technology.

### Polymerisation Techniques

The process by which the composite paste turns into a hard material is the *polymerisation* of the resin matrix.

With the early composites, this was achieved by supplying two pastes, a mixture of which would contain the necessary ingredients for polymerisation. There would be an activator, such as a tertiary amine, in one paste, and an initiator, usually benzoyl peroxide, in the other.

Then, the ultraviolet light activated composites became available, and the practice of having a single paste which would set hard on demand was readily adopted by the dental profession. This opened the way for the introduction of the visible light activated composites, particularly as there were some serious drawbacks with the use of the ultraviolet light cured systems. The methods are summarised in *Table 11*.

**Table 10** The chemical structure of some monomers.

| | |
|---|---|
| Methyl methacylate | $CH_2 = \overset{\overset{\displaystyle CH_3}{\vert}}{\underset{\underset{\displaystyle O}{\parallel}}{C}} - C - O - CH_3$ |
| Bis-phenol-A | $HO - \langle\rangle - \overset{\overset{\displaystyle CH_3}{\vert}}{\underset{\underset{\displaystyle CH_3}{\vert}}{C}} - \langle\rangle - OH$ |
| Glicydal methacrylate | $CH_2 = \overset{\overset{\displaystyle CH_3}{\vert}}{\underset{\underset{\displaystyle O}{\parallel}}{C}} - C - CH_2 - \overset{\overset{\displaystyle O}{\diagup \ \diagdown}}{CH} - CH_2$ |
| Bis-GMA | $CH_2 = \overset{\overset{\displaystyle CH_3}{\vert}}{\underset{\underset{\displaystyle O}{\parallel}}{C}} - C - O - CH_2 - \overset{\overset{\displaystyle OH}{\vert}}{CH} - CH_2 - O - \langle\rangle - \overset{\overset{\displaystyle CH_3}{\vert}}{\underset{\underset{\displaystyle CH_3}{\vert}}{C}} - \langle\rangle - O - CH_2 - \overset{\overset{\displaystyle OH}{\vert}}{CH} - CH_2 - O - \overset{\overset{\displaystyle CH_3}{\vert}}{\underset{\underset{\displaystyle O}{\parallel}}{C}} - C - CH_2$ |
| Triethylene Glycol Dimethacrylate | $CH_2 = \overset{\overset{\displaystyle CH_3}{\vert}}{\underset{\underset{\displaystyle O}{\parallel}}{C}} - C - O - (CH_2)_2 - O - (CH_2)_2 - O - \overset{\overset{\displaystyle CH_3}{\vert}}{\underset{\underset{\displaystyle O}{\parallel}}{C}} - C - CH_2$ |
| Hydroquinone | $HO - \langle\rangle - OH$ |

**Table 11** Methods of polymerisation.

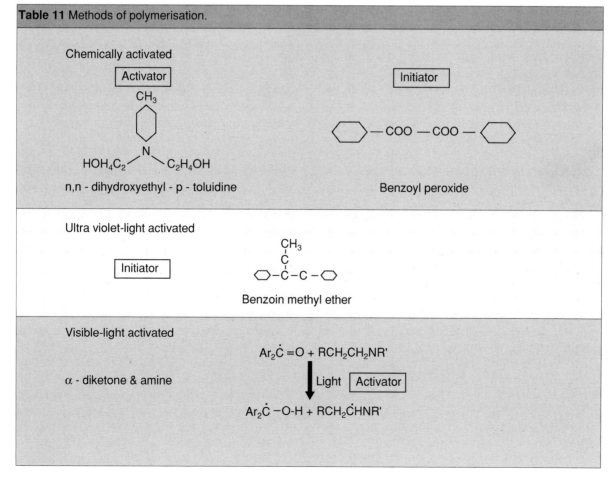

Chemically activated

Activator

n,n - dihydroxyethyl - p - toluidine

Initiator

Benzoyl peroxide

Ultra violet-light activated

Initiator

Benzoin methyl ether

Visible-light activated

α - diketone & amine

$Ar_2\dot{C} = O + RCH_2CH_2NR'$

Light   Activator

$Ar_2\dot{C} - O\text{-}H + RCH_2\dot{C}HNR'$

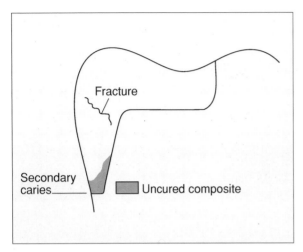

**91** Lack of cure of light-activated composite material at the base of a proximal box.

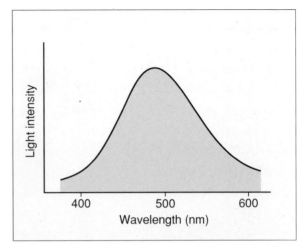

**92** Light spectrum for a visible-light curing unit.

### Safety

Concern has been expressed about the safety aspects of the use of high intensity ultraviolet light, and avoidance of these problems has been facilitated by the new visible light activated systems. There is still a need to be cautious in the use of this system however, as it may not be as safe as might be thought.

The use of the phrase 'visible light' instils a feeling of safety, since it is something that we are exposed to all the time. Nevertheless, it is not advisable to expose oneself unnecessarily to the light from the visible-light production units.

The use of high-intensity light itself can have a harmful effect on the retina, and there is also the potential of damaging the retina due to the 'blue light hazard'. Little is known about the blue light hazard and how serious a problem it might be.

These potential problems are readily resolved by using suitable eye protection, and it is better to err on the side of caution in these matters.

Another difficulty that the discerning dentist needs to be aware of is that caused by a long period of exposure to high intensity light. Such exposure can upset one's colour perception, meaning that the selection of suitable shades of composites then becomes a real problem, especially when performing multiple restorations or when applying composite veneers.

### Limited Depth Of Cure

Another reason why the visible light activated (VLA) composites have replaced the ultraviolet (UV) systems is that the depth of cure that can be achieved with ultraviolet light is considerably less than that obtained with visible light.

In particular, there is a danger of incomplete curing with the UV systems when it is used for deep restorations, which would be a serious drawback in posterior applications. For the UV cured composites, the maximum depth of cure is little more than 2.0 mm while for the VLA composites, a depth of cure of 3–4 mm is possible with a *good light source* and *good technique.*

However, the depth of cure is limited for both systems, and there is always the danger that deeper parts of the restoration will not be fully cured. This is especially problematic with the proximal boxes of posterior composites (**91**). All can appear perfectly satisfactory on the surface, but the bases of the boxes of composite may not be fully cured, particularly when metal matrix bands are being used.

Any lack of cure provides a poor foundation for the restoration and may lead to fracture. This is due to a lack of support or secondary caries at the cervical margins, caused by wash-out of the uncured restorative material.

There are a number of points that need to be emphasised. The light source used with VLA composites is more accurately described as *blue light* rather than *visible light of extremely high intensity.* The typical output from a good quality, visible-light source would produce a spectrum as shown in **92**. The selectivity is necessary to ensure optimumal degree and depth of cure.

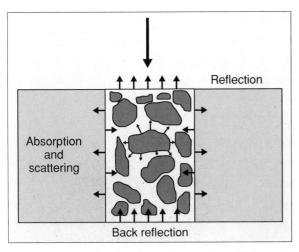

**93** Reflection, scattering and absorption of light as it enters the composite.

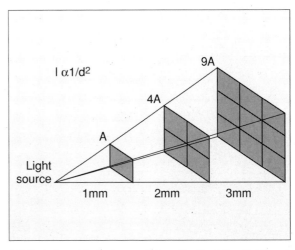

**94** Relationship between intensity (I) of the light and the distance (d) from the light source to the surface.

For all light-activated composites, the conversion from a paste to a solid material relies on the ability of the light to access and initiate the curing in all parts of the restoration. The degree to which the light can penetrate the composite is limited, so the depth to which the material can be cured is limited. A number of factors affect the depth of cure:

- *The type of composite* – As light hits the composite, it is reflected, scattered and absorbed as shown in **93**, and this limits the amount of penetration that is achieved. This is a particular concern for the darker shades of composite, and special care should be taken that these are cured to the full depth of the restoration, using an incremental technique and long exposure times.
- *The quality of the light source* – The cure of the resin in VLA composites is most effectively initiated by light in the wavelength range 450–500 nm. The light source should be designed so as to produce its maximum light output at approximately 480 nm (**92**). Thus, it is not enough simply to have a high light output, but it must also be of the correct wavelength. Deterioration of the light source also occurs, and it is important that the quality of the output is checked at regular intervals. A variety of inexpensive light meters are now available for this purpose.
- *The method used* – The tip of the light guide should be placed as close as possible to the surface of the restoration, as the curing efficiency drops off dramatically when the tip is moved away from the surface. In fact, the light intensity on unit surface area drops off with the inverse square of the distance between the light source and the resin, as shown in **94**. Every effort must be made to ensure that the light tip does not become contaminated with composite as this will reduce the curing efficiency on subsequent use. The material should be exposed to the light for no less than the recommended time, so that there is no danger of under-curing. For large restorations, the light tip may not be large enough to cover the whole of the restoration and there may be a tendency to fan the surface. This should not be done, as it is impossible to tell how long any particular area of the surface has been exposed. If fanning is carried out, it must be followed up with further curing, one spot at a time. For large surfaces, it must be ensured that the spots overlap.

There is a tendency on the part of some manufacturers to recommend curing times of as little as 20 seconds, as this obviously reduces the time it takes to complete a particular procedure. This may be sufficient for applications where only a very thin layer of the composite is to be applied, but will be insufficient when adopted for extensive restorations. Curing times should be at least 40–60 seconds.

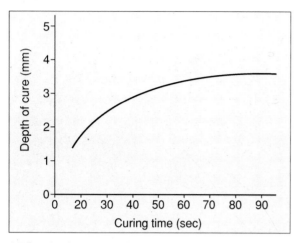

**95** Depth of cure as a function of curing time.

In situations where light access presents a problem, such as distal boxes of an MOD restoration in a posterior composite, aids to curing such as light conducting wedges and transparent matrices must be considered. Curing for excessively long times is, however, not a means of getting greater depths of cure.

The depth of cure for a particular composite used in conjunction with a particular light source reaches a limit which can not be exceeded (**95**). Thus, curing times of more than 60 seconds tend to be inefficient.

The interpretation of the values for the depths of cure that are quoted in the literature is fraught with difficulty. As yet, there is no recommended definition of depth of cure, and since it is highly technique dependent, comparison of data from different sources is virtually impossible. The general rule that should be followed is that curing to a depth of greater than 2 mm should be avoided, and exposure to the light source should be for at least 40 seconds. If the cavity to be filled is deeper than 2 mm, an incremental packing technique must be employed.

## New Filler Technology

Criticisms of the early composites were that they had rough surface finishes and a disappointing resistance to wear. Both of these are directly affected by the choice of filler used in the composite. The factors of interest in the selection of the filler are:

- Composition.
- Particle size.

**Composition**

The filler most used until quite recently was quartz, but today most composites employ one or other of a variety of glass fillers, including colloidal silica, lithium–aluminium silicate glass and silica glasses containing barium or strontium.

The glass formulation is critical because it has a major effect on the colouring of the composite. Its refractive index must closely match that of the resin to avoid excessive scattering of incoming light occurring, which would result in poor aesthetics.

The inclusion of barium or strontium provides radio-opaque versions of the composites, and this aids the detection of recurrent caries. Quartz is by far the hardest material used as a filler but composites formed in this way are not radio-opaque. The silica glasses are considerably softer, which some argue improves the surface finish of the composite.

**Particle Size**

The particle size of the filler is important as it determines the amount of filler that can be added to the resin, without the necessary handling characteristics being lost. Particle size also has a pronounced effect on the final surface finish of the composite restoration, in that the smaller the filler particle size the smoother the composite will be. (It should be said that the hardness of the filler, relative to the matrix, is another factor that should be considered when talking about the quality of the finish.)

The earliest filler used in composites was quartz, which has a particle size of up to 70 μm. Changing to the softer glasses has allowed a reduction in the size of the filler particles, and by choosing a suitable combination of sizes, it has been possible to increase the filler loading of the resins considerably in the last few years.

A filler loading as high as 74% by volume has been claimed for some of the posterior composites, which is well above the usual 55–60% volume obtained for many anterior composites. Of course, such high filler loadings may not be desirable with the anterior composites, as the quality of the aesthetics would be compromised; this is clearly not of the same importance for the posterior composites.

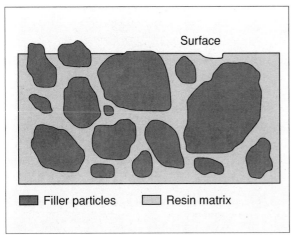

**96** Filler particles protruding from the surface due to preferential removal of the resin matrix.

**97** A homogeneous microfilled composite.

# Classification Of Composites

It is possible to categorise dental composites into five main groups, according to the nature and the particle size of the filler.

## *Traditional Composites*

These are composites which contain glass filler particles with a mean particle size of 10–20 µm, and a largest particle size of 40 µm.

These composites had the disadvantage that the surface finish was very poor, with the surface having a dull appearance due to filler particles protruding from the surface as the resin was preferentially removed around them, as shown in **96**.

## *Microfilled Resins*

The first microfilled resins were introduced in the late 1970's, and contain colloidal silica with an average particle size of 0.02 µm.

The small size of the filler particles means that the composite can be polished to a very smooth surface finish, and provides a very large surface area of filler in contact with the resin. This high surface area (compared to that of the filler used in the traditional composites), means that it is very difficult to obtain a high filler loading, as a large amount of resin is required to wet the surfaces of these filler particles. If the filler is added directly to the resin and a reasonably fluid consistency is to be maintained, then the maxi-

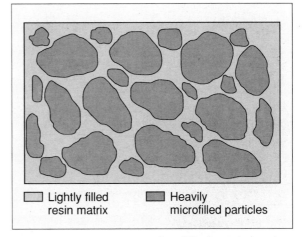

**98** A heterogeneous microfilled resin, using prepolymerised particles which are added to the resin containing a small amount of colloidal silica.

mum filler loading that can be achieved is only of the order of 20% (**97**).

To ensure an adequate filler loading, a two-stage procedure for the incorporation of the filler has been developed. A very high filler loaded material is first produced by one of a variety of techniques. This material is then polymerised and ground into particles of 10–40 µm in size. This is then used as a filler for more resin.

Thus, what is finally obtained is a composite containing composite filler particles (**98**). Although the filler loading of the prepolymerised particles can be as high as that of the large

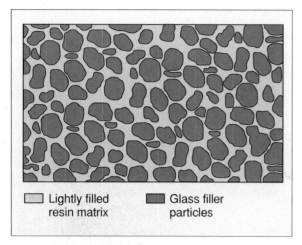

Lightly filled resin matrix
Glass filler particles

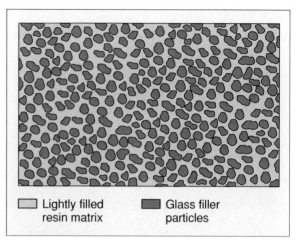

Lightly filled resin matrix
Glass filler particles

**99** Structure of a hybrid composite, consisting of large filler particles in a resin matrix containing colloidal silica.

**100** A small particle filled composite.

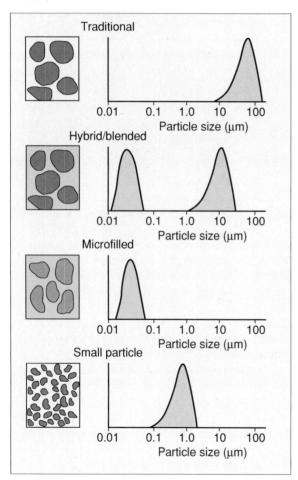

**101** A classification of composites based on filler type, with the horizontal axis as the logarithmic scale of the particle size.

particle composites, the overall filler loading is still considerably less.

## *Hybrid Or Blended Composites*

These are composites which contain large filler particles, of an average size of 15–20 µm and also a small amount of colloidal silica, which has a particle size of 0.01–0.05 µm (**99**).

It should be noted that virtually all composites now contain small amounts of colloidal silica, but their behaviour is very much determined by the size of the larger filler particles.

## *Small Particle Composites*

Improved methods have allowed the grinding of glasses to particle sizes smaller than had been previously possible. This has led to the introduction of composites having filler particles with an average particle size of around 1 µm, and a typical range of particle sizes of 0.1–6.0 µm (**100**). The smaller sized filler particles allow composites to be polished to a smoother surface finish than the larger particle sizes, but this is at the expense of lower filler loading, which may have an adverse effect on the wear resistance.

The classification proposed above is shown schematically in **101** in terms of the particle size distributions. In order to increase the filler loading to its maximum, it is possible to select fillers with two or more complementary particle size distributions. The filler with the smaller particle size distribution fills in the spaces left

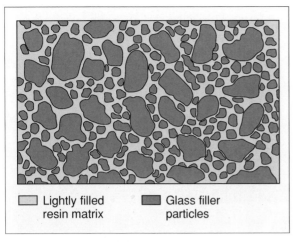

Lightly filled resin matrix    Glass filler particles

**102** Bimodal particle size distribution.

**Table 12** Polymerisation shrinkage of various composites.

| Material | Polymerisation Shrinkage | |
|----------|------------|------------|
| | Linear (%) | Volume (%) |
| Traditional | 0.2–0.5 | 1.2–2.1 |
| Hybrid | 0.4–1.2 | 1.3–3.5 |
| Microfilled | 0.3–1.9 | 2.0–4.5 |
| Unfilled resin | 1.7 | 5.2 |

between the larger filler particles (**102**). This has meant that the packing density of composite restorative materials has been increased, while the size of the filler has been reduced.

By ensuring that the aesthetics are not compromised, composites can be used for both anterior and posterior applications. There is a trend towards the use of universal composites, rather than specific composites for anterior and posterior use.

# Physical Properties

## *Polymerisation Shrinkage*

A long recognised and serious drawback with composites has always been the polymerisation shrinkage. In a sense, the whole field of adhesive restorative dentistry grew from this limitation of composites, because there would invariably be a marginal gap as the composite shrunk away from the cavity wall on setting.

The polymerisation shrinkage of a composite is dependent upon the type of resin employed and the amount of resin present in its unpolymerised form. Most dental composites use resins with comparable polymerisation shrinkages. In general, a higher proportion of glass filler results in a lower final shrinkage. Such highly filled composites do not necessarily have lower shrinkages than the microfilled resins, as the latter use prepolymerised particles which may themselves be as highly filled as the glass particle systems.

Typical values for polymerisation shrinkage are shown in *Table 12*.

Ideally, the polymerisation shrinkage of the composite should be as low as possible, since this enhances marginal adaptation and so reduces the possibility of recurrent caries. The traditional amalgams minimise this problem because they show a slight expansion on setting, and, in due course, the gap fills with corrosion products.

The use of varnishes and liners provides a barrier to leakage (see section II.IV).

Although there have been major advances in the field of adhesive dental materials, the polymerisation shrinkage has been implicated as a primary source of interfacial breakdown. During the setting process, shrinkage stresses develop because the material is constrained by the adhesion to the cavity walls. These stresses can be sufficient to cause breakdown of the interfacial bond, whereby the advantage of the adhesive procedure is lost. This is particularly so for the bond to dentine (for the bonding agents currently available), which is considerably less strong than that achieved to acid-etched enamel.

Another potential problem is that the shrinkage will cause the cusps of the tooth to be pulled inwards so that they become highly stressed. This effect has been suggested as a source of pulpal sensitivity following the placement of posterior composites. This effect can be exacerbated if a rigid tightly bound matrix band is used during placement of a posterior composite.

## *Water Sorption*

The water sorption should be kept low for composites, because excessive water sorption has a detrimental effect on the colour stability and the

**Table 13** Equilibrium water uptake for a number of composites, adapted from data of Oysaed and Ruyter (1986).

| Material (Manufacturer) | On Material ($\mu$g/mm$^{-3}$) | On Resin* ($\mu$g.mm$^{-3}$) | Volume of Resin (%) |
|---|---|---|---|
| Occlusin (ICI Dental) | 12.9 | 41.6 | 31 |
| P-10 (3M Dental) | 16.0 | 44.4 | 36 |
| Profile (SS White) | 16.3 | 37.0 | 44 |
| Ful-Fil (LD Caulk) | 20.3 | 63.4 | 32 |
| Heliomolar (Vivadent) | 20.6 | 43.6 | 47 |
| Estilux (Kulzer) | 23.1 | 82.4 | 28 |
| P-30 (3M Dental) | 36.9 | 119.0 | 31 |

*The uptake of water by the resin was based on the assumption that the glass does not absorb water and worked out using the volume % resin shown in the last column.

wear resistance. If the composite can absorb water, then it is also able to absorb other fluids from the oral cavity which results in its discoloration.

Water sorption occurs mainly as a direct absorption by the resin. The glass filler will not *absorb* water into the bulk of the material, but can *adsorb* water onto its surface. Thus, the amount of water sorption is dependent on the resin content of the composite and the quality of the bond between the resin and the filler. As such, it would perhaps make more sense to relate the value for the water sorption to the resin content of the composite. This would show whether or not the amount of water sorption is that predicted from a knowledge of the water sorption characteristics of the resin alone or if it is unduly high.

Data shown in *Table 13* indicate that when the filler content of the restorative material is taken into account, marked differences between the water sorption values for a range of composites become apparent.

The intrinsic water sorption for the resin appears to be around 40–45 $\mu$g.mm$^{-3}$, but for two of the composites in the table, the water sorption is two to three times what might have been expected. The question is, 'Where does this extra water go?'

A high water sorption value for a composite (when corrected for the amount of filler present), may indicate that the material has a high soluble fraction, which dissolves and leaves a space into which the water can flow (this is possibly due to incomplete cure of the resin), or that the glass may be partially dissolved. In addition, the resin

may contain air voids, introduced during mixing or placement. Another contributory factor may be hydrolytic breakdown of the bond between the filler and the resin, allowing adsorption onto the surface of the filler particles. This has two important consequences.

Firstly, as the bond between the filler particles and the resin is lost, the filler will lose its effectiveness as a reinforcing agent, resulting in a rapid deterioration of the restoration. Secondly, the filler particles lose their surface cohesion, resulting in a high rate of wear. Thus, a worrying combination of features for a composite would be a high filler loading combined with a high value for water sorption.

It is often suggested that the water sorption may, to some extent, compensate for the polymerisation shrinkage, but water sorption is a gradual process taking many months to complete. This can readily be shown from a knowledge of the diffusion coefficient, D, of water in a composite, which is typically of the order of $1.25 \times 10^{-9}$ cm$^2$.s$^{-1}$.

For a sample of 2mm thickness, the material would require 166 days to reach equilibrium, and if the sample is 5 mm thick, the time taken to reach equilibrium is in excess of three years.

Thus, water sorption cannot prevent interfacial debonding, since it cannot counteract the instantaneous shrinkage that occurs on setting. In due course, the slight swelling may well improve the marginal adaptation of the restoration, but the chances are that by then it will be too late.

It is important to realise that if measurements of the water sorption characteristics are to be undertaken, it is necessary for samples to be ex-

**Table 14** The coefficient of thermal expansion (α) and the differential expansion factor (D) for some composites compared with enamel.

| Material (Manufacturer) | Type | $\alpha$ (ppm.$^\circ$C$^{-1}$) | D |
|---|---|---|---|
| Enamel | | 11.4 | 1.00 |
| Miradapt (J&J) | Hybrid | 21.4 | 1.88 |
| P-10 (3M) | Hybrid | 22.5 | 1.97 |
| Adaptic (J&J) | Traditional | 25.7 | 2.25 |
| Finesse (Caulk) | Microfilled | 51.3 | 4.50 |
| Delton (J&J) | Unfilled | 90.3 | 7.92 |

tremely thin to be able to reach equilibrium water sorption in a realistic time.

## Coefficient Of Thermal Expansion

To minimise the possibility of stresses being developed due to differential expansion and contraction, the coefficient of thermal expansion of the composite needs to be as close as possible to that of tooth tissue. The glass fillers have a low coefficient of expansion while the resin has a high coefficient of expansion so that the higher the inorganic filler loading, the lower the coefficient of expansion will be. Since the microfilled resins have a high resin content, with resin being present in both the matrix and the prepolymerised filler particles, these tend to have a high coefficient of expansion compared to the glass filled composites.

Examples of the coefficient of expansion of some commercially available composites are presented in *Table 14*, which also shows the differential expansion factors when compared with enamel.

## Radio-Opacity

When composites are used as a posterior restorative material, their radio-opacity is of the utmost importance. The detection of caries under a non-radio-opaque composite is virtually impossible, and would allow the caries process to continue undetected for far too long. Some composites have a radio-opacity lower than that of dentine, which is inadequate because an X-ray would not reveal the presence of caries. However, it is not clear what the optimum radio-opacity for a composite is, since excessive radio-opacity can potentially mask out caries lying behind the restoration. Nevertheless, the composite should at least be as radio-opaque as the enamel. Some

composites fall far short of this requirement, and should not be used for posterior restorations.

## Colour Match

The aesthetic qualities of composites are now well recognised. The earliest composites suffered from discoloration, which can manifest itself in one of three ways:

- Marginal discoloration.
- General surface discoloration.
- Bulk discoloration.

Marginal discoloration is usually due to the presence of a marginal gap between the restoration and the tooth tissues. Debris penetrates the gap and leads to an unsightly marginal stain; elimination of the marginal gap would completely avoid this staining. If the margin is in enamel, it is possible to overcome this problem by employing the acid-etch technique of bonding to enamel. The bond between acid-etched enamel and composite is sufficiently strong and durable to achieve a good marginal seal which avoids the ingress of debris. The use of an unfilled bonding resin is generally recommended, as this helps marginal adaptation.

General surface discoloration may be related to the surface roughness of the composite, and is more likely to occur with those composite resins employing large filler particles. Debris gets trapped in the spaces between the protruding filler particles and is not readily removed by tooth brushing. Polishing with a suitable abrasive, such as one of the aluminium oxide pastes available commercially, should remove this surface stain. Sometimes a dark pitted discoloration can be observed, which is due to the exposure of trapped air bubbles as the composite wears

**Table 15** Compressive strength data for a variety of materials.

| Material (Manufacturer) | Compressive strength (MPa) |
|---|---|
| Molar enamel | 260 |
| Molar dentine | 305 |
| Sybralloy (Kerr ) | 500 |
| Dispersalloy (Johnson & Johnson) | 440 |
| Adaptic (Johnson & Johnson) | 250 |
| Silux (3M Dental Products) | 286 |
| Aurafil (Johnson & Johnson) | 345 |
| Occlusin (ICI Dental Products) | 310 |
| P-30 (3M Dental Products) | 393 |

away. Such discoloration can not easily be removed, and it may be better to replace the restoration with a light activated composite, which will have virtually no air trapped in it if it is placed sufficiently carefully.

Bulk, or deep, discoloration is a particular problem with the two-paste amine-cured composites. The colour of the restoration changes slowly over a long time period, giving the restoration a distinctly yellow appearance. This type of discoloration arises due to both the chemical breakdown of components within the resin matrix and the absorption of fluids from the oral environment. The new, visible light activated composites seem to have much better colour stability.

# Mechanical Properties

## Compressive Strength

If one compares the compressive strengths of a number of composites and amalgams with those of enamel and dentine, the indications are that these materials are quite adequate (*Table 15*).

It is interesting to note that an anterior composite can have a similar compressive strength as a posterior composite, yet the recommendations for their uses are quite different. It is important to know the significance of this value.

Being relatively easy to measure, the compressive strength of a material is quoted frequently. Unfortunately, it is also a property that is difficult to interpret due to the possible modes of failure under compression:

- Ductile materials can spread sideways, rather like putty.
- Brittle materials, like glass and stone, can explode in all directions.
- Buckling can occur in long, thin samples.

As can be imagined, highly complex stresses are generated in the specimen when testing compressive strength.

If we ask ourselves whether restorations fail in any of the modes described above, then the answer is that this would seem unlikely. It is much more likely that the restorations will fail under tension (due to the application of bending forces), as composites have a very low tensile strength.

Thus the compressive strength is but a poor indicator of a material's resistance to failure, as there is no simple relationship between a material's compressive and tensile strengths.

## Diametral Tensile Strength

If restorative materials *are* more likely to fail in a tensile mode, then it would make more sense to measure their tensile strength than their compressive strength.

Unfortunately, the measurement of the tensile strengths of brittle materials is extremely difficult, and gives rise to a great deal of scatter in the data. The reason for this is that such materials are highly susceptible to the presence of internal flaws or small cracks in their surfaces, which are impossible to eliminate. As a consequence, the tensile strengths of composites are dependent upon the quality of surface finish.

The *diametral tensile test* is an alternative method for measuring the tensile strength of a material. Again, complex stress patterns arise in the material, but the results are reasonably reproducible and it is an easy property to measure. For these reasons, the diametral tensile strength is often quoted for dental materials.

It is interesting to note that this test is usually applied to brittle materials. Hence, if the diametral tensile strength is quoted rather than conventional tensile strength, this indicates that the material is brittle and therefore suffers from a lack of toughness.

Typical values for the diametral tensile strength of a number of composites are given in *Table 16*. From these figures it can be seen that the traditional anterior composite has a similar diametral tensile strength to that of the current posterior composites. Yet, clinical experience has shown us that traditional composites do not perform well in the posterior situation. Thus, as for the compressive strength, it would seem that the diametral tensile strength alone gives no direct indication as to the particular use of a composite or its potential clinical performance.

As composites are used more and more widely for the restoration of posterior teeth, fracture of the restorations is likely to become an increasingly significant cause of failure; it may be that the above properties will then provide a useful indicator of the resistance to such fractures.

## Hardness

The surface hardness of a dental material can be measured readily by a number of techniques, resulting in a hardness value that can then be used to compare different composites. At one time, it was thought that the hardness would provide a good indicator of the wear resistance of a composite, and this is true up to a point.

The original acrylic resins were very soft materials, but their hardness and wear resistance were much improved by the addition of a filler. Measurement of the hardness initially gave some indication of the wear resistance, but this relationship unfortunately breaks down at the high filler loadings used in the current generation of composites (see below).

## Wear

Wear is the process by which material is displaced or removed by the interfacial forces which are generated as two surfaces rub together. Types of wear that occur in the oral environment are as follows.

### Abrasive Wear

When two surfaces rub together, the harder of the two materials may indent, produce grooves in, or cut away material from the other surface. This direct contact wear is known as *two-body abrasion*, and occurs in the mouth whenever there is direct tooth-to-tooth contact, in what most dentists would call *attrition*.

**Table 16** Diametral tensile strength of some composite restorative materials.

| Material (Manufacturer) | Diametral tensile strength (MPa) |
|---|---|
| Adaptic (Johnson&Johnson) | 51 |
| Aurafil (Johnson&Johnson) | 52 |
| Occlusin (ICI Dental) | 54 |
| P-30 (3M Dental Products) | 67 |

Abrasive wear may also occur when there is an abrasive slurry interposed between two surfaces such that the two solid surfaces are not actually in contact. This is called *three-body abrasion*, and occurs in the mouth during mastication, with food acting as the abrasive agent. (Tooth pastes act as abrasive slurries between the toothbrush and the tooth.)

### Fatigue Wear

The repeated loading of teeth produces cyclic stresses that can in time lead to the growth of fatigue cracks. These cracks often form below the surface, and initially grow parallel to it before veering towards the surface or coalescing with other cracks.

### Corrosive wear

Chemical attack on composites can occur either as the hydrolytic breakdown of the resin or the breakdown of the resin-filler interface.

It is likely that all of the above mechanisms are involved in wear of the composites. In occlusal contact areas, the main wear mechanisms are two-body abrasion and fatigue, whereas three-body abrasion dominates in non-contact areas. Corrosive wear can occur in either situation, and, when in combination with stressing conditions, can lead to stress corrosion cracking. This process involves the slow growth of a crack, which will eventually become sufficiently large to cause catastrophic fracture.

Since wear is a such a multifaceted process, it does not lend itself to being measured by any single parameter. The poor correlation between mechanical properties and wear has already been noted, and some of the physical properties such as a low water sorption can only give an indication of potential wear resistance, particularly in relation to corrosive wear.

In general, a high filler loading, a smooth surface finish, a hydrolytically stable resin and a strong bond between the filler and the resin are desirable attributes in a posterior composite, but it must be recognised that these by themselves do not guarantee that a material will be resistant to wear.

An alternative approach is the laboratory simulation of the clinical condition. Unfortunately, it is very difficult to simulate all of the conditions in the mouth that contribute to the wear process. Although a wide variety of *in vitro* methods for measuring the wear rate have been tried, none have been found to predict with any measure of certainty the *in vivo* rate of wear of the posterior composites.

Another major stumbling block in the development of a reliable laboratory wear test is that one needs to be able to correlate the results with clinical wear data, which, in itself is extremely difficult to acquire and interpret. From the many variables that have to be taken into account, the variation in wear from patient to patient is one of the more difficult to understand.

However, it has been shown that there is a marked difference in wear rates between occlusal contact areas and non-contact areas. Thus, any value quoted for a wear rate is meaningless unless it is supported with information on the methods used in determining it.

The size of the restoration can also affect the rate of wear, perhaps due to there being a greater likelihood of direct tooth-to-restoration contact with larger restorations. It must also be considered that larger restorations tend to occur more posteriorly, where the occlusal loads are higher.

Thus, even *in vivo* wear data are only a guide to the ability of posterior composites to resist wear. The situation is further complicated at present by the lack of a generally accepted method for the measurement of *in vivo* wear, and data have to be interpreted with a great deal of caution.

The best measure of the wear resistance of a posterior composite is its clinical performance.

# Composite Inlays

Composite inlays are composite restorations that are constructed in the dental laboratory by a dental technician, based upon an impression prepared by the dental surgeon. (There are a number of systems that allow the construction of such inlays at the chairside.)

Composite inlays are ideally suited to those situations where there is a need to carry out multiple posterior restorations in a single quadrant. The clinical placement of multiple direct composites poses a number of problems, such as the time consuming nature of the placement itself, the difficulty of ensuring good tooth-to-tooth contact, the problems of marginal adaptation caused by polymerisation shrinkage, and the risk of incomplete curing of the restoration due to the limited depth of cure. One way to overcome these problems is to use composite inlays.

The advantage with this type of restoration is that much of the work of achieving good anatomical contour and tooth-to-tooth contact is done by the technician. Full depth of cure is assured, and, since the curing process is carried out in the laboratory and not *in situ*, problems associated with polymerisation shrinkage are much reduced.

However, it has been suggested that even the thin layer of resin cement used to fix the restoration to the tooth tissue can cause sufficiently high shrinkage stresses to cause failure of the adhesive bond, especially that to the dentine. Thus, problems with polymerisation shrinkage are not totally eliminated. There is also some doubt as to the quality of the bond between the resin cement and inlay itself. The laboratory curing process for the composite inlays is so effective that there are few methacrylate groups left on its surface to react with the resin luting cement.

Many laboratory and chairside inlay systems use the same composites that are used for direct placement. Consequently, they suffer from many of the same shortcomings as direct composites, which therefore limits their range of applications. Thus composite inlays should only be used in those situations where a direct composite would also be considered acceptable.

# Clinical Considerations

The indications for the use of composite restorations are primarily associated with their ability to achieve an excellent aesthetic result. These materials are therefore ideally suited for anterior applications, such as the restoration of proximal lesions, abrasion and erosion lesions and incisal tip fractures.

For the posterior region, the application of composites tends to be more limited due to such potential problems as a lack of marginal seal, wear and fracture; they should ideally be considered only as primary restorative materials for small early carious lesions.

The composite restoration should, at all times, be considered as an adhesive restoration. The advantages are manifold, but, principally, the reliance on adhesion rather than retention helps to conserve tooth structure, to improves the strength of the tooth crown and to provide a barrier to marginal leakage. It is therefore important that these materials are used only in situations where a good quality adhesive bond can be achieved; the following contraindications are suggested:

## *Avoid Large Restorations*

This problem is most likely to occur in the posterior application of composites, where these materials are frequently considered as a replacement for failed amalgam restorations. Since such cavities are generally much bigger than those of primary caries lesions, this is not the ideal circumstance in which to use composites. For a start, the cavity design has been largely dictated by the amalgam to be replaced, and was designed with retention in mind, rather than adhesion.

The larger the restoration, the greater the problem of polymerisation shrinkage, and the lower the chances of achieving a good marginal seal. The shrinkage on polymerisation causes the composite to pull away from the cavity walls, and, although acid-etch bonded enamel is sufficiently strong to resist the shrinkage forces generated, dentine bonding agents may not have a sufficiently strong bond to dentine to do likewise. This can give rise to marginal leakage and post-operative sensitivity. Even when most or all of the margins are in enamel (where a good

bond and seal is possible), the breakdown of the bond to dentine will result in a fluid filled gap beneath the restoration. This too can give rise to post-operative sensitivity, due to the movement of the fluid up and down the dentinal tubules when the restoration is subjected to a load or a change in temperature.

Another contributory factor to lack of marginal seal is the mismatch in the coefficient of expansion of the restorative material and the tooth tissues. This is a problem with all composites, and, although it is minimised by having high filler loadings of low expansion glasses, it has not yet been resolved.

With larger restorations, it is more likely that there will be occlusal contact between the restoration and the opposing tooth. As composites suffer from considerably higher rates of wear in contact areas than in contact-free areas, occlusal contact combined with the higher loads that are experienced posteriorly can give rise to unacceptable rates of wear. Hence, only non-functional cusps should be involved.

Composites are low strength, brittle materials, and do not have properties much better than amalgams in this respect. The restoration derives its strength from the ability to bond to the tooth tissues. If this bond breaks down, the potential for fracture is much increased, even more so if the occlusal loads are high. The reliability and durability of the adhesive bond is much reduced as the size of the restoration is increased.

## *Avoid Deep Gingival Preparations*

Proximal restorations, whether anterior or posterior, can extend sub-gingivally such that the base of the box extends into root dentine. In such circumstances, it is extremely difficult, if not impossible, to ensure close marginal adaptation and to obtain a perfect marginal seal, even with the use of dentine bonding agents.

Microleakage and the associated problems of staining, caries and sensitivity are therefore likely to be a problem. Although it has been suggested that the base of such a box may first be filled with a glass–ionomer cement, there is the possibility that the cement will eventually erode, leaving the marginal ridge of the composite restoration unsupported and possibly causing it to fracture.

## Lack Of Peripheral Enamel

The acid-etch bond to enamel of composites is extremely effective such that breakdown of these margins is unlikely.

When a tooth is badly broken down, there will be little enamel left to bond to and the restoration has to rely more and more on the bond to the remaining dentine. This bond is as yet highly unreliable and thus increases the possibility of a breakdown of the marginal seal when subjected to stresses generated by polymerisation shrinkage, thermal mismatch and occlusal loading.

Ideally resin composites should only be used when all the margins are in enamel. The only exception to this are restorations of abrasion/erosion lesions, which tend not to be subjected to high stressing conditions and have proved reasonably effective clinically, although adhesive failures remain a problem.

## Replacement Or Onlays Of Load Bearing Cusps

As noted earlier, composites suffer from much higher rates of wear when thay are in occlusal contact with opposing teeth.

Anteriorly this has not proved a major problem, but posteriorly, where the loads are generally much higher, excessive wear of the composite is likely to occur. This becomes more of a problem the further posterior the restoration is placed. The increased loads experienced by the restoration will also increase the chances of cuspal fracture, especially if preceded by the breakdown of the adhesive bond.

## Poor Moisture Control

Since it is impossible to obtain an adhesive bond between tooth tissues and composites when the tooth surfaces are contaminated with moisture, any situation in which moisture control is not possible should be avoided and an alternative approach must be adopted.

## Habitual Bruxism/Chewing

The aggressive wearing action associated with bruxism will cause any composite restoration that is in occlusal contact or one that is in contact with an implement such as a pipe, to wear down extremely rapidly. Thus, even incisal tip restorations, which do not normally suffer from high rates of wear, are contraidicated unless the patient can be weaned off their habit.

# Summary

The introduction of resin-based composite restorative materials has had a major impact on the practice of restorative dentistry.

Many of the advances in new techniques have the composite materials as their basis. Their clinical applications are many and varied, and will continue to grow as further improvements in their properties are achieved. However, there are certain limits to the use of this group of materials and it is important that these are not exceeded.

# Further Reading

Asmussen E. A.(1983) Factors affecting the color stability of restorative resins. Acta Odont. Scand. **41**, 11–18

Asmussen E. A.(1985) Clinical relevance of physical, chemical and bonding properties of composite resins. Oper. Dent. **10**, 61

American Dental Association Committee on Dental Materials, Instruments and Equipment (CDMIE). (1983) Status report on posterior composites. J. Amer. Dent. Assoc. **107**, 74–77

CDMIE (1986) The effects of blue light on the retina and the use of protective filtering glasses J. Am. Dent. Assoc. **112**, 533–535

Davidson C. L.& de Gee A. J. (1984) Relaxation of polymerization contraction stresses by flow in dental composites. J. Dent. Res. **63**, 146–148

Eliades G. C., Vougiouklakis G. J., & Caputo A. A. (1987) Degree of double bond conversion in light-cured composites. Dent. Mater. **3**, 19–25

Gilbert J. A. (1987) Posterior composites: an ethical issue. Oper. Dent. **12**, 79–81

Jorgensen K. D. (1980) Restorative resins: abrasion vs mechanical properties. Scand. J. Dent. Res. **88**, 557–568

Lambrechts P., Braem M. & Vanherle G. (1987) Evaluation of clinical performance for posterior composite resins and dentine adhesives. Oper. Dent. **12**, 53–78

Leinfelder K. F.,(1985) Composite resins. Dent. Clin. N. Am. **29 (2)**, 359–371

Lutz F., Phillips R. W., Roulet J. F. & Setcos J. C. (1984) *In vivo* and *in vitro* wear of potential posterior composites. J. Dent. Res. **63**, 914–920

Morin D., de Long R. & Douglas W. H. (1984) Cusp reinforcement by the acid-etch technique. J. Dent. Res. **63**, 1075–1078

Omer O. E., Wilson N. F. & Watts D. C. (1986) Radio-opacity of posterior composites. J. Dent. **14**, 178–179

Oysaed H. & Ruyter I. E. (1986) Water sorption and filler characteristics of composites for use in posterior teeth J. Dent. Res. **65**, 1315–1318

Van Dijken J. W. V. (1986) A clinical evaluation of anterior conventional, microfiller and hybrid composite resin fillings. Acta Odont. Scand. **44**, 357–367

Van Noort R. (1983) Controversial aspects of composite restorative materials. Brit. Dent. J. **155**, 380–384

Watts D. C., Amer O., Combe E. C. (1984) Characterisation of visible-light-activated composite systems. Brit. Dent. J. **156**, 209–215

# II.III

# GLASS–IONOMER CEMENTS

## Introduction

Glass–ionomer cements (GICs) are restorative materials that consist of a powder and a liquid which are mixed to produce a plastic mass that subsequently sets to a rigid solid.

The glass–ionomer cements were first described by Wilson and Kent in 1971, and, at the time, presented a natural extension to the zinc polycarboxylate cements that had become available in the late 1960s. The advantage they provided was that the phosphoric acid was replaced by polyacrylic acid.

The glass–ionomer cements were immediately seen as a potential replacement for the silicate cements that had been around for some 80 years and that were gradually being ousted by the resin-based composites.

The two main features of glass–ionomer cements that have allowed them to become one of the accepted dental materials are their ability to bond to dentine and their ability to release fluoride from the glass component of the cement. Thus, the glass–ionomer cements combine the adhesive qualities of the zinc polycarboxylate cements with the fluoride release of the silicate cements. The relationship between the different materials is shown in **103**.

Until recently, the glass–ionomer cements have been used mainly for the restoration of erosion lesions and as a luting agent for crown and bridge reconstruction. Their clinical application is now being extended by the introduction of a wide variety of new formulations which has given rise to some interesting new uses. Thus, this group of materials deserves closer attention.

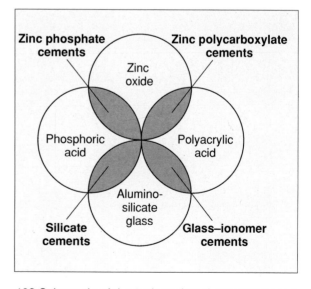

**103** Schematic of the various dental cements based on powders of zinc oxide and alumino-silicate glass, and liquids consisting of phosphoric acid and polyacrylic acid

# Chemistry Of Glass–Ionomer Cements

## Composition

What makes the glass–ionomer cement such an interesting material compared to the zinc phosphate cements is the enormous variety of compositions that can be achieved.

The composition of the glass can be varied widely, giving many different properties, and, to add to this, there are numerous combinations of polyacids that are suitable for copolymerisation. (In contrast, for the zinc phosphate cements, once the composition is optimised in terms of the powder–liquid ratio and the concentration of the phosphoric acid, there is little scope for improvement.)

Of course, such a variety can be as much of a hindrance as a help, and this is reflected in the development of the glass–ionomer cements which began in the early 1970s.

It could never be claimed that the glass–ionomer cements have had a smooth passage since their inception. The proof of this statement is in the observation that the materials currently marketed are quite different from those originally made available for clinical use. The early materials consisted of a glass powder to which a concentrated solution of a polyacrylic acid was added. ASPA (De Trey) was the first commercial product, and was made available in 1976.

### The Glass

The glasses for the glass–ionomer cements contain three main components: silica ($SiO_2$) and alumina ($Al_2O_3$) mixed in a flux of calcium fluoride ($CaF_2$), as shown in **104**. The composition of the glass is largely restricted to the central region of the phase diagram by the desire to have a translucent glass.

The mixture (which also contains sodium and aluminium fluorides and calcium or aluminium phosphates as additional fluxes) is fused at a high temperature, and the molten mass is then shock-cooled and finely ground to a powder before use.

The particle size of the powder is dependent upon its intended application. For filling materials, the maximum particle size is 50 μm, while

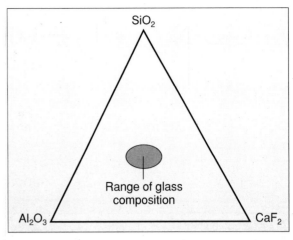

**104** Composition of glass used in glass–ionomer cements.

for the luting and lining materials it is reduced to less than 20 μm.

The rate of release of ions from the glass (which is an important factor in determining the setting characteristics, the solubility, and the release of fluoride), is a function of the type of glass employed (see below). The glass also plays a major role in the aesthetics of the restoration, as this is dependent on both the refractive index of the glass and the presence of pigments within it.

### Polyacid

There are a wide range of polyacrylic acid analogues, which, when combined with variations in molecular weight and configuration, means that a large variety of formulations are possible. The polyacids most used in current formulations are copolymers of acrylic and itaconic acid or acrylic and maleic acid (**105**).

There is an optimum acid concentration in the case of the silicate cements, but the glass–ionomer cements are not so dependent upon this. The strength and the resistance to aqueous attack both steadily increase with polyacid concentration, so the limiting factor is the consistency of the cement paste. The viscosity of the liquid depends both upon the polyacid concentration and the molecular weight, which can vary from 10 000 to 30 000, depending upon the formulation selected.

Tartaric acid is an important hardener, and controls the pH during the setting process which in turn controls the rate of dissolution of the glass.

**Acrylic acid**

$$-CH_2-\underset{\underset{\textstyle COOH}{|}}{\overset{\overset{\textstyle HC}{|}}{C}}$$

**Itaconic acid**

$$-CH_2-\underset{\underset{\textstyle COOH}{|}}{\overset{\overset{\textstyle COOH}{|}}{\underset{\textstyle CH_2}{C}}}$$

**Maleic acid**

$$-CH_2-\underset{\underset{\textstyle COOH}{|}}{\overset{\overset{\textstyle HC}{|}}{C}}\!\!-\!\!\underset{\underset{\textstyle COOH}{|}}{\overset{\overset{\textstyle HC}{|}}{C}}\!-$$

**Tartaric acid**

$$H\underset{\underset{\textstyle COOH}{|}}{\overset{\overset{\textstyle OH}{|}}{C}}\!\!-\!\!\underset{\underset{\textstyle COOH}{|}}{\overset{\overset{\textstyle OH}{|}}{C}}H$$

**105** Acid components used in a glass–ionomer cement.

## *Presentation*

### Powder/liquid

Many glass–ionomer cements consist of a glass powder to which is added a proprietary liquid. The powder is much as described above, and the liquid is an aqueous solution of polyacrylic or polymaleic acid and tartaric acid. A number of deficiencies were soon recognised with this mode of presentation and brought about a change in formulation.

One of the problems is the excessive solubility of the cement in saliva coupled with the slow setting reaction, and another is concerned with judging the correct powder to liquid ratio. There is a tendency to reduce the powder content of the cement in order to obtain a smooth creamy paste, but this results in a slower-setting, weaker cement that is even more susceptible to dissolution.

### Anhydrous Cements

Nowadays, many glass–ionomer cements are of a water-hardening type, and the cement is formed by the addition of the correct amount of distilled water. The glass powder is blended with freeze dried polyacid and tartaric acid powder.

The first product that used this approach became available commercially in 1981. The new formulations, described as the *anhydrous systems*, present as a powder and a liquid. The powder contains alumino-silicate glass, polyacid powder and tartaric acid, and the liquid is just distilled water.

### Capsules

It is well recognised that achieving the correct powder to liquid ratio can still be a problem, and one way in which this may be overcome is by the use of preproportioned capsules.

The contents of different capsules do not necessarily have the same constituents, so it is inadvisable to mix them. For example, to ensure the most appropriate handling and physical properties, the filling materials have much larger glass filler particles than the luting agents. Similarly, the liquids used can vary in composition to suit the particular glass formulation and to give the correct working and setting times. This is dealt with in some detail later, in relation to the application of the different formulations.

## *Setting Reaction*

The setting reaction of the glass–ionomer cements is via an acid-base reaction:

$$\underset{\text{glass}}{MO.SiO_2} \; + \; \underset{\text{acid}}{H_2A} \; \rightarrow \; \underset{\text{salt}}{MA} \; + \; \underset{\text{silica gel}}{SiO_2 + H_2O.}$$

The setting process of a glass–ionomer cement involves three overlapping stages:

- Dissolution.
- Gelation.
- Hardening.

This happens because of the different rates at which the ions are released from the glass and the rate at which the salt matrix is formed (**106**);

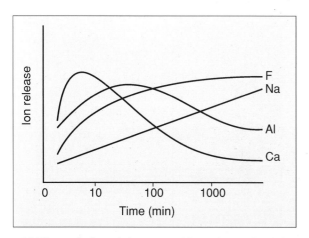

**106** The variation of the rates of ion release from the glass.

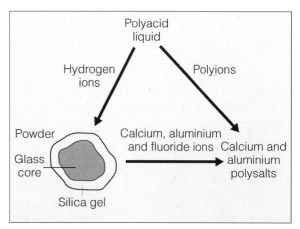

**107** The initial stages of the setting reaction in a glass–ionomer cement.

as is apparent from this curve, the calcium ions are more rapidly released than the aluminium ions. It is the calcium and the aluminium ions which will eventually form the salt matrix. The sodium and fluorine ions do not take part in the setting process but combine to be released as sodium fluoride.

### Dissolution

When the proprietary solution or the water is mixed with the powder, the acid goes into solution and reacts with the outer layer of the glass. This layer becomes depleted in aluminium, calcium, sodium and fluorine ions, so that only a silica-gel remains (**107**).

The hydrogen ions that are released from the acid diffuse to the glass, and make up for the loss of the calcium, aluminium and fluoride ions. The setting reaction for the cement is a slow process, and it takes some time for the material to stabilise; the final translucency of the material is not apparent until 24 hours after placement.

Although the material appears hard after its required setting time (usually 3 to 6 minutes, depending on whether it is a filling or a luting cement), it has still not reached its final physical and mechanical properties.

### Gelation

The initial set is due to the rapid action of the calcium ions, which, being divalent and more abundant initially, react more readily with the carboxyl groups of the acid than do the trivalent aluminium ions (**108**). This is the *gelation phase* of

the setting reaction. The efficiency with which the calcium ions crosslink the polyacid molecules is not as good as it might be, because they are also able to chelate carboxyl groups on the same molecule.

Various things can happen if the restoration is not protected from the outside environment during this critical phase. Aluminium ions may diffuse out of the material and be lost to the cement, thereby being unable to crosslink the polyacrylic acid chains. If the water is lost, the reaction can not go to completion. In both instances, a weak material will result. Alternatively, additional moisture may be absorbed, and may be contaminated with blood or saliva, leading to poorer aesthetics, with the restoration looking exceptionally dull and white. The contaminating moisture will also weaken the material and may even cause it to crumble. Hence, it is essential that contamination by moisture and drying of the restoration are both

**108** Gelation phase of the setting process.

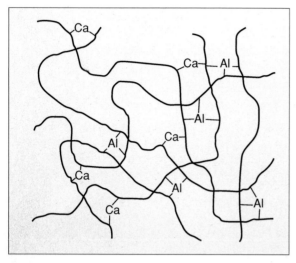

**109** Hardening phase of the setting process.

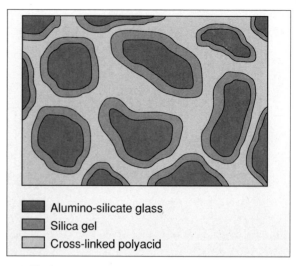

Alumino-silicate glass
Silica gel
Cross-linked polyacid

**110** The structure of a glass–ionomer cement.

avoided, at least during the initial period of setting when the material is at its most vulnerable.

It has been suggested that some of the newer formulations of the luting cements do not need the protection of a surface coating because they have a more rapid set. Although the solubility (measured as the water-leachable component at 7 minutes) has been reduced from approximately 2% to 1% in the transition from a conventional to a water-hardened cement (would appear to be even less for the maleic acid-based cements), it may be as well to continue to offer some initial protection, since the dissolution due to erosion will continue to be a problem. In any case, it still takes some time for these materials to reach their final set.

### Hardening

After the gelation phase there is a hardening phase that can last as long as seven days. It takes some 30 minutes for the uptake of aluminium ions to become significant, but it is the aluminium ions which provide the final strength to the cement as they are responsible for the introduction of the cross-links. In contrast to the calcium ions, the trivalent nature of the aluminium ions ensures that a high degree of cross-linking of the polymer molecules takes place (**109**).

There is a continuation of the formation of aluminium salt bridges, and water becomes bound to the silica gel which now surrounds the residual core of each of the glass particles. Once the cement has fully reacted, the solubility is quite low. The final structure is as shown in **110**, and consists of glass particles, each of which is surrounded by a silica gel in a matrix of crosslinked polyacrylic acid.

Whereas normally it is desirable for glasses to resist ion release, in the case of the glass–ionomer cements a controlled release of the ions of calcium and aluminium is essential. The skill in choosing the correct glass and the correct formulation is to balance the various requirements of good handling characteristics, low solubility and adequate fluoride release.

# Properties

## *Handling Characteristics*

The effects of the composition of the glass on the setting process are very pronounced and of considerable importance in determining the acceptability of the final handling characteristics of the cement. The Al:Si ratio of the glass for the glass–ionomer cements is higher than that for the silicate cements, because the polyacrylic acid and its analogues are much weaker than phosphoric acid. One of the effects of this increased ratio is that the working time is reduced.

However, glass–ionomer cements were inclined previously to have prolonged working

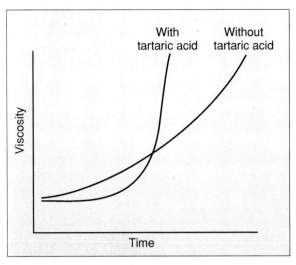

**111** The effect of tartaric acid on the viscosity–time curve for a setting glass–ionomer cement.

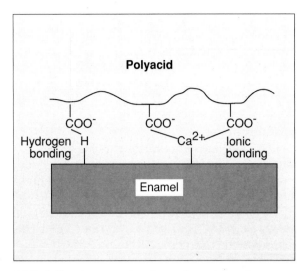

**112** Adhesive mechanisms for glass–ionomer cements.

and setting times. This was certainly one of the problems with the earliest formulations of this cement until it was overcome by the inclusion of the optimum concentration of tartaric acid; by adding the correct amount of tartaric acid it is possible to achieve longer working times while the setting time remains virtually unchanged (**111**).

By manipulation of the glass composition and particle size, and the incorporation of tartaric acid, the handling characteristics have been much improved over the years, and are now far superior than those of the first commercially available products. These improvements are shown in *Table 17*. As a consequence of these changes, the glass–ionomer cements now have a much better defined snap set.

## Adhesion

Glass–ionomer cements are able to bond to dentine and enamel. It has been suggested that the polyacrylate ions react with the apatite structure (displacing calcium and phosphate ions, and creating an intermediate layer of polyacrylate, phosphate and calcium ions) or bond directly to the calcium in the apatite as shown in **112**.

The bond to dentine may be a hydrogen-bond type of adhesion to the collagen combined with an ionic bond to the apatite within the dentine structure. The bond is not particularly strong (2–7 MPa), but clinical experience would indicate

that it is durable when the material is used for the restoration of erosion lesions. The major limitation on the bond strength of the glass–ionomer cements appears to be the low tensile strength, which is only of the order of 7 MPa, due to the brittle nature of these materials.

To obtain a good bond to dentine, the surface must first be treated with a conditioner. The best conditioner appears to be polyacrylic acid, although tannic acid has also proved to be effective. Typical bond strengths that have been measured for the bond to dentine are presented in *Table 18*.

**Table 17** Handling characteristics of old and new glass–ionomer cements.

| Material | Mixing | Working | Setting | Finishing |
|---|---|---|---|---|
| ASPA | 60 s | 90 s | 6 min | 24 hrs |
| Modern GIC | 20 s | 75 s | 2 min | 7 min |

**Table 18** The effects of surface treatments on the tensile bond strength of glass–ionomer cements to enamel and dentine.

| | Surface treatment | Bond strength (MPa) |
|---|---|---|
| **Enamel** | None | 3.2 |
| | Citric acid | 5.6 |
| | Polyacrylic acid | 7.1 |
| **Dentine** | None | 3.1 |
| | Citric acid | 3.7 |
| | Polyacrylic acid | 6.8 |

The major purpose of the surface treatment is to remove debris and to produce a smooth, clean surface. Citric acid should not be used as it opens up the dentinal tubules, increasing the dentine permeability and the potential for pulpal reaction. Additionally, it demineralises the dentine which may compromise the bond to the apatite component.

With the move towards the use of glass–ionomer cements as cavity bases under composites (where the glass–ionomer cement bonds to the dentine and the composite is bonded to the glass–ionomer cement), it has become important to know what quality of bond between the glass–ionomer cements and the composites can be achieved.

At one time, the etching of the glass ionomer base with phosphoric acid was considered to be beneficial to the bond with the resin composite. However, acid-etching of glass–ionomer cements causes extensive fracture and is best avoided. It is advisable to use a low-viscosity resin in order to obtain a good bond between the composite and the glass–ionomer cement.

## *Aesthetics*

A major requirement on any restorative material intended for use in anterior teeth is that it must blend in well with the surrounding tooth tissues, so as to be barely distinguishable. The factors which govern this are the colour and the translucency of the restorative material.

In glass–ionomer cements, the colour is produced by the glass, and the selection of additives of colour pigments such as ferric oxide or carbon black.

Whereas colour does not present a major problem, the translucency of the glass–ionomer cements was inadequate in the early materials. This lack of translucency has meant that the aesthetic appearance of glass–ionomer cements has always been considered inferior to that of many composite resins. The cements appeared dull and lifeless, and this limited their application to that of a filling material for the treatment of erosion lesions and non-critical class III cavities. In fact, the translucency of the glass–ionomer cement was more closely matched to that of dentine than that of enamel. There are essentially two causes for the opacity of glass–ionomer cements:

- *Phase separation of the glass* – To some extent this problem can be overcome by reducing the aluminium, calcium and fluorine content of the glass, but this reduces the strength of the material and extends the working and setting times.
- *Mismatch of refractive index* – This problem can be minimised by reducing the aluminium content and increasing the fluorine content; however, the latter leads to phase separation. In general, optically good glass–ionomer cements tend to have poor setting characteristics.

The translucency of a restorative material can be described and measured by considering its inverse – *opacity*. Opacity is defined as being zero for a transparent material and 1.0 for a white opaque material. The opacity, or *contrast ratio*, is defined as the ratio between the intensity of the reflected light from the material when placed against a dark background and that obtained for a white background of known reflectivity (70% in the case of dental cements).

This is not an absolute property of the material as it depends upon the thickness of the material and the spectral distribution of the incident light. This property, denoted by $C_{0.70}$ (for a thickness of 1mm), gives mean values for enamel and dentine of 0.39 and 0.70 respectively. The early formulations of the glass–ionomer cements gave $C_{0.70}$ values in the range 0.7–0.85. These have been improved and are now approaching those of enamel with $C_{0.70}$ values of 0.4 for some formulations.

The opacity is affected by the absorption of water, causing a decrease in the opacity. Thus, clinically, the restoration can darken when it comes in contact with water.

Selecting the appropriate colour and translucency is a difficult problem as they are affected by the optical properties of the underlying material. On some occasions, the translucency has to be forsaken, and a relatively opaque material must be used in order to mask out a particularly dark substructure. In these cases, the glass–ionomer cements can prove to be particularly suitable.

While the initial match in colour and translucency between the enamel and the glass–ionomer cement is important, it is also important that this close match is maintained in the severe environment of the oral cavity. A loss of aesthetic quality of the restoration can arise from staining, and, if excessive, would be considered a clinical failure and would need replacement.

The glass–ionomer cements appear less susceptible to staining than the silicate cements which preceded them. The staining of glass–ionomer cements has also been found to be far less pronounced than that of the composite resins. This has been ascribed to the superior adhesion between the matrix and the glass in the glass–ionomer cement when compared to the bond between the resin and filler in the composite.

## Solubility

Due to their high solubility, the dental silicates had a reputation for loss of material in the mouth. To some extent this can be attributed to incorrect preparation and handling, but it is an inherent feature of all dental cements, and, as such, the glass–ionomer cements are no exception.

Nevertheless, this negative aspect of the material's behaviour can be minimised by an appreciation of the mechanisms involved and the adoption of proper clinical technique. The processes giving rise to loss of material are complex as there are many variables involved, such as the cement composition, the clinical technique used and the nature of the environment. The loss of material from a glass–ionomer cement can be classified into three main categories:

- Dissolution of the immature cement.
- Long-term erosion.
- Abrasion.

Dissolution of the immature cement occurs before the material is fully set, which can take up to 24 hours. The temporary protection of a layer of nitro-cellulose, methyl methacrylate or amide resin acting as a varnish should be sufficient to minimise this effect. This protection must survive for at least one hour, as it takes this much time for the glass–ionomer cement to approach the properties that are achieved when it is fully set. At present, there is some controversy as to the quality and duration of protection offered by the different varnishes available, and

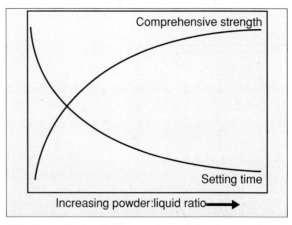

**113** The effects of changes in powder:liquid ratio on the properties of glass–ionomer cements.

some clinicians advocate the use of an unfilled light-activated resin, as this will give longer protection. A high powder-to-liquid ratio helps, because it accelerates the setting process, whereas a thin mix has the opposite effect, and also adversely affects the mechanical properties (**113**).

Once the cement has fully set (usually within two to three days; manifested by a dramatic drop in the amount of water-leachable material) this particular form of material loss will stop. From this point onwards, loss of material can be considered long term, and is a function of the conditions in the oral environment.

Loss of material in the long term may arise either from acid attack or mechanical abrasion. This is hardly surprising, given that the main application of glass–ionomer cements is the restoration of lesions which have themselves arisen because of the combined effect of acid and abrasion. The potential for acid attack tends to be very marked in stagnation regions such as around the gingival margin. Here, plaque accumulates and a highly acidic environment develops due to the formation of lactic acid. The glass–ionomer cements are more resistant to this form of attack than the silicate cements, as indicated by a reduction in the extent of surface markings.

Glass–ionomer cements are extensively used in applications where they will be subject to mechanical abrasion, such as tooth brushing. Their resistance to abrasion is poor, which limits their application to low stressing conditions and certainly prevents their use as permanent posterior restorative materials.

**Table 19** Clinical applications of glass–ionomer cements.

| Tooth coloured filling materials |
| --- |
| • Abrasion and erosion lesions |
| • Class III lesions involving exposed root dentine |
| • Occlusal lesions on deciduous dentition |
| • Temporary anterior and posterior restorations |
| • Repair of crown margins |
| **Cavity bases and liners** |
| • Cement base under composites, amalgams and ceramics |
| • Blocking out undercuts |
| **Luting cements** |
| • Cementation of crowns and bridges |

An *in vitro* test, in which cement samples are arranged in small holders and subjected to a jet of liquid consisting of a dilute acid, attempts to assess loss of material by a combination of abrasion and acid attack. Using this method, the indications are that the polyacrylic acid-based cements are more resistant to abrasion/erosion than the polymaleic acid-based cements. However, it should be remembered that this observation is based on a laboratory test and would need to be confirmed clinically before its validity can be established.

## Fluoride Release

The fact that dental cements dissolve in the oral environment is usually regarded as an adverse effect, since it leads to degradation of the material. However, fluoride is also released, and it is believed that this significantly increases the caries resistance of enamel adjacent to the restoration. Whether fluoride release or other factors (e.g. the release of other ions, antibacterial properties and adhesive capabilities) have a role to play in the anti-carcinogenic characteristics of glass–ionomer cements is still a matter of debate. Nevertheless, attempts have been made to impart this property to amalgams and composites as well as the glass–ionomer cements.

This presents the dentist with an interesting dilemma in making the choice between a glass–ionomer cement or a composite, with the former being most definitely weaker but providing some protection of the surrounding tissues, and the latter being more stable and stronger but not providing such protection.

# Clinical Applications

It must be appreciated from the outset that the glass–ionomer cements are designed to suit a wide variety of applications, their range encompassing materials with widely different properties.

Hence, although they are all based on the same principles outlined above, each formulation has features which make it more suited to a particular application, and it is important that these are not confused. The various applications are listed in *Table 19*.

## Tooth-Coloured Filling Materials

### Presentation

The materials are available in three formulations:

- The traditional powder/liquid systems with the polyacids in an aqueous solution.
- The anhydrous systems with the dried acid incorporated in the powder.
- Encapsulated versions.

The latter requires activation of the capsule, and the mixing in of an amalgamator, which ensures an accurate powder:liquid ratio, not unlike the amalgam capsules.

Some of the properties of a number of tooth-coloured glass–ionomer cements are presented in *Table 20*. The differences are not really sufficient to suggest that one material is superior to another.

The main feature of all of these materials is their low diametral tensile strength, which is an indication of the low tensile strength of these materials. Thus, glass–ionomer cements should not be used where they are going to be subjected to high tensile loads, such as incisal tip restorations, cuspal replacement or pin retained cores. In situations where the restoration is supported all around by tooth tissue, the glass–ionomer cement is protected (to some degree) from tensile loading conditions.

The size of the glass powder particles ensures that a very high powder:liquid ratio can be achieved, and this is reflected in the compressive and diametral tensile strengths of these materials. (These strengths are much higher than for the luting and lining cements described later.) It also affects the solubility, which is reduced as the powder:liquid ratio is increased.

There are differences in the working and setting times of the different cements: some have much shorter setting times than others (which is desirable in limiting the early solubility), but the working time is also much reduced, which may present a problem to some clinicians.

### Shade Selection

The aesthetic quality of the tooth-coloured glass–ionomer cements has long been considered a drawback, but recent changes in formulation have resulted in a marked improvement.

The choice of shade of the restorative material should be carried out prior to the isolation of the tooth or any other form of preparation. The colour of rubber dam, if used, alters the colour of the tooth. This change in shade is increased still further when the enamel is allowed to dehydrate during isolation.

For the restoration of lesions that involve an extensive amount of the labial surface, the use of glass–ionomer cements may not give an aesthetically adequate result, and the use of composites should be considered. Nevertheless, for those patients who are known to have a high caries rate, it may be better to forsake some of the aesthetic quality of the composites in preference to the fluoride protection provided by the glass–ionomer cements.

Another aspect of the aesthetics of glass–ionomer cements is the observation that there is a colour change during the setting process. Generally, the shade is somewhat darker after the material has fully set than at the time of placement. This darkening is believed to be associated with an increase in translucency on setting and may take up to 24 hours to develop.

### Cavity Preparation

The adhesive quality of the glass–ionomer cements dictates that an ultra-conservative approach should be adopted. This means that minimal removal of tooth substance is required, and it should be stressed that the excessive removal of tooth tissues for the provision of undercuts or dovetails is not necessary. However, for situations where the restoration may be subjected to high stresses, some undercut may be advantageous. In the case of a replacement

**Table 20** Compressive and diametral tensile strengths of a range of commercially available glass ionomer cement filling materials.

| Material (Manufacturer) | Compressive Strength (MPa) | Diametral Tensile Strength (MPa) |
|---|---|---|
| Chemfill-II (De Trey) | 230 | 19 |
| Ketac-Fil (ESPE) | 170 | 10 |
| Legend (SS White) | 220 | 16 |
| Opus-Fil (DSD) | 220 | 18 |
| RGI (Rexodent) | 220 | 16 |

restoration, the original restoration should be carefully removed without removing any tooth tissues unless it is carious. The cavo-surface margins should be butt jointed and not bevelled.

### Isolation

Although the glass–ionomer cements are hydrophilic materials, it is recommended that careful isolation of the field of operation is carried out. The presence of blood or saliva will not only impair the formation of a strong bond but may also lead to contamination of the restoration, thereby reducing both bond strength and aesthetics. A well placed glass–ionomer cement should not fail adhesively, as the bond to dentine and enamel is at least as strong as the cohesive strength of the cement.

### Preparation Of The Dentinal Surfaces

The nature of the dentine surface varies from site to site, with the major distinction being between cut dentine after caries removal and sclerotic dentine.

- *Abrasion/erosion lesions* – Lesions at the cervical margin need to be restored to provide direct protection of the pulp, to prevent the development of pulpal sensitivity and to improve appearance. Since the glass–ionomer cements are adhesive, it should not be necessary to cut any finishing lines or undercuts in the dentine. Preparation prior to placement of the material should only involve the cleaning and conditioning of the dentine surface. The cleaning procedure should be carried out by scrubbing for a few seconds only with a slurry of pumice and water in a soft rubber cup or bristle brush, and is aimed at removing any surface contaminants such as plaque or pellicle which obscure the dentine surface. The surface should be thoroughly washed to remove any debris. A conditioner consisting of an aqueous solution of polyacrylic acid may then be applied to the surface for 30 seconds, using a pledget of cotton wool and a light rubbing action. This procedure will ensure that the surface is clean, but will also result in some opening of the dentinal tubules. Some argue that exposure of the dentinal tubules is contraindicated, as it increases the dentine permeability and thus raises the likelihood of a pulpal reaction. This is probably not a problem in the case of patients who have no history of sensitivity, since the tubules will have sclerosed, and secondary dentine will have been laid down. However, for those patients with sensitivity, acid treatment of the dentine surface should not be undertaken. There is still some controversy as to the need for the prior application of polyacrylic acid to the dentine surface. Some studies have shown that this will improve the dentine bond strength, whereas others have shown that it has no effect.

- *Class III , Class V and other carious lesions* – It is not necessary to clean the cavities with pumice and water in the case of carious lesions, as the surface will consist of freshly exposed dentine. However, there is still the dentine smear layer to consider, which is present in any cavity preparation. While the smear layer is strongly bonded to the underlying dentine, surface debris needs to be removed in such a way as to avoid opening of the dentinal tubules. Again, the use of polyacrylic acid is recommended. A variety of other dentine conditioners have been advocated from time to time (e.g. citric acid, EDTA and ferric chloride), but these should not be applied to freshly cut dentine for the reasons already mentioned. The simplest and most effective dentine surface conditioner appears to be polyacrylic acid.

**Pulpal Protection**

The increased application of glass–ionomer cements in recent years has raised some interesting problems, not least being the pulpal toxicity associated with these materials and whether or not a lining material should be used. If the cement is in direct contact with the pulp, this will result in a localised zone of pulp necrosis which inhibits calcific repair. However, in those instances where there is a residual dentine layer, dentine bridge formation will occur. It is recommended that a calcium hydroxide lining is placed on the pulpal aspects of mechanically prepared cavities prior to the insertion of the glass–ionomer cement.

The potential cause of pulpal sensitivity when using glass–ionomer cements has been suggested to be due to differences in techniques of manipulating the cement, or some other, unknown patient-related factors. As yet, it is not clear what gives rise to the small number of cases of pulpal sensitivity, nor is it clear what the role of bacterial contamination or invasion may be.

Lower levels of bacteria are associated with glass–ionomer cements than with zinc phosphate or zinc polycarboxylate cements. This may be because glass–ionomer lining cements have a pronounced antimicrobial effect. Nevertheless, for all types of glass–ionomer cement ( including the silver cermets) lining the dentine is recommended, especially if the tooth is symptomatic or the cavity preparation is particularly deep.

There are situations where a small amount of caries may be left in the deepest portions of the preparation since there is the danger of a microscopic pulpal exposure if it were removed. The ability of calcium hydroxide to activate the formation of secondary dentine and its alkalinity are of great value under these circumstances. However, this material should be used sparingly to ensure that the maximum amount of dentine remains exposed for bonding to the glass–ionomer cement.

In general, if there is any doubt about the thickness of the remaining dentine, it is advisable to line the cavity of freshly prepared dentine with calcium hydroxide. For sclerotic dentine, it is not usually necessary to use a calcium hydroxide cavity base, but the use of citric or phosphoric acid should be avoided.

**Dispensing, Mixing and Insertion**

For the powder/liquid systems, great care must be exercised to ensure that the correct amount of powder is mixed with the liquid. It is important that the manufacturer's instructions are carefully followed.

Tapping the bottle prior to use will ensure that the powder is not compacted. Any excess powder should be scraped off with a spatula and not against the side of the bottle. The powder should be spatulated quickly into the liquid in no more than two increments. The maximum mixing time is 20 seconds. The incorporation of a large amount of powder initially should be avoided, as this will appear to give a satisfactorily thick mix even though the powder:liquid ratio may be too low.

In the case of the preproportioned capsules, the capsule should be shaken before activation. The mixing should be carried out in a high speed amalgamator, typically operating at around 4000rpm, for a period of 10 seconds. The whole process of activation, mixing and application should be carried out without any delays.

Contamination of the filling materials with saliva should be avoided during insertion, setting and finishing. The cavity and surrounding area should be dry, although excessive dessication must not occur.

**Finishing and Polishing**

After the material has been allowed to set for the required time, the matrix can be removed and the restoration should be protected immediately from contamination or dehydration, by placing a waterproof varnish. The best surface finish is achieved at this stage, and the removal of excess material will be detrimental to the finish. However, it is virtually impossible to place a glass–ionomer cement without having to do some trimming and polishing.

Gross excess may be trimmed with a sharp blade. As the material is still fairly weak and the bond to the tooth tissues tenuous, the trimming process should be performed from the restoration towards the tooth and not the other way round. It has been shown that the use of hand instruments for carving can damage the marginal integrity of the restoration. In fact, one manufacturer specifically recommends that hand instruments are not used.

It has been suggested that after the initial set, finishing may be performed with rotary instruments such as a white stone or with flexible discs lubricated with a grease such as vaseline or petroleum jelly. The use of a water spray at this stage is not recommended since the material is still highly soluble. Final finishing should not be attempted, and is best left to a later visit by the patient, preferably within 24 hours.

A number of studies have shown that if finishing is carried out after only eight minutes, the resultant surface finish is very poor when using either abrasive discs, impregnated rubber wheels, tungsten carbide blanks or white stones, even in the presence of petroleum jelly. This situation may change with the more recent rapid-setting materials, but so far the early finishing of glass–ionomer cements is contraindicated.

After 24 hours the material is set sufficiently for final finishing to be carried out using either a fine diamond or a 12-bladed tungsten carbide bur. This should be carried out in the presence of a copious supply of water to avoid dehydration, and is now possible as the early susceptibility to dissolution in water has subsided. Final polishing can be performed with the range of abrasive discs, again in the presence of water.

Whichever method is used, it is not possible to obtain a smooth surface finish for a glass–ionomer cement.

**Surface Protection**

The use of a varnish is extremely important. Solutions of natural (Copal) and synthetic resins (cellulose acetate) dissolved in an organic solvent such as ether, acetone or chloroform are generally recommended. Polyurethane varnishes, which polymerise on contact with water and nitro-cellulose (nail varnish), are a less permeable and less soluble alternative.

The light activated enamel bonding resins or dentine bonding agents that are supplied with the composites provide an particularly effective seal and last sufficiently long to offer the necessary protection. The disadvantage with their use is that a small ledge may be left, especially at the gingival margin, which has to be dealt with at a later stage. Also, they suffer from an oxygen inhibited set, so that the surface layer remains tacky. However, if only a thin layer is applied it is too readily removed. The problem can be overcome by the use of a matrix strip but this is very cumbersome to use. Further finishing should be carried out within 24 hours.

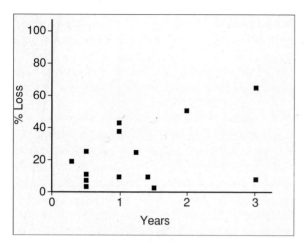

**114** A compilation of survival data for class V restorations restored with ASPA cement taken from publication during the period 1977–1983.

The use of greases or gels such as Vaseline offers little protection, as these are rapidly removed by the action of the lips and the tongue.

Glass–ionomer restorations which have been in place for some time still need to be protected from dehydration during any prolonged isolation of the dentition during other restorative procedures. This is especially the case when using rubber dam. Thus, all known or suspected glass–ionomer cement restorations, crowns, inlay margins and cermets should be protected with a layer of varnish.

### Clinical Performance

The primary applications of the glass–ionomer cements have always been as a filling material for the treatment of abrasion and erosion lesions, and as a luting agent for crowns, bridges and inlays. With the advent of newer and better materials, their use is being extended to include class III restorations, occlusal restorations (particularly in deciduous teeth), action as a core material, and, very much in the forefront now, action as a dentine adhesive lining cement under composite restorations.

Most of the interest in the clinical evaluation of glass–ionomer cements has centred around their use as restorative filling materials. Their ease of placement in bulk, their adhesive qualities and their fluoride protection are seen as important advantages over the aesthetically more pleasing composites.

Whilst there have been quite a few publications on the clinical performance of glass–ionomer cements for class III and class V restorations, it would be difficult, if not impossible, to draw many conclusions from the data. A compilation of results for the performance of class V restorations is given in **114**.

In many of the studies undertaken, there was little appreciation of the exacting requirements of the early materials in terms of powder:liquid ratio or the need for protection during the long setting period. Thus, high failure rates reported in these studies may have been a consequence of techniques inappropriate or inadequate for these particular materials.

We will need to await the results of reasonably long-term studies with the newer formulations before their clinical performance can be judged with any degree of certainty.

Although not recommended for class II restorations for adults, glass–ionomer cements have been used with some success in deciduous posterior teeth. Minimal cavity preparation is required, and the marginal seal and the release of fluoride compensate adequately for the limited life span of such restorations, which is acceptable when used to fill a short term need.

## Luting Cements

The requirements of the glass–ionomer luting cements are quite different from those of the filling material. For example, since the space between the restoration and the tooth tissues is only of the order of 20–50μm, it is important that the luting agent has a very thin film thickness. For this reason, the glass powder has a smaller particle size than that for the filling materials.

The film thickness is important because a luting agent needs to be sufficiently thin to both fill the space between the crown or bridge and the tooth and to ensure proper seating of the restoration. A thick film would be unacceptable, as the restoration may end up higher than originally intended, causing occlusal problems and a need for it to be ground down. Also, a poor marginal fit would result in more cement being exposed at the surface than necessary. As the cements are soluble in the oral environment and prone to erosion, this will cause the loss of material at the margin which can lead to plaque accumulation, staining and secondary caries.

**Table 21** Physical and mechanical properties of two glass–ionomer luting cements.

|  | Aqua-Cem (De Trey) | Ketac-Cem (ESPE) |
| --- | --- | --- |
| Radio-opaque | No | No |
| Solubility in water |  |  |
| 7 minutes | 0.90% | 1.00% |
| 1 hour | 0.46% | 0.40% |
| Solubility in lactic acid solution | – | 0.57% |
| Compressive strength at 24 hours | 82 MPa | 105 MPa |
| Diametral tensile strength at 24 hours | 7.6 MPa | 5.3 MPa |
| Flexural strength at 24 hours | 15.2 MPa | 4.1MPa |
| Creep at 24 hours | 1.37% | 0.63% |

The working time can also affect the film thickness. Longer working times allow more flow and will aid seating of the restoration. Once the material begins to set, the viscosity rises rapidly and flow becomes impossible. Thus, it is extremely important that the mixing and placement of the cement is completed within 2–2.5 minutes, since, after this time, the material becomes stiff and a thicker film will result. It is a matter of preference and familiarity whether a short or slightly longer working time is desired.

It is best to use a purpose-made cement for luting, as changing the powder:liquid ratio of a glass–ionomer filling material in order to modify the working and setting times or film thickness will result in a material with inferior properties.

Not only do the handling properties of different luting cements vary, but so do the physical and mechanical requirements. A comparison of a number of properties of two commercially available cements is presented in *Table 21*.

As far as the mechanical properties are concerned, the results would indicate that Aqua-Cem has a lower stiffness (which would account for the higher diametral and flexural strength), but this is at the expense of the compressive strength and creep resistance. Ketac-Cem is slightly more brittle than Aqua-Cem. In both instances, the materials have little resistance to fracture and need to be well supported by the surrounding structures. Clinically, it has been noted that it is easier to remove Ketac-Cem from the soft tissues than Aqua-Cem. This is probably because the former is more brittle immediately after placement.

## Base/Lining Cements

In recent years, the concept of using glass–ionomer cements as a lining under composite restorations has gained widespread acceptance. The glass–ionomer liner is able to bond to the dentine, and the composite can be bonded to the glass–ionomer cement. The ability to release fluoride gives added protection to the enamel and dentine that is adjacent to the restoration.

A wide selection of glass–ionomer lining cements are now available. These materials are all radio-opaque, which is especially important when used in the posterior situation. They tend to have shorter working and setting times, that are appropriate to their application as a base under composites or amalgams, as the rapid set reduces the waiting time before placing the restorative material. A slow set would be a disadvantage, especially in the case of the composite placement technique which is already quite time consuming.

For those liners which need to be etched to bond to the composite resin, the etching process should be undertaken for no more than 20 seconds. The best method of etching is to employ a viscous etchant gel in a syringe. This can then carefully be applied to the enamel surfaces for a period of 20 seconds; thereafter the whole surface (including the glass–ionomer cement) is exposed to the etchant for an additional 20 seconds.

Excessive exposure of the glass–ionomer cement to etching will cause crazing of the surface and acid penetration that is impossible to remove on washing; this may develop into pulpal pain or sensitivity. The move is now towards glass–ionomer liners which do not require etching in order to achieve a bond to the composite resin.

# Silver Cermets

By its nature, glass is extremely brittle, and tends to fracture relatively easily compared to metals. The idea is that the incorporation of silver in the glass will increase the toughness of the resultant material by acting as a stress absorber and will improve wear characteristics. This has been attributed both to the increase in toughness of the material and to the very low coefficient of friction of the surface, with the silver imparting a polished metallic finish.

In terms of the other properties of the material, such as compressive strength, flexural strength and solubility, the silver cermets seem no better than the glass–ionomer cements.

Naturally, the silver cermets have the ability to bond to enamel and dentine to the same degree as the glass–ionomer cements. As with the glass–ionomer cements, it is recommended that a surface conditioner such as polyacrylic acid is applied to the dentine before placing the cement.

## *Composition And Presentation*

The silver cermets are available either as a powder/liquid composition, presented in two separate bottles which have to be mixed by hand, or are dispensed in a preproportioned capsule which has to be placed in a high speed amalgamator. In some formulations, the powder is presented as a simple mixture of glass and silver, whereas in others the silver is incorporated in the glass powder.

The latter is produced from a mixture of glass and silver of equal volumes (17.5/82.5 wt%). The particle size of the silver is approximately 3–4 μm. The mixture is formed into pellets and then sintered at 800°C until the glass and the silver fuse together and form an intimate mixture. The sintered solid substance is then ground to produce the right particle size for mixing and manipulation. The particles are rounded by the grinding process which aids mixing with the polyacid.

Thus, each particle consists of a mixture of glass and silver particles tightly bonded to each other by the sintering process. In addition, approximately 5% $Ti_2O$ is added to improve the aesthetics by acting as a whitening agent. The liquid consists of an aqueous solution of a copolymer of acrylic and/or maleic acid (37%) and tartaric acid (9%).

The wear resistance of the silver cermets is adequate for small class I cavities, but anything bigger should be treated with caution. Unpublished information would suggest that the cermets do not stand up to the wear in large multiple surface restorations. Thus, its use is very much limited to the treatment of the early carious lesion. Because of the large amount of silver in the powder particles, the final restoration is sufficiently radio-opaque to allow ready detection of recurrent caries.

As with the glass–ionomer cements, the release of fluoride also occurs with the cermets, which should provide protection to the enamel adjacent to the restoration. Silver cermets may be used under posterior composites where the radiopacity is an advantage.

# GIC–Resin Hybrids

Some of the major disadvantages of glass–ionomer cements are:

- Short working time and long setting time.
- Cracking on dessication.
- Poor resistance to acid attack.

Recently, a new group of materials have appeared on the market. They are glass–ionomer cements that can be light cured.

Using this approach, the advantages of glass–ionomer cements, such as the ability to bond to dentine and enamel and to release fluoride, are combined with a prolonged working time and a rapid set, once irradiated with visible light.

Their strength, and their resistance to dessication and acid attack is believed to be much improved. The bond to enamel and dentine is as good, if not superior, to that of the glass–ionomer cements, since the resin component imparts additional tensile strength to the set cement.

## Composition

The material is presented either as a powder / liquid system, with the powder consisting of a radio-opaque fluoroaluminosilicate glass and a photo-active liquid kept in a dark bottle (to protect it from ambient light) or in capsule form. The liquid composition varies from product to product, but in general it is an aqueous solution of hydroxyethyl methacrylate (HEMA), poly-acrylic acid or a copolymer of polyacrylic acid with some pendent methacryloxy groups, tartaric acid and a photo-initiator.

## Setting Reaction

The acid-base setting reaction is essentially the same as for the glass–ionomer cements, and is initiated when the powder and liquid are mixed. The material differs from other glass–ionomer cements is that this reaction is much slower, giving a considerably longer working time.

The rapid set is provided by the light activation mechanism, causing polymerisation of the HEMA, and, for the copolymer containing materials, additional cross-linking through the pendant methacrylate groups as shown in **115**. Once mixed, the material can be made to set hard after just 30 seconds of exposure to light. If not exposed to the light, the material will eventually set in some 15–20 minutes.

One system is also known to contain a redox reaction curing process, using micro-encapsulation technology. This has the advantage that if the light from the curing unit is not able to penetrate to the full depth of the restoration, the redox reaction will ensure full depth of cure of the resin component. It should be appreciated that the light activated curing reaction precedes the formation of the aluminium salt bridges.

## Applications

The visible-light activated glass–ionomer cements have only recently been introduced, and have been designed specifically as direct restorative materials or as bases or liners for use under composites, amalgams and ceramic restorations. When used in conjunction with composites, a strong bond is obtained between the liner and the composite and there is no need to etch the surface of the VLC-GIC hybrid glass–ionomer cement.

**115** Combined light activated cross-linking and hardening during the setting process for a GIC–resin hybrid.

These materials have become very popular, and have the potential to replace many other types of cavity bases and liners. Whether or not they are superior to and will replace the glass–ionomer bases and liners only time will tell.

# Summary

Glass–ionomer cements have had a major impact on restorative dentistry. A wide variety of formulations are now available designed for specific applications. The material has been much improved compared to the original ASPA cements. Glass–ionomer cements have shown themselves to be efficacious dental restorative materials and are still evolving dental materials which suggests that more improvements can be expected.

# Further Reading

Atkinson A. S. and Pearson G. J. (1985) The evolution of glass–ionomer cements. Brit. Dent. J. **159**, 335–337

Croll T. P. & Phillips R. W. (1986) Glass–ionomer-silver cermet restorations for primary teeth. Quint. Int. **17**, 607–615

Fukazawa M. *et al.* (1987) Mechanism of erosion of glass–ionomer cements in an acid buffer solution. J. Dent. Res. **66**, 1770

Knibbs P. J. (1988) Glass–ionomer cement; 10 years of clinical use. J. Oral. Rehab. **15**, 103

Knibbs P. J., Plant C. G. & Shovelton D. S. (1986) The performance of zinc polycarboxylate and glass–ionomer luting cements in general dental practice. Brit. Dent. J. **160**, 13–15

McKinney J. E., Antonucci J. M. & Rupp N. W. (1988) Wear and microhardness of a silver-sintered glass–ionomer cement. J. Dent. Res. **67**, 831

McLean J. W., Wilson A. D. & Prosser H. J. (1984) Development and use of water-hardening glass–ionomer luting cements. J. Prosthet. Dent. **52**, 175–181

Paterson R. C. and Watts A. (1987) Toxicity to the pulp of a glass–ionomer cement. Brit. Dent. J. **162** 110–112

Phillips R. W. & Lund M. S. (1987) *In vivo* disintegration of luting cements. J. Am. Dent. Assoc. **114**, 489

Setchell D.J., Teo C.K. & Khun A.T. (1985) The relative solubilities of four modern glass–ionomer cements. Brit. Dent. J. **158**, 220–220

Smales R. J. (1981) Clinical use of ASPA glass–ionomer cement. Brit. Dent J. **151**, 58

Smith D. C. (1968) A new dental cement. Brit. Dent. J. **125**, 381–384

Walls A. W. G. (1986) Glass polyalkeonate (glass–ionomer ) cements: a review. J. Dent. **14**, 231–246

Wilson A.D. & Kent B.E. (1972) A new translucent cement for dentistry. Brit. Dent. J. **132**, 133–135

# INTERMEDIATE RESTORATIVE MATERIALS

## Introduction

A wide variety of restorative materials (e.g. amalgams, composite resins, glass–-ionomer cements and gold) are placed in dentine in close proximity to the pulp.

The presence of a restoration may have an adverse effect on the pulp (for reasons that will be considered at the end of this section), so a range of materials, termed *intermediate restorative materials* (IRMs) has been developed to be applied to the dentine prior to the placement of the restorative material. These materials include cavity varnishes, bases and liners.

The distinction between cavity bases and liners is that the former consists of a thick mix of material which is placed in bulk in the cavity while the latter is only applied as a thin coating over the exposed dentine. As they are intended to remain in place permanently, these materials should not be confused with temporary restorative materials. Their role may be protective, palliative or therapeutic when they are applied to vital dentine.

We will first discuss the chemistry of these materials and then consider which may be the most appropriate for various clinical applications.

The main groups of materials that fall into the category of cavity bases and liners are:

- Varnishes.
- Calcium hydroxide cements.
- Zinc oxide-based cements.
- Glass–ionomer cements.
- Visible-light cured resins.
- GIC–resin hybrids.

On this list the glass–ionomer cements have already been dealt with in section II.III.

## Cavity Varnishes

### *Presentation And Constituents*

Cavity varnishes consist of a clear or yellowish liquid that contains natural resins such as copal, colophony and sandarac or synthetic resins such as polystyrene. The resins are dissolved in a solvent such as alcohol, ether or acetone, and are applied to the cavity floor with a brush or cotton pledget. The solvent is allowed to evaporate, leaving behind a thin coating of the resin. This process may have to be repeated up to three times to ensure a uniform coating of resin.

## Applications

Their main uses are:

- To present a barrier to the penetration of chemicals.
- To act as a temporary barrier to the loss of constituents from the surface of a filling material.

# Calcium Hydroxide Cements

## Presentation And Constituents

This material is supplied as two white or light yellow pastes. One paste consists of a mixture of calcium hydroxide (50%), zinc oxide (10%) and sulphonamide (40%). The other paste consists of butylene glycol disalicylate (40%) with varying amounts of titanium dioxide and calcium sulphate.

## The Setting Process

Equal volumes of the two pastes are mixed together for about 30 seconds; the cement will then set in approximately two minutes. The setting process for these materials have not been fully elucidated but is believed to involve a chelating reaction between the zinc oxide and butylene glycol disalicylate.

## Properties

These materials have a low compressive strength, typically 20 MPa, but this is sufficient to withstand the condensation pressures of dental amalgam filling materials.

The freshly mixed cement is highly alkaline, with a pH of 11–12. It is believed that this is responsible for an important feature of calcium hydroxide cements: their ability to cause the pulp of the tooth to lay down secondary dentine. When the paste is placed in contact with the pulp, possibly in the presence of a microexposure, it will cause a three-layer necrosis of some 1.5mm thickness. This eventually develops into a calcified layer.

Once the bridge becomes dentine-like in appearance and the pulp has been isolated from any irritant, hard tissue formation ceases.

# Zinc Oxide-Based Cements

The zinc oxide-based cements used in dentistry are powder/liquid systems, with the powders being bases and the liquids being acids. When they are mixed, there is an acid-base reaction with the general formula:

$$MO + H_2A \rightarrow MA + H_2O$$
$$\text{base} \qquad \text{acid} \qquad \text{salt} \qquad \text{water}$$

In these dental cements there is a surplus of powder, such that the final material consists of unreacted powder particles held together by a salt matrix.

There are three major types of cements used in dentistry which use zinc oxide as the powder component. These are:

- Zinc oxide–eugenol.
- Zinc oxide–phosphoric acid.
- Zinc oxide–polyacrylic acid.

# Zinc Oxide–Eugenol Cements

Within the group of zinc oxide–eugenol cements, there are a wide variety of different formulations for different applications.

## Unmodified Zinc Oxide–Eugenol

This comes as a white powder which is mainly zinc oxide, but contains up to 10% magnesium oxide, that is mixed with a clear liquid, which is eugenol mixed with either olive oil or cotton seed oil. The oils are added to mask the taste of the eugenol and modify the viscosity.

### Setting Process

The cement is mixed by adding the powder to the liquid in small increments until a thick consistency is obtained; this should take about one minute, and the powder:liquid ratio is about 3:1.

The zinc oxide initially absorbs some eugenol, which is confined to the surface layer of the powder particles and reacts to form an amorphous zinc eugenolate as shown in **116**. This binds

**116** Chelating reaction of zinc oxide with eugenol to form a zinc eugenolate.

the unreacted portion of the powder together. A trace of water is needed to initiate the reaction, but, once started, it is a by-product of the setting reaction. The set material contains both unreacted zinc oxide and eugenol.

The material is available as a slow setting or a fast setting cement. The slow setting cement takes some 24 hours to set hard, with the fast setting cement taking as little as 5 minutes, although this depends on the nature of the powder, its particle size and the addition of accelerators such as zinc acetate or acetic acid.

### Properties

The set cement has a pH of 6.6–8.0, and has little or no effect on the pulp when placed in deep cavities. The presence of free eugenol has an obtundent effect on the pulp, and reduces pain that may be associated with the antibacterial properties of the cement. However, its use is not recommended when there is a suspected pulpal exposure, since it is mildly irritant to the pulp when in direct contact with it.

One of the main failings of zinc oxide–eugenol cements is their high solubility in the oral environment. Eugenol is constantly released, and, as it dissolves, the cement gradually disintegrates. It also has poor mechanical properties, with a compressive strength of only 15 MPa. This, combined with the high solubility, makes it unsuitable as a cavity base or liner material. The eugenol is also known to inhibit the set of resins, so eugenol containing cements can not be used in conjunction with resin-based restorative materials.

### Applications

The slow setting version is most commonly used as a root canal sealing material, with its various modifications being discussed in more detail in section II.VI. The fast setting version is mainly used in periodontal dressings.

## Modified Zinc Oxide–Eugenol

In order to overcome some of the short-comings of the above cement, modified versions have been introduced. These are aimed at raising the compressive strength and reducing the solubility. These modifications take the form of resins added to the powder and/or the liquid, such as:

- Hydrogenated rosin 10%, which is added to the powder.
- Polystyrene or methyl methacrylate, which is dissolved in the liquid.

### Properties And Applications

The added resin raises the compressive strength to 40 MPa. This is sufficiently high for the material to be used as a cavity base or liner. The material can also be used as a temporary filling material since it is less soluble in the oral cavity than the unmodified cements.

## EBA Cement

EBA cement is another modified zinc oxide eugenol cement, presented as a white powder and a pinkish coloured liquid. The powder consists of zinc oxide (60–75%), fused quartz or alumina (20–35%) and hydrogenated rosin (6%). The liquid is 37% eugenol and 63% ethoxy-benzoic acid (EBA). The EBA encourages the formation of a crystalline structure which imparts greater strength to the set material.

### Properties And Applications

With the above additions and modifications, a considerable improvement in the compressive strength (60MPa) and a reduction in the solubility is achieved. This makes EBA cements suitable as liners and temporary filling materials.

# Zinc Phosphate Cements

These come as a white powder that is mixed with a clear liquid. The powder consists of mainly zinc oxide, with up to 10% magnesium oxide included, and the liquid is an aqueous soluion of phosphoric acid of 45–64% concentration.

## *Powder*

The powder is fired at a temperature in excess of 1000 °C for several hours in order to reduce its reactivity and provide a suitable working and setting time for the cements; the material would set far too rapidly without this firing process.

The magnesium oxide is added as it helps maintain the white colour of the cement. It has the additional advantages of making the pulverisation process of the zinc oxide somewhat easier, and also increases the compressive strength of the cement. Other oxides (such as silica and alumina) have been added in small quantities of up to 5% to improve the mechanical properties of the set material and to provide a variety of shades.

Some formulations include fluorides (usually in the form of a few percent of stannous fluoride), and are generally recommended for situations where fluoride release is going to be particularly beneficial, such as for the cementation of orthodontic bands.

## *Liquid*

The liquid is buffered with a combination of the oxides that are present in the powder and with aluminium hydroxide, which acts to form phosphates in the liquid. The aluminium is essential to the cement-forming reaction, producing an amorphous zinc phosphate, while the zinc helps to moderate the reaction, making sure that the cement has the appropriate working time. This control over the working time also helps to ensure that an adequate amount of the powder is incorporated into the liquid.

## *Setting Reaction*

When zinc oxide is mixed with an aqueous solution of phosphoric acid, the superficial layer of the zinc oxide is dissolved by the acid. In the case of pure zinc oxide mixed with phosphoric acid, the acid–base reaction first involves the formation of an acid–zinc phosphate:

$$ZnO \quad + \quad 2H_3PO_4 \quad \rightarrow \quad Zn(H_2PO_4)_2 \quad + \quad H_2O$$

This is followed by a further reaction, where, in this second phase of the process, a hydrated zinc phosphate is produced:

$$ZnO + Zn(H_2PO_4)_2 + 2H_2O \quad \rightarrow \quad Zn_3(PO_4)_2.4H_2O$$
$$\text{(hopeite)}$$

This substance is virtually insoluble, and crystallises to form a phosphate matrix, which binds together the unreacted parts of the zinc oxide particles. The reaction is slightly exothermic and some shrinkage of the cement takes place.

It is thought that in the commercial materials the presence of the aluminium prevents the crystallisation process, so producing a glassy matrix in the form of an alumino-phosphate gel. This lack of crystallisation is exacerbated by the presence of magnesium which delays the development of any crystallinity. Some crystallisation, resulting in the formation of hopeite, may occur with time.

Unbound water forms globules within the material and makes the cement highly permeable, resulting in a porous structure when the material is dry. The final structure is that of particles of unreacted zinc oxide in a matrix consisting of phosphates of zinc, magnesium and aluminium.

## *Properties*

As a general observation, it is worth noting that zinc phosphate cements have been around for some considerable time and have provided excellent clinical service. This may be related to the general ease with which the material can be used, as well as the wide range of applications available. They have a well defined working time and a rapid setting time.

## Working And Setting Time

The working time for most brands of zinc phosphate cement, when used with the consistency of a luting agent, is usually within the region of 3–6 minutes. The corresponding setting time can vary from 5–14 min utes. Both of these times depend upon the mixing procedure adopted.

Depending upon the application, the material is mixed either to a thick consistency for cavity bases or a thinner consistency when used as a luting agent. The mixing process is carried out by the slow incorporation of the powder into the liquid. The recommended procedure is that initially only small increments are added to the powder, followed by a couple of larger increments. Finally, smaller increments are again added, as this will ensure that the desired consistency is not exceeded.

Extended working and setting times can be achieved by mixing the powder into the liquid in increments over a large area of the mixing slab. This helps to dissipate the heat of reaction that would otherwise speed up the setting process. Conversely, the rapid mixing of powder into the liquid will shorten both the working and setting time. This will have the result that a thick mix is obtained, with a low powder to liquid ratio, because of the early initiation of the setting process. The low powder content will mean that an inferior material is obtained.

By using a cooled glass slab for the mixing procedure, it is possible to extend the working time without simultaneously increasing the setting time. This also has the benefit of allowing more powder to be added to the liquid, so raising the strength and reducing the solubility. However, great care must be exercised when using this technique, as there is a danger of water contamination either from the slab not having been dried properly or due to condensation. Both will have the effect of reducing the working time. The combination of the cool glass and the incremental process ensures that an adequate working time is maintained. The mixing procedure should be completed within about 60–90 seconds.

The setting time can be extended by a process known as *slaking the fluid*, in which a small quantity of the powder is added to the liquid about a minute before the main mixing procedure is started.

The consistency of the paste depends upon the powder to liquid ratio, and it is important that the correct powder to liquid ratio is used for the particular application.

For instance, too low a powder to liquid ratio would produce a weak and highly soluble material with an unacceptably low pH. Whilst the manufacturers suggest optimum powder to liquid ratios for their products, these are difficult to adhere to in practice since the dispensing system is not very accurate. Consequently, most dentists prefer to mix sufficient powder into the liquid until a consistency is obtained which is suitable for the particular application. This makes it all the more important that a consistent and reproducible procedure is adopted.

The liquid is kept in a stoppered bottle. If the top is kept off the bottle, the loss of water by evaporation will lower the pH of the liquid as it becomes more concentrated; this will slow down the setting process. If a lot of water is lost the phosphoric acid will begin to separate out and the liquid will take on a cloudy appearance. Should this occur, the liquid must be discarded.

When the cement is used as a luting agent, it is important that the powder and liquid are not dispensed until just prior to when they are needed, as evaporation of the water may occur which will slow down the setting reaction.

Neither should the material be left for any length of time once mixed, because the setting reaction takes place virtually immediately on mixing. If the paste is left for too long, the viscosity will have increased to such an extent that the material will no longer have adequate flow characteristics.

## Biocompatibility

A freshly mixed zinc phosphate cement will have a pH in the region 1.3–3.6. This low value tends to persist for some considerable time, and it can take up to 24 hours for the cement to return to a near neutral pH.

When placed in a particularly deep cavity, the initial pH is sufficiently low to induce an inflammatory response in the pulp. This is especially so if a pulpal microexposure is present. It should be remembered that the thinner the mix, the lower the pH will be, and the longer it will take for the cement to return to a neutral pH. Thus, the general recommendation is that, for deep cavities, a sublining should be used of a less irritant material that will provide some pulpal protection. The most commonly used sublinings in these situations are the calcium hydroxide cements.

Zinc phosphate cement has no antibacterial properties, and this, combined with the slight shrinkage on setting, means that it does not provide an ideal barrier to the ingress of bacteria. Thus, the pulpal sensitivity associated with the material may be due to a combination of shrinkage, a lack of antibacterial behaviour and the high acidity when freshly mixed, rather than just the high acidity as is generally thought.

The patient may experience some pain during a cementation procedure. This can arise as a result of both the low pH of the cement and the osmotic pressure developed by the movement of fluid through the dentinal tubules. Such an experience is usually only transient, and should subside within a few hours. If there is a persistent pulpal irritation, it may have been caused by using too thin a mix of the cement.

The hardening process for a zinc phosphate cement takes a considerable time, and during the first 24 hours there is a significant release of magnesium with lower amounts of zinc. What biological effects the presence of these various ions might have on the surrounding tissues is not known.

## Mechanical Properties

As with all other properties, the mechanical properties are very much dependent upon the powder to liquid ratio of the final cement. The compressive strength can vary from as low as 40 MPa up to 140 MPa. The relationship between the powder to liquid ratio and the compressive strength is virtually linear.

The cement shows an initially rapid rise in strength, reaching 50% of its final strength within the first 10 minutes. Thereafter, the strength increases more slowly, reaching its final strength after approximately 24 hours. The cement is extremely brittle, and this is reflected by its very low tensile strength, which is of the order of 5–7 MPa. The modulus of elasticity is approximately 12 GPa, which is similar to that of dentine.

## Consistency And Film Thickness

To ensure the proper seating of the restoration when zinc phosphate cement is being used as a luting agent, it is important that the cement is capable of forming a very thin film .

On mixing, the powder is partially dissolved in the acid, such that the final size of the remaining powder in the set structure ranges from 2–8 µm. As the mix flows readily, a film thickness of less than 25 µm can be achieved. This is adequate for cementation purposes, but the thickness of the layer is very much dependent on the procedure adopted.

The viscosity of the mix increases quite rapidly with time. Within a couple of minutes the viscosity can already be quite high, although the material itself is still quite manageable. Nevertheless, it is recommended that no undue delay is allowed to occur when cementing a restoration, as the reduced viscosity can result in a significantly higher film thickness for the cement and thus a poorly seated restoration.

## Solubility

The solubility of a cement is an important consideration, particularly when it is being used as a luting agent. Dissolution contributes to marginal leakage around the restoration and results in bacterial penetration. This may either cause loosening of the restoration, or, what is more likely, the induction of recurrent caries which may undermine the whole tooth.

The cement is highly soluble in water for the first 24 hours after setting, and the loss of material can range from 0.04–3.3%; an acceptable upper limit is 0.2%. After this time, the solubility is much reduced.

The solubility is highly dependent upon the powder to liquid ratio achieved for the cement, with a high ratio being desirable. Once the material has fully set, it remains only slightly soluble in water (with some release of zinc and phosphates), but is still susceptible to acid attack in the presence of lactic acid. As the final set takes some time to achieve, it is important that the cement is not unduly exposed to the oral fluids.

The fluoride containing cements show a continuous release of fluoride over a long period. The fluoride uptake by the surrounding enamel should reduce the likelihood of decalcification, especially when used for the cementation of orthodontic bands.

## Applications

The most common applications for zinc phosphate cements are their uses as cavity bases and as luting agents. Other applications include the cementation of orthodontic bands and use as a temporary restoration.

These cements exhibit several advantages:

- They are easy to mix.
- They have a sharp, well-defined set.
- They have a sufficiently high compressive strength to resist the forces of amalgam condensation.

However, they also have disadvantages:

- They have a potential for pulpal irritation due to low pH.
- They have no antibacterial action.
- They are brittle.
- They have no adhesive qualities.
- They are susceptible to acid attack.

# Zinc Polycarboxylate Cements

These cements come as a white powder and a clear, syrupy liquid. The constituents of the powder are zinc oxide and magnesium oxide, and the liquid is a 30–40% aqueous solution of polyacrylic acid.

## Powder

The powder is based on the same formulation used for the zinc phosphate cements, containing zinc oxide with approximately 10% magnesium oxide, or, sometimes, tin oxide. In addition there may be other additives such as silica, alumina or bismuth salts. The powder is fired at a high

**117** Formation of cross-links between polyacrylic acid polymer chains.

temperature to control the rate of reaction and is then ground to the appropriate particle size. Some brands also contain stannous fluoride to impart the benefits of fluoride release. Pigments may be present to provide a variety of shades.

## Liquid

The liquid is usually a copolymer of polyacrylic acid with other unsaturated carboxylic acids, such as itaconic and maleic acid. (The structures of polyacrylic acid and itaconic acid were presented in section II.III.) The molecular weight of the copolymer is in the range of 30 000–50 000.

In more recent formulations, the acid is freeze dried and then added to the powder, in which case, the liquid component is distilled water. This method was developed in order to simplify the achievement of the correct ratio between the components, which was difficult beforehand because of the high viscosity of the liquid. The pH is adjusted by the addition of sodium hydroxide, and tartaric acid is added to control the setting reaction.

## Setting Reaction

The basic setting reaction of these cements involves a reaction between the zinc oxide and the ionised copolymer of acrylic acid and itaconic acid.

Upon mixing the powder and the liquid, the acid attacks the powder and causes a release of zinc ions. This is followed by the formation of cross-links (in the form of salt bridges), in the same way as occurs for the glass–ionomer cements, except that in this case the zinc provides the cross-links rather than calcium and aluminium, as shown in **117**.

The result of the reaction is a cored structure in which the unreacted powder particles are bound by a matrix of zinc polyacrylate.

## Properties

### Working And Setting Times

When compared to the zinc phosphate cements, the setting reaction proceeds rapidly; mixing should be completed within 30–40 seconds to ensure an adequate working time.

The viscosity of these cements does not rise as rapidly as for the zinc phosphate cements. This has the effect that, after a couple of minutes, the viscosity of the zinc polycarboxylate cement is less than that of the zinc phosphate cement, even though the viscosity of the zinc polycarboxylate cement was initially higher. In addition, the freshly mixed zinc polycarboxylate cement has the property of being pseudoplastic, and shows shear thinning on mixing. This means that although the material may appear to be too thick to flow properly whilst it is being placed, the pressure that is exerted makes it flow quite satisfactorily.

This property is not always appreciated by the dentist, who will be inclined to produce a thinner mix by reducing the powder to liquid ratio under the misapprehension that this will make the cement flow more readily. However, in doing so, the properties of the cement are considerably impaired.

In general, the higher the powder to liquid ratio or the higher the molecular weight of the copolymer, the shorter the working time will be. The recommended powder to liquid ratio for luting purposes is 1.5:1 by weight, which, will give a working time at room temperature of 2.5–3.5 minutes, and a setting time at 37°C of 6–9 minutes.

As with the zinc phosphate cements, the working time can be extended by using a cooled glass slab or by refrigerating the powder. It is not recommended to refrigerate those liquids which still include the polyacrylic acid, as this leads to gelation of the polymer due the hydrogen bonding.

The ability to extend the working time is particularly useful for mixes that have a higher powder to liquid ratio when they are being used as cavity bases. Nevertheless, the short working times of the zinc polycarboxylate cements have been recognised as a potential problem.

This has been overcome with more recent formulations by optimising the amount of tartaric acid in the material. Tartaric acid has the beneficial property of extending the working time without markedly affecting the setting time of the cement.

### Biocompatibility

The presence of zinc polycarboxylate in contact with either the soft or hard tissues has been found to result in only a very mild response. Although it has a low pH initially (in the range of 3.0–4.0), this does not appear to have the same adverse affect as the zinc phosphate cements. It is suggested that this may be due to a combination of a rapid rise to neutrality of the pH on setting and a limited ability of the polyacid to penetrate the dentine.

The zinc polycarboxylate cements have been found to have some antibacterial properties, which means that a better barrier to the ingress of bacteria is provided than by zinc phosphate cements; this resistance to the penetration of bacteria is augmented by its adhesive quality.

It is probably these factors that are responsible for the lack of pulpal response, rather than the higher pH and the high molecular weight of the acid compared to the zinc phosphate cements, although these latter factors *will* contribute to the blandness of the material.

Stannous fluoride is frequently incorporated into the cements, and this does not appear to affect the biological response. The fluoride release appears to be sufficient to have a genuinely beneficial effect on the neighbouring enamel and dentine.

### Mechanical properties

When the cement is prepared to a consistency suitable for luting purposes, the compressive strength of the fully set cement is in the region of 55–85 MPa. This strength depends upon the powder to liquid ratio achieved, and is somewhat lower than that of the zinc phosphate cements.

The tensile strength is higher, however, being in the range of 8–12 MPa. The elastic modulus is around 4–6 GPa, which is about half that of the zinc phosphate cement.

As already mentioned, the zinc polycarboxylate cements set quite quickly, and this is reflected in the time it takes to reach its full strength; the cement will reach 80% of its final strength within one hour. Long-term storage in water does not appear to have an adverse effect on the mechanical properties.

### Solubility

The solubility in water has been measured to be from 0.1–0.6% by weight, with higher values for solubility seeming to occur with the cements containing stannous fluoride.

As with the zinc phosphate cements, these cements are susceptible to acid attack, but as yet this does not appear to be sufficiently serious to be of any clinical significance, as indicated by the good clinical results obtained when using this cement. When failure has occurred this is more often than not due to the improper handling of the material. This is usually related to the use of a powder to liquid ratio that is too low, possibly in an attempt to extend the working time.

### Adhesion

A feature of the zinc polycarboxylate cements that sets them apart from the zinc phosphate and zinc oxide–eugenol cements is their ability to adhere to enamel and dentine.

The bonding mechanism is the same as that of the glass–ionomer cements, and has already been described in section II.III. The quality of the bond is such that it is maintained *in vivo* and can be good enough to exceed the cohesive strength of the cement. That being the case, the bond strength is in fact limited by the poor tensile strength of the cement, and is thus not likely to exceed 7–8 MPa.

Bonding to some metallic surfaces is possible with the zinc polycarboxylate cements, and this can be very beneficial when it is used as a luting agent with cast restorations. This again involves specific ions binding to the metallic surface.

Bonding to pure gold is not good, usually resulting in an adhesive failure of the interface due to the highly inert nature of the gold's surface. This can be improved by sandblasting or abrading the surface, thus providing some mechanical adhesion.

Superior bond strengths are obtained with the base metal alloys (giving rise to cohesive rather than adhesive failures on testing the bond strength), and is probably related to the presence of an oxide layer that provides the necessary metallic ions.

## Applications

By using the appropriate powder to liquid ratio, the zinc polycarboxylate cements can be used as cavity bases, as luting agents, and for the cementation of orthodontic bands.

They have the advantages that:

- They bond to enamel and dentine as well as some of the metallic cast restorations.
- They have a low irritancy.
- Their strength, solubility and film thicknesses are comparable to that of zinc phosphate cement.
- They have an antibacterial action.

They have disadvantages as well, however:

- Their properties are highly dependent upon handling procedures.
- They have short working times.
- An exacting technique is required to ensure bonding.

# Visible-Light Cured Resins

A variety of resin-based cavity bases and liners have appeared on the market, whose role is somewhat obscure. The objective with these materials seems to be to combine the advantages of light activation with some of the therapeutic effects of calcium or fluoride release.

Materials included in this group are Bis–GMA resins containing calcium hydroxide, phosphonated resins containing a fluoride releasing glass, and Bis-GMA resins containing calcium hydroxide and a fluoride releasing glass. How these materials differ from light activated composites (other than in the nature of the filler) is not clear.

Since the fillers are encased in resin, their effect on the surrounding tissues is debatable, although the resins may be sufficiently permeable to allow the release of some fluoride and calcium hydroxide. As yet, these materials have not shown any particular advantage over the many other cavity bases and liners available, and it is unlikely that they will replace them, especially since these have been superseded by the GIC-resin hybrids which were discussed in section II.III.

# Choice Of Intermediate Restorative Material

The choice of cavity varnish, base, or liner requires an appreciation of the need for pulpal protection, and how the agents may interact with the restorative material chosen for a particular clinical situation.

## *Pulpal Protection*

In order to make the correct choice of which intermediate restorative material to use for a particular restorative procedure, it is important to understand the nature and mechanisms by which adverse factors affect the pulp. Three possible sources of pulpal irritation have been identified:

- Thermal stimuli.
- Chemical stimuli.
- Bacteria and endotoxins.

The importance of the first two factors has been well recognised for some time, but more recently it has been shown that the latter factor is probably the most important in producing pulpal irritation.

### Thermal Stimuli

In the intact tooth, temperature changes are conducted through the enamel and dentine to the pulp. Here, nociceptive afferent fibres may be thermally stimulated, eliciting a painful response. When dentinal tubules are exposed, it is possible for fluid to flow into and out of the pulp. This mechanism is almost certainly responsible for the short latency pain produced by thermal stimulation of some minimal-amalgam restorations.

Direct thermal stimulation of pulpal nerves is only likely to occur in deep cavities that have been restored entirely with a metallic restoration, and that contain little or no lining. The placement of a thin lining in a shallow cavity is done in order to protect against fluid movement through the dentine, and not to act as a thermal insulator, as is most commonly thought.

### Chemical Stimuli

Many of the dental materials that come into contact with dentine may release compounds which are thought to be toxic to the pulp, either because of their organic structure or their pH.

Acrylic resins have been cited as examples of materials that will cause a pulpal reaction when placed without a lining. However, toxicity tests suggest that these materials are well tolerated by the soft tissues. (Acrylic resins are extensively used as bone cements in hip replacements without any adverse inflammatory reaction. This would suggest that other factors are responsible for the pulpal reaction associated with these materials.)

Until recently, most studies of pulpal toxicity of restorative materials have not considered the influence of bacterial contamination, which is now believed to play a major role in the production of pulpal inflammation, as considered below. This does *not* mean that we need not worry about chemical toxicity, as the low pH of some materials, such as zinc phosphate cements and zinc polycarboxylate cements, may well have an effect on the pulp.

### Bacteria And Endotoxins

A matter of considerable interest and debate is the effect of *microleakage*. This term loosely describes the penetration of oral fluids and small numbers of bacteria and their toxic byproducts between the filling material and the cavity walls. This percolation has been shown to be a potential source of pulpal irritancy.

In experiments that use germ-free animals, it has been shown that the pulpal response to some materials is considerably different to that which is seen in animals with a normal microbiological flora.

For example, zinc phosphate cements do not show pulpal inflammation (and may even show some dentine bridge formation) when placed on exposed pulps in the absence of bacteria. In contrast, control animals showed severe pulpal inflammation and abscess formation. Other materials do show an inflammatory response, even in the germ-free animals, demonstrating that chemical toxicity may still be an important factor in some instances.

Our increased understanding of the mechanism of pulpal toxicity does not change the fact that some materials will damage the pulp if not separated from the overlying dentine by a suitable lining. However, whereas in the past it was thought that the primary role of a lining material was to protect the pulp from the toxic action of restorative materials, this view has had to be modified to take account of the role of bacterial toxins. The use of cavity bases and liners is now aimed at either eliminating the potential for bacterial microleakage (by the use of adhesive techniques so that no gap exists between the restorative material and the tooth) or to present an antibacterial barrier to the infiltrating bacteria so as to protect the pulp from their toxins.

## Amalgams

The choice of cavity base or liner for an amalgam restoration depends on whether the cavity is a minimal, moderate or deep caries cavity.

### Minimal Depth Cavities

For minimal depth caries, the cavity should be prepared only to a depth sufficient to provide adequate bulk of amalgam. Dentine should not be removed (to create space for a lining material) unnecessarily, as there is sufficient dentine to act as thermal insulator. Neither should a lining material be placed in the cavity in such bulk that the amalgam will be thin in section which will make the amalgam prone to gross fracture.

In this situation, the pulp requires protection only from fluid movement down the dentinal tubules arising from occlusal pressure, from thermal expansion of the metal, and from the ingress of bacteria down the dentinal tubules.

The most common method is to apply a thin layer of calcium hydroxide cement to the floor of the cavity. However, this does not offer complete protection as only part of the exposed dentine is covered. A varnish is then placed over the whole of the dentine surface. The varnish effectively seals the dentinal tubules, preventing fluid movement, and also reducing the potential for microleakage. Although the varnish will eventually dissolve (being only a few microns thick), the gradual deposition of corrosion products from the amalgam helps to seal the margins.

### Moderately Deep Dentine Caries

When the caries extends beyond what can be considered a minimal cavity, there is the possibility of direct thermal stimulus of the pulp; this is especially so in the case of an inflamed pulp as temperature thresholds are reduced.

There is no need to encourage the growth of reparative dentine, as this will have occurred in response to the caries attack. Also, any inflammation will subside if the irritating stimulus (i.e. bacteria and toxins in the caries) is removed. A modified zinc oxide–eugenol cement would be a good choice in such situations, because the eugenol has an obtundant effect on the inflamed pulp and kills off any residual bacteria in the cavity. The thermal insulating properties of these materials are adequate. Finally, a cavity varnish is applied, as not all the exposed dentine is necessarily covered by the lining material.

### Deep Caries

In situations of a near exposure of the pulp, it is generally considered desirable to leave some caries in the floor of the cavity rather than risking an exposure. However, this is not possible if the caries has progressed to the stage where it can not remineralise. (It is possible to distinguish between caries dentine that will remineralise and irreversible dentine caries as the former is more difficult to remove with hand instruments.) Calcium hydroxide cement must first be placed in the deepest parts of such a cavity. This will encourage the formation of reparative dentine and help to remineralise the caries dentine. A thermal insulating base of zinc oxide–eugenol is then placed over the top, followed by a cavity varnish.

## Composites

A fully set composite has little cytotoxicity, and pulpal inflammation under restorations of these materials is due primarily to the leakage of organisms and endotoxins. To overcome the problem of microleakage, a variety of adhesive techniques have been developed, three of which are in current use:

- Acid-etching of enamel.
- Glass–ionomer bonded base.
- Dentine bonding agents.

Of these, the first two are probably the most reliable.

### Incisal Tip Restorations And Fissure Sealants

If the restorative procedure involves enamel only, such as for small incisal tip restorations or fissure sealants, a cavity base or liner is not necessary. The cavity preparation involves only the use of the acid-etch technique, which virtually eliminates any microleakage and is described in more detail in section II.V.

### Preventive Resin Restoration

This is a minimal restoration, where there may be small amount of exposed dentine. As the margins of this restoration are wholly within enamel, the use of the acid-etch technique will ensure that there is a good marginal seal. There would therefore appear to be no need to protect the dentine surface from the effects of microleakage. In addition to this, the composite is an excellent thermal insulator, so there is no need to worry about thermal stimulus of the pulp. However, the use of phosphoric acid-etchant on exposed dentine is not recommended, as the protective smear layer that is formed on cut dentine (blocking many of the dentinal tubules) is removed by the acid solution, re-opening the tubules. The consequence of this is a greatly increased permeability of the dentine. It is therefore wise to protect the dentine surface from the acid. A number of choices are available for achieving this.

Natural resin varnishes and zinc oxide–eugenol cements may *not* be used, since they interfere with the set of the composite resin. In contrast, synthetic varnishes (such as polystyrene) *can* be used. If a bevelled, acid-etched cavity is prepared, the whole cavity and tooth surface may be coated with a thin layer of varnish. The bevel is then cut, leaving only this cut surface to be exposed to the acid.

More commonly, nowadays, a dentine bonding agent may be employed. This acts in a manner similar to the varnishes (in that it protects the dentine from the acid), but a bond to the dentine is also achieved. The combination of enamel bonding with the acid-etch technique and dentine bonding with a dentine bonding agent should eliminate any possibility of microleakage occurring in these minimal restorations.

The different types of dentine bonding agents and their modes of action are dealt with in more detail in section II.IV.

A third possibility is the use of a glass–ionomer cement lining material – the so-called *sandwich technique*. Here, use is made of the ability of glass–ionomer cements to bond to dentine and to composite. It is important that the glass–ionomer cement that is selected is radio-opaque. These techniques are dealt with in more detail in section II.III.

### Proximal And Occlusal Caries Lesions

Due to the size of these restorations and the fact that not all of the margins may be confined to enamel, there is a strong likelihood of microleakage leading to pulpal inflammation.

Whilst the acid-etch technique for enamel bonding of composites is very effective, the same can not be said for dentine bonding procedures. Thus, it would be unwise to rely solely on the adhesive bond of dentine bonding agents to provide a hermetic seal around all of the margins of the restoration. In fact, it has to be assumed that microleakage *will* occur and is unavoidable. Calcium hydroxide is the best lining material to use in such situations. However, it should be used sparingly so that only a small amount of dentine is covered, leaving more available for bonding.

Glass–ionomer lining materials present a problem, as they may produce a mild pulpal inflammation in freshly cut cavities. Although the adhesive bond to dentine limits microleakage, bacteria have been found in voids beneath the material. These bacteria are not affected by the material, as it has little or no antibacterial action. It is therefore prudent to protect any areas close to the pulp with a calcium hydroxide cement prior to the placement of the glass–ionomer liner and the composite restorative material.

### Abrasion/Erosion Lesions

Since this type of lesion involves a large expanse of dentine, the composite resin needs to be bonded to the dentine via a dentine bonding agent or a glass–ionomer cement liner. When a glass–ionomer liner is applied to dentine that has been exposed for some time (as in abrasion lesions), the secondary dentine that is laid down seems to protect the pulp. In this situation, glass–ionomer cement can be applied directly to the dentine and then overlaid with composite resin in the so-called sandwich technique. From clinical studies, this would appear to be a more effective means of bonding composite resin to dentine than the use of a dentine bonding agent. It should be noted, however, that there are rapid improvements in dentine bonding agents, so this situation will have to be reviewed very regularly.

## Glass–Ionomer Cements

The same arguments as outlined above for glass–ionomer lining materials apply to the filling materials.

## Gold Inlays/Onlays

With the exception of gold foil, all gold restorations are cast and cemented in the tooth. Microleakage is minimised by the accurate fit of these restorations, which is enhanced by burnishing the margins after placement. Thermal insulation is only necessary in deep cavities, and the main effects on the pulp are as a result of the cement used and the quality of the marginal seal obtained.

Zinc phosphate cement may be irritant to the pulp, and requires the prior protection of the pulp with a calcium hydroxide cement. Zinc polycarboxylate cement is a possible choice for this, as it is less irritant to the pulp and has the advantage of being adhesive to enamel and dentine, so reducing the likelihood of microleakage. An alternative would be EBA cement, but this material has a long setting time and is difficult to place.

# Further Reading

Fisher F. J. and McCabe J. F. (1978) Calcium hydroxide base materials: an investigation into the relationship between chemical structure and antibacterial properties. Brit. Dent. J. **144**, 341

Øilo G. (1984) Early erosion of dental cements Scand.J.Dent.Res. **92**, 539

Smith D. C. (1971) Dental cements Dent. Clin. N. Am. **15**, 3

Wilson A.D. (1978) The chemistry of dental cements Chem. Soc. Revs **7**, 265

# II.V

## ENAMEL AND DENTINE BONDING

## Introduction

The development of an adhesive approach to restorative dentistry has brought many advantages, such as:

- Better aesthetics.
- Conservation of tooth tissue.
- Improved crown strength.
- A wider range of techniques.
- Reduced potential for pulpal sensitivity.

A wide variety of adhesive systems have been introduced in recent years, many of which have not survived the test of time. Such adhesives were unable to satisfy the stringent requirements that are placed upon a dental adhesive.

A dental adhesive should:

- Provide a high bond strength to enamel and dentine.
- Provide an immediate and durable bond.
- Prevent of the ingress of bacteria.
- Be safe to use.
- Be simple to use.

The bonding systems that have survivedthe test of time include:

- The acid-etch technique for bonding resins to enamel, now extensively used in the placement of anterior and posterior composites, resin-bonded bridges, veneers and orthodontic brackets.
- The glass–ionomer cements, with their abilities to bond to both enamel and dentine as direct adhesive restorations, to act as dentine bonded bases under composite restorative materials and as ceramic inlays and onlays.

By comparison, the dentine bonding agents have had a turbulent history. Many have come and gone, but at each stage of their development there has been an encouraging improvement. Perhaps some of the dentine bonding agents now being marketed will survive the test of time.

Why some materials and techniques should have survived and others waned is due to the complex requirements that the adhesive need to bond a variety of materials (e.g. composites, metals, ceramics) to two very different substrates namely (e.g. enamel and dentine).

In this section, the methods of bonding composites and resins to enamel and dentine will be considered. The adhesive aspects of glass–ionomer cements have already been dealt with in sections II.III and II.IV.

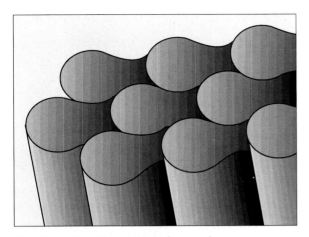

**118** The prismatic structure of enamel.

# Enamel Bonding

## *The Structure Of Enamel*

Enamel is the most densely calcified tissue of the human body, and is unique in the sense that it is formed extracellularly.

It is a heterogeneous structure, with mature human enamel consisting of 96% mineral, 1% organic material and 3% water by weight (89%, 2% and 9% by volume respectively). The mineral phase is made up of millions of tiny crystals of hydroxyapatite $[Ca_{10}(PO_4)_6(OH)_2]$, which are packed tightly together in the form of prisms, held together by an organic matrix. Due to ionic substitution (e.g. fluoride), the enamel apatite does not have the calcium:fluoride ratio of theoretically pure hydroxyapatite (1.6:1) and is usually in the ratio 2:1 by weight.

The prisms are long, rod-like shapes of approximately 5 μm in diameter, having a distinctive keyhole cross-section with a head and a tail. The prisms are aligned perpendicular to the tooth surface as shown in **118**.

The crystals of hydroxyapatite are flattened hexagonals, as shown in **119**, and, because of their structure, it is not possible to obtain a perfect packing. The spaces left between the crystals is occupied by water and organic material. Much of the water is tightly bound within the enamel structure and not easily removed on drying.

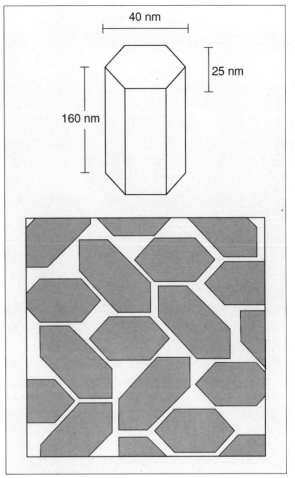

**119** Structure and packing of the enamel apatite crystals.

The surface layer of enamel tends to have a higher organic content than the deeper layers, and is protected by a layer of pellicle which is about 1 μm thick.

## *The Acid-Etch Technique*

Due to its composite structure, the surface of enamel can be modified by the application of acid primers. The importance and potential exploitation of this was first appreciated by Buonocore in 1955, when he found that he could make the surface of enamel more amenable to adhesive techniques by modifying it with the application of a solution of phosphoric acid. Thence, the acid-etch technique for the bonding of composite restorative materials to enamel was developed.

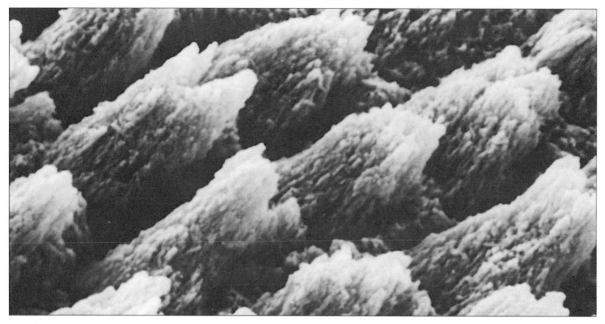

**120** SEM micrograph of the enamel surface after etching for 40 seconds with 35% phosphoric acid solution.

Its main effect is that of increasing the surface roughness of the enamel at the microscopic level (**120**). A major shortcoming of composites is that they have no intrinsic adhesive qualities to tooth tissues, as the resins are essentially non-polar. The acid-etch modification of the enamel surface allows the formation of an intimate micromechanical bond between enamel and the resin component of the composite.

This discovery has allowed the introduction of a wide variety of restorative techniques that were not previously possible, such as fissure sealants, directly bonded orthodontic brackets, resin-bonded bridges and laminate veneers. Many studies have contributed to our understanding of the relationship between etched enamel and resins, such that now the acid-etch technique forms an integral part of restorative procedures using composites.

As mentioned, the application of a strongly acidic solution (such as phosphoric acid) to enamel has the effect of modifying the surface characteristics. It does this in two important ways.

Firstly, the etching process increases the surface roughness of the enamel. When the phosphoric acid is applied to the enamel surface, the hydroxyapatite goes into solution and different

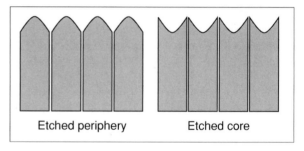

Etched periphery          Etched core

**121** The effect of phosphoric acid on enamel in removing prism periphery or core.

topical features can develop. These include a predominant loss of enamel prism periphery, a predominant loss of prism core constituents, and a pattern in which there is no specific evidence of a prism structure. These are shown schematically in **121**. The overall effect is that of increasing the surface roughness and hence the bonding area. It is possible to bond to this surface by a process of micromechanical interlocking. The increased surface roughness provides the added advantage that the surface area for bonding by chemical means, be it only through secondary bonding, is much enhanced.

Secondly, the acid has the effect of raising the surface energy of the enamel by removing surface contaminants. This provides for a better wettability of the enamel by the adhesive (see section I.X). Typically, the surface tension of an adhesive resin is in the range of 34–38 mJ.m$^{-2}$. Untreated enamel has a surface energy lower than this, and thus the conditions for perfect wetting to take place are not complied with.

Normally, the surface of enamel is covered with a layer of pellicle which has an extremely low surface energy (28 mJ.m$^{-2}$). This layer is removed by the acid and exposes the underlying surface of the enamel with its high surface energy and thus high reactivity (42 mJ.m$^{-2}$). The resin will adapt well to this high surface energy surface, as long as it is thoroughly dry. The micromechanical interlocking will ensure that the resin will not separate from the enamel. Thus, the acid-etch bond to enamel is essentially mechanical in nature.

## Clinical Procedure

The features of increased surface roughness and raised resin wettability using the acid-etching of the enamel surface combine to offer the opportunity for an excellent bond between a composite and the enamel. However, as with any seemingly simple techniques, mistakes are easily made unless the operator adheres strictly to the rules for achieving a bond. The various stages of the acid-etch technique can be identified as follows:

- Patient selection.
- Enamel prophylaxis.
- Application of the etchant.

### Patient Selection

The first rule of achieving a good adhesive bond is that the surfaces to be bonded to must be kept free of contaminants. If the surface becomes contaminated with water or saliva, a good bond between the composite and enamel will not be obtained. The highly polar nature of the surface contaminants will prevent the non-polar resin from closely adapting to the enamel surface.

The best approach to the prevention of contamination of the surface of the enamel is to use rubber dam. This may not always be possible, and in those cases where rubber dam can not be used, it is inadvisable to adopt an adhesive approach.

Appropriate patient selection can avoid these problems. In particular, the use of the enamel acid-etch technique should not be used in mentally handicapped patients, difficult children and very elderly patients. These patients find the use of the acid-etch technique too time-consuming and are unable to sit still for the required time.

### Enamel Prophylaxis

As with any other adhesive joint, it is important that the surface of the substrate is thoroughly cleaned. The surface of enamel is covered with a layer of pellicle and possibly a layer of plaque as well. Such layers need to be removed before the etching process.

Whereas a thin layer of pellicle may be stripped off by the acid, it is not possible to remove any deposits of plaque in this way. If this cleaning is not done, the resin will effectively bond to the surface contaminants and not the enamel. Cleaning of the enamel surface is best performed with a slurry of pumice and water, applied with a bristle brush for some 30 seconds. It is best to avoid proprietary brands of prophy pastes, as these may contain components, such as oils, which are left behind on the enamel surface. These will have the effect of reducing the wettability of the enamel surface by the resin.

Once the surface has been cleaned, it should be thoroughly washed and dried to remove all the debris.

### Application Of The Etchant

Considerable research has been undertaken to evaluate the best method of etching the surface of enamel.

With the teeth dried and properly isolated from the saliva, the aqueous solution of phosphoric acid-etchant can be applied to the enamel with a cotton pledget. An interesting and important observation is that there is an inverse relationship between the etching efficiency and the concentration of the phosphoric acid. High concentrations of phosphoric acid are not as effective at producing the ideal etch pattern as low concentrations. The optimum concentration appears to be in the range of 30–50% percent. Excessively high concentrations of phosphoric acid tend to show minimal change of the enamel surface, possibly because the low concentration of the water causes a rapid saturation of the water with the reaction by-products, slowing down the rate of dissolution. Hence, the use of phosphoric acid solutions supplied with zinc phosphate cements should not be used, as the concentration is too high (approximately 65%).

The resin applied after this etching process will readily invade all the surface irregularities and form resin tags that penetrate the enamel to a depth of up to 30 μm. This produces a very effective bond, by the mechanism of micromechanical interlocking.

It is important that the surface of the enamel is not rubbed during the etching process as the enamel prisms that stick up from the surface are extremely friable and will break under even the slightest load. A rubbing action will have the effect of breaking all of these prisms, and the crevices and cracks for resin tag formation will be lost.

It is important that all of the phosphoric acid and the reaction products produced during the etching process are removed. Too often this is dealt with in a cursory and dismissive manner. The procedure to adopt is first to wash the enamel surface with copious amounts of water, and to follow this with a water-air spray for no less than 20 seconds. If cotton rolls are used to isolate the teeth, these will have to be replaced in order to ensure a dry field.

The drying process is equally critical, as the objective is to achieve a perfectly dry enamel surface. (Since water is highly polar, the non-polar resin will not adapt to a wet surface.) The removal of surface hydroxyl groups in the drying procedure will enhance the wettability of the resin on the surface and allow it to flow readily over the surface and into all the little cracks and crevices generated by the etching process. It is important to ensure that the air-hose that is used for drying is free of any contaminants such as oils and water.

The etched and dried enamel should have the appearance of a dull, white, slightly frosted surface finish.

## Intermediate Resins

Although opinions are divided, it is recommended, on balance, that a low viscosity resin (i.e. either an unfilled Bis-GMA resin or one of the many dentine adhesive resins) is applied to the enamel surface prior to the placement of the composite. The rationale for the use of such an intermediate bonding resin is that the low viscosity of the bonding agent facilitates a better penetration into the microscopic spaces in the etched enamel than would be achieved by the direct placement of the composite.

The wettability of the resin composite is as good as that of the low viscosity resin, but the high viscosity of the composite prevents it from spreading easily over the surface of the enamel.

Also, the viscosity of the composite is sufficiently high that it can actually bridge across the recesses in the enamel and cause entrapment of air. This has the dual effect of creating a zone of inhibition of the cure of the resin, and an interfacial defect which may be the source of subsequent bond breakdown.

## Bond Strength

If the above procedure is carried out with diligence, an extremely effective bond between the enamel and the composite is created. In those situations where failure of the adhesive bond has occurred, it can usually be ascribed to poor clinical technique.

Clinically, bonding to enamel should not present a problem. However, this does not mean that failure of enamel bonded restorations will not occur, since cohesive failure of the adhesive or the restoration can still take place. Equally, metallic or ceramic restorations can fail adhesively due to a lack of bonding between the resin and these restorative materials.

# Dentine Bonding

## The Structure Of Dentine

Dentine is composed of approximately 70% inorganic material, 20% organic material and 10% water by weight (45%, 33%, and 22% respectively by volume).

The inorganic material is mainly hydroxyapatite and the organic material is predominantly collagen. A characteristic feature of dentine is the arrangement of dentinal tubules that traverse its entire thickness. The presence of these tubules makes the dentine permeable to drugs, chemicals and toxins, which can diffuse through the dentine and injure the pulp.

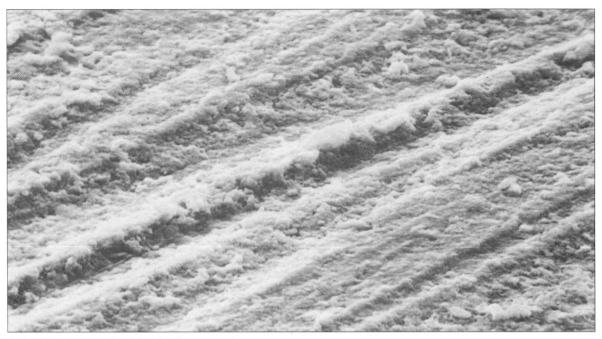

**122** SEM micrograph of the dentine smear layer.

The heterogeneous composition of dentine makes it a particularly difficult substrate to bond to with an adhesive. In the case of an abrasion/erosion lesion, the dentine surface usually consists of sclerotic dentine that is covered with a layer of pellicle, plaque and possibly calculus. It is important that these surface contaminants are removed prior to the use of a dentine bonding procedure. This removal is very readily achieved with the application of pumice and water. A surface is then available that should be free of any contaminants and ready for the bonding procedure. However, the dentine surface is still covered with a layer of disorganised dentine known as the smear layer (**122**).

The smear layer consists essentially of a gelatinous surface layer of coagulated protein, some 0.5–5 µm thick. It is generally highly contaminated with bacteria from the caries process and contains cutting debris. The problems with dentine bonding can thus be summarised as follows:

- Dentine is hydrophilic whereas most adhesives are hydrophobic.
- Dentine is a vital tissue.
- Dentine consists of both inorganic and organic material.
- Dentine is covered by a smear layer.

## Dentine Bonding Mechanisms

With the exception of glass–ionomer cement, which is an adhesive bulk filling material, the primary role of a dentine adhesive is to provide a means of bonding hydrophobic composites to hydrophilic dentine. Thus, they act as an intermediary, and can be considered to be coupling agents in the sense that they are bifunctional and can combine with two distinctly different materials. The situation is analogous to that of bonding resin to glass in the composites, where a silane coupling agent is used (see section I.X). The general formula for the coupling agent in resin-based dentine adhesives is as follows:

Methacrylate group – Spacer group – Reactive group

$$M \quad - \quad O \quad - \quad R$$

The methacrylate group has the ability to bond to the composite and provide a strong covalent bond. The methacrylate group must be able to provide a satisfactory means for polymerisation with the resin of the composite. The spacer group must be able to provide the necessary flexibility to the coupling agent to enhance the potential for bonding of the reactive groups. If the molecule is excessively rigid (due to steric hindrance), the ability of the reactive group to

141

**Table 22** Polarity patterns in some common functional groups.

| Compound type | Functional group structure |
|---|---|
| Alcohol | $-\overset{\displaystyle \mid}{\underset{\displaystyle \mid}{C}}-OH^{\delta-}$ with $\delta+$ on C |
| Amine | $-\overset{\displaystyle \mid}{\underset{\displaystyle \mid}{C}}-NH_2{}^{\delta-}$ with $\delta+$ on C |
| Carboxylic acid | $-\overset{\displaystyle O^{\delta-}}{\underset{\displaystyle OH^{\delta-}}{C^{\delta+}}}$ |
| Aldehyde | $-\overset{\displaystyle O^{\delta-}}{\underset{\displaystyle H}{C^{\delta+}}}$ |

**Table 23** Coupling agents used for dentine bonding.

Hydroxy Ethyl Methacrylate (HEMA)

$$\underset{H}{\overset{H}{C}}=\underset{O}{\overset{CH_3}{C}}-C-O-CH_2-CH_2-OH$$

Dimethacryloxyethyl Phenol Phosphate (MEP-P)

$$\underset{H}{\overset{H}{C}}=\underset{O}{\overset{CH_3}{C}}-C-O-CH_2-CH_2-O-\overset{O}{\underset{OH}{P}}-C-\langle O \rangle$$

NPG-GMA

$$\underset{H}{\overset{H}{C}}=\underset{O}{\overset{CH_3}{C}}-C-O-CH_2-\underset{OH}{CH}-CH_2-\underset{\langle O \rangle}{N}-CH_2-C-OH$$

find a satisfactory conformational arrangement may be jeopardised, leading at best to a strained bond arrangement and at worst to only limited sites for bonding being available.

The reactive groups are polar pendent- or end-groups. A variety of polar bonds are shown in *Table 22*. The bond polarity is a consequence of asymmetric electron distribution in the bond. Polar reactions occur as the result of attractive forces between positive and negative charges on the molecules. Thus, the polar pendent- and end-

groups on the coupling agent can combine with similar polar molecules in the dentine. The attraction may be purely physical, but can in some instances result in the formation of a chemical bond.

Although all of the coupling agents used in dentine adhesives have reactive groups, these vary from dentine bonding agent to dentine bonding agent. All have the objective of producing a strong bond to the dentine. The nature of this reactive group will determine whether the bond will be to the apatite in the dentine or to the collagen. In some cases, both may be involved. A variety of examples of these coupling agents are shown in *Table 23*.

The resin-based dentine bonding agents are believed to rely on a combination of physical attraction, mediated by the polar end-groups and the penetration into the dentine, creating a molecular entanglement network.

## Composition Of Dentine Bonding Agents

Based on the concepts of primers and coupling agents as discussed in I.X, dentine bonding agents can be considered to consist of three essential components, namely:

- A primer.
- A coupling agent.
- An unfilled resin.

In the dental field, the primers are commonly called *dentine conditioners*, and consist of a variety of acids that alter the surface appearance and characteristics of the dentine. The coupling agents have already been mentioned, and are frequently incorporated with the acidic primers, with such mixtures also being described as primers. Similarly, the unfilled resins are often combined with the coupling agent with the mixture being referred to as a *dentine sealer*.

This mixing of components and terminology adds to the general confusion surrounding dentine bonding agents. In *Table 24*, the various components of a number of commonly used dentine bonding agents are identified by their correct terms, although they may be presented to the user in a variety of mixtures, which are attempts by manufacturers to reduce the number of steps involved in the bonding procedure.

**Table 24** Components of a number of commercially available dentine bonding agents.

| Product | Primers | Coupling Agents | Resins |
| --- | --- | --- | --- |
| XR-Bond (Kerr) | None | Phosphonated ester | UDMA |
| Scotchbond Multipurpose (3M Dental) | Maleic acid | HEMA | Bis-GMA |
| Mirage ABC (Chameleon) | Nitric acid | NTG-GMA and PMGDM* | Bis-GMA |
| Gluma 2000 (Bayer) | EDTA and glutaraldehyde | HEMA | Bis-GMA |
| Clearfill New Bond (Kuraray) | Phosphoric acid | Phosphonated ester | Bis-GMA |
| Prisma Universal Bond 3 (LD Caulk) | Glutaraldehyde | HEMA and phosphonated ester | UDMA & TEG-DMA |
| Syntac (Vivadent) | Maleic acid and glutaraldehyde | None | Bis-GMA and TEG-DMA |

*NTG-GMA:N-tolyglycine-glycidyl methacrylate; PMGDM: pyromellitic acid glycidyl dimethacrylate

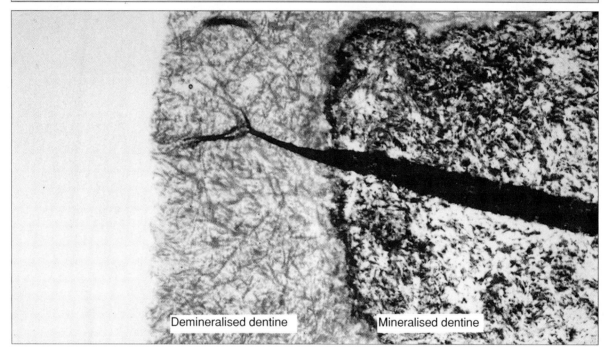

Demineralised dentine    Mineralised dentine

**123** Transmission electron micrograph of dentine after application of a nitric acid primer to the surface.

## Adhesive Mechanisms

One of the major distinguishing features of the dentine bonding agents is the variety of dentine primers that can be used in some situations, whereas in some other situations no primers are used at all. In the case of the latter the coupling agents bond directly to the dentine smear layer.

### Action Of Acidic Primers

Those bonding systems with acidic primers, such as maleic acid, EDTA, phosphoric acid and nitric acid, seek to modify the smear layer to varying degrees. The application of an acid to the dentine smear layer results in an opening of the dentinal tubules and a demineralised surface layer of dentine that is up to 4 µm deep (**123**). The stronger the acid, the more pronounced this effect is. Thus, for EDTA, which is a mild acid, only partial opening of the tubules occurs, whereas for nitric acid, which is a strong acid, extensive opening of the dentinal tubules occurs (**124**).

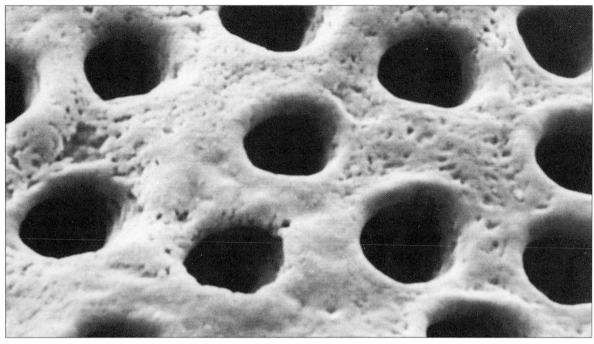

**124** SEM micrograph of the dentine surface after application of a nitric acid primer.

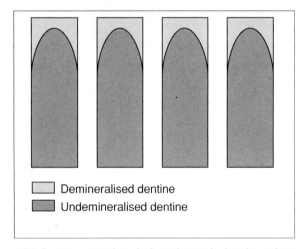

Demineralised dentine
Undemineralised dentine

**125** A cross-sectional view through dentine after application of an acid primer.

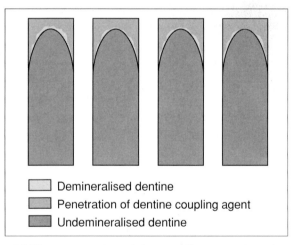

Demineralised dentine
Penetration of dentine coupling agent
Undemineralised dentine

**126** The penetration of the coupling agent into the demineralised dentine.

With EDTA, the demineralised zone is less than 2 µm deep. The effect of this is shown for a cross-sectional view of the dentine in **125** .

The use of glutaraldehyde as a primer is also aimed at modifying the dentine, whether it is the smear layer or the peritubular dentine (if an acid is used in conjunction with the glutaraldehyde). Glutaraldehyde is a cross-linking agent which is said to produce a stronger dentine substrate. The glutaraldehyde forms intermolecular cross-links that provide excellent stability to the collagen. A reservation about the use of glutaraldehyde is that tissue necrosis has been observed in other areas where it has been used.

**Coupling Agents**

The action of the coupling agent is to penetrate into the demineralised dentine layer and create a molecular entanglement network. The depth of penetration is usually aided by the use of a solvent carrier, such as ethanol or acetone, which is extremely effective at seeking out water and displacing it, carrying the coupling agent along as it goes (**126**).

Although the application of an unfilled resin, such as Bis-GMA, directly to an acid-treated dentine surface would result in the formation of resin tags, this has been shown not to result in an adequate bond between the resin and the dentine. The major difference being that the unfilled resin will adapt poorly to the dentine. When a coupling agent is employed, it makes the dentine surface more hydrophobic, thus preventing the resin from shrinking away from the walls within the dentinal tubules, and ensures the formation of a tightly fitting resin-tag structure.

For example, HEMA is able to penetrate the demineralised dentine and bond to the collagen through the hydroxyl groups, forming a molecular entanglement network. The methacrylate ends of the HEMA are available for bonding to the sealer when this is subsequently placed onto the prepared surface of the dentine.

Some penetration of the sealer down the dentinal tubules will occur, providing additional micromechanical bonding.

The dentine surface is thus thoroughly sealed with a resin, which is bonded to the dentine via the HEMA entangled within the cross-linked collagen. This sealer will readily bond to the composite. The resulting interpenetrating layer of dentine and resin is commonly referred to as the *hybrid zone* as shown schematically in **127**.

## Wet Dentine Bonding

The coupling agent component of the dentine bonding agents is carried in a volatile solvent such as ethanol or acetone. Such solvents are very effective at displacing the water in the dentine, and, in the process, pull the adhesive into the dentine with them.

It is not necessary (in fact it would be detrimental) to dehydrate the dentine surface excessively, as this will reduce the penetration of the solvent carrier. Therefore it is only necessary to remove excess surface moisture.

## Total-Etch Systems

The concept of the total-etch systems is a very aggressive preparative procedure that involves etching both the enamel and the dentine simult-

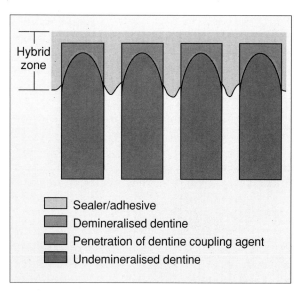

**127** The hybrid zone created with a dentine bonding agent.

aneously. This is only applicable to freshly cut enamel, and unprepared enamel still needs to be etched in the conventional way.

## Read The Instructions

It should be clear from the above description of dentine bonding agents that:

*There is no universal technique for producing a bond to dentine; each system has its own unique procedure.*

It is therefore extremely important that careful note is taken of the instructions for use of individual products, as these will differ widely, depending upon the components used and how these are presented to the user.

## Selection Of A Dentine Bonding Agent

The choice between the many different bonding agents is determined by two factors:

### Pulpal Response

The way in which the pulp may react to the procedure adopted (particularly the application of acid to dentine) is the first consideration. It is apparent that these dentine adhesives rely to varying degrees upon the formation of resin tags in order to achieve a bond to dentine. One potential problem is that opening the dentinal tubules can cause fluids from within the tubules to rise to the surface under the influence of the pulpal pressure. This will prevent good bonding, as it prevents the adhesive from penetrating the dentinal tubules and from adapting to the dentine surface. Whilst this may be overcome by thorough drying of the dentine surface prior to the application of the bonding agent, excessive desiccation of the dentine is likely to result in post-operative pulpal sensitivity.

There is a considerable degree of reticence within the dental profession to the use of these adhesive systems, since the opening of dentinal tubules and the consequent increase in dentine permeability can present a problem.

Concern has also been expressed about the possible pulpal response to the application of acids to the dentine surface. Also, should the adhesive bond fail, there is a ready route for bacterial invasion through the permeable dentine.

In the case of sclerotic dentine, as is found in cervical abrasion lesions on mature patients, the application of acids to the dentine is felt to be acceptable as the dentine is highly mineralised and an open pathway to the pulp is not created. This would not be so in the case of carious dentine, although a number of studies have indicated that dentine bonding agents and their associated acid primers will not have an adverse affect on the pulp.

Thus, pulpal inflammation will only recur if there is a bond failure resulting in bacterial leakage. Whether or not this is likely to happen depends upon the second set of factors, i.e. the strength and durability of the bond to dentine, how easy it is to achieve this bond clinically, and the restorative material used.

### Strength And Durability Of The Dentine Bond

A breakdown of the adhesive bond can have serious consequences as it allows the reintroduction of bacteria and debris into the cavity margins. This will cause unsightly marginal staining and can result in the development of pulpal sensitivity.

Alternatively, the restoration may just simply be lost due to a lack of adhesion, unless some form of retention has been provided.

There are a number of potential causes for breakdown of the bond between the restoration and the dentine:

- Polymerisation shrinkage.
- Differential thermal expansion and contraction.
- Internal stresses from occlusal loading.
- Chemical attack, such as hydrolysis.

The possible consequences of polymerisation shrinkage of the composites has been widely reported already.

As it can take up to 24 hours before the full bond strength for the dentine bonding agents is achieved, the polymerisation shrinkage may cause disruption of the bond before it has had a chance to establish itself. The breakdown of the dentine bond due to polymerisation shrinkage is also dependent on the cavity shape. If the free surface for contraction is very small compared to the surface area of the interface between the tooth and the restoration, then disruption of the composite/dentine bond is favoured over contraction towards the surface. This means that a bond may only be achievable on a flat surface or in very shallow cavities, unless the bond is sufficiently strong to resist the stresses generated by the polymerisation contraction of the resin. Should this be the case, then the cusps of the tooth will need to deform to compensate for the shrinkage effect.

In situations of heavily undermined cusps, as may be the case in large MODs, this could result in fracture at the base of the cusp. Even if this does not occur, the stress generated within the tooth crown may give rise to pulpal sensitivity.

## Clinical Use Of Dentine Bonding Agents

For small restorations with margins wholly in enamel, direct composites with dentine bonding agents are acceptable as long as suitable techniques are adopted to minimise the effects of polymerisation shrinkage. For larger restorations involving extensive areas of exposed dentine, and especially where the cavity extends sub-gingivally, the use of direct composites in conjunction with dentine bonding agents is contraindicated. The problem of polymerisation shrinkage can be overcome, to some degree, by the use of composite inlays. However, the mismatch in the coefficient of expansion still presents a problem, and resin-bonded ceramic restorations may be preferred since these will place less stress on the dentine bond.

It is in the particular area of bond durability that dentine bonding agents still need to prove their clinical efficacy. Unfortunately, the *in vitro* measurement of tensile or shear bond strength has been shown to be a poor indicator of clinical performance. Only few dentine adhesives being promoted have been adequately evaluated clinically and they cannot as yet be recommended for widespread clinical use.

The alternative is to use glass–ionomer cements as a dentine bonded base underneath the composites, which have been shown to be effective in a number of clinical studies, not withstanding their low dentine bond strength.

# Conclusions

There are many different dentine adhesives and each appears to be unique in its properties. The latest generation of dentine bonding agents are very promising, but more clinical data are required before they can be recommended for widespread use. The alternative is to use the glass–ionomer cement as a dentine bonded base underneath composite restorative materials.

# Further Reading

Council for Dental Materials, Instruments and Equipment (1987) Dentine bonding systems: an update. J. Am. Dent. Assoc. **114**, 91–95

Davidson C. L. *et al.* (1984) The competition between the composite-dentin bond strength and the polymerisation contraction stress. J. Dent. Res. **63**, 1396–1399

Duncanson M. G. *et al.* (1984) Resin dentin bonding agents – rationale and results. Quint. Int. **17**, 625–629

Fan P. L. (1984) Resin dentin bonding systems. J. Am. Dent. Assoc. **108**, 240–241

Johnson G. H., Powell L. V. and Gordon G. E. (1991) Dentin Bonding Systems: a review of current products and techniques. J. Am. Dent. Assoc., **122**, 34–41

Paterson R. C. and Watts A. (1990) The dentine smear layer and bonding agents. Restorative Dent. **Aug**, 19–25

Tyas M. J. *et al.* (1989) Clinical evaluation of Scotchbond: three-year results. Aust. Dent. J. **34**, 277–279

Tyas M. J. *et al.* (1988) Bonding - retrospect and prospect. Aust. Dent. J. **33**, 364–374

van Noort R., Northeast S. E. (1986) The potential clinical consequences of dentine bonding resins. Brit. Dent. J. **161**, 437–443

van Noort R. *et al.* (1989) A critique of bond strength measurements. J. Dent. **17**, 61–67

Watts A. and Paterson R. C. (1991) A review of current proprietary bonding systems. Restorative Dent. **Aug**, 56–61

# II.VI

## ENDODONTIC MATERIALS

## Introduction

Endodontics is concerned with the morphology, physiology and pathology of the human dental pulp and periradicular tissues. Endodontic treatment is aimed at saving the tooth when injury to the pulp and associated periradicular tissues has occurred. Treatments involving the use of dental materials include capping of an exposed pulp or sealing of the root canal space when the pulp has had to be removed.

## Pulp Capping

The two main causes of pulpal exposure are:

- Dental caries.
- Accidental exposure during operative procedures.

In each of the above instances the pulp is exposed, and remedial treatment is necessary to save the tooth. The nature of this treatment depends upon which of the above causes of pulpal injury applies.

### Indirect Pulp Capping

Sir John Tomes stated in 1859 that 'It is better that a layer of discoloured dentine be allowed to remain for the protection of the pulp rather than run the risk of sacrificing the tooth.' He had observed that discoloured and demineralised dentine could be left behind in deep cavities of the tooth before restoration, often with highly satisfactory results. This is especially applicable if microexposures of the pulp are suspected. The procedure is now commonly called *indirect pulp capping*. It has been shown that demineralised dentine, if it is free of bacteria, will remineralise once the source of the infection has been eliminated. The removal of this dentine would have undoubtedly have led to the exposure of the pulp, thus impairing its prognosis.

### Direct Pulp Capping

If obvious pulpal exposure *does* occur as a consequence of tooth preparation, as long as steps are taken to avoid bacterial contamination, the procedure of direct pulp capping carries a good prognosis for saving the pulp. A pulp capping material can be used as a wound dressing for the exposed pulp. Such a material can either passively wall off the pulp from the outside environment or can induce some change in the pulp.

There is evidence to suggest that the pulp has the capacity to wall itself off by forming a connective tissue barrier that eventually changes into hard tissue. The induction of hard tissue formation needs to be preceded by a low grade irritation that results in superficial coagulation necrosis. On this basis, a pulp capping material must:

- Have a superficial effect on the pulp tissue, thereby inducing a biological encapsulation process that results in hard tissue formation.
- Cause no adverse effects, whether systemically or locally, such that the pulp is kept alive.

In other words, a pulp capping material needs to be able to interact with the pulp to initiate hard tissue formation, and, once this process has been triggered, should adopt a passive role.

If the pulp is exposed due to the presence of caries, the procedure for pulp capping is contra-indicated; the infiltration of bacteria that will have occurred into the pulp cannot be reversed, and the only solution is a full pulpectomy.

## Pulp Capping Materials

The only materials that appear to satisfy the requirements for pulp capping are calcium hydroxide cements. These are available in both setting and non-setting versions.

The non-setting versions are slurries of calcium hydroxide and water or methyl cellulose, with the versions containing methyl cellulose being somewhat easier to handle. The setting pastes are either two-paste systems (as described in section II.IV), or are single paste systems consisting of calcium hydroxide-filled dimethacrylates, and polymerised by light.

The problem with the non-setting versions is that they will gradually dissolve and disappear from underneath the restoration, which can undermine the restoration's function. The setting versions are therefore generally preferred. The difficulty for the manufacturer is to achieve a balance between a material that is sufficiently soluble to be therapeutic and not so soluble as to dissolve away. This would suggest that the VLC cements are contraindicated for pulp capping.

When the paste is brought in contact with the pulp it causes a layer of necrosis of some 1.0–1.5 mm thick, that eventually develops into a calcified layer. Experiments using radioactive calcium in the paste have shown that the calcium salts necessary for mineralisation of the bridge are not derived from the cement, but are instead supplied by the tissue fluids of the pulp. Once the bridge has become dentine-like in appearance, and the pulp has been shut off from the source of the irritation, the hard tissue formation ceases. It is believed that the high pH of the calcium hydroxide cement is responsible for this type of pulpal response, and that this is also closely associated with its antibacterial properties.

Failure after capping with calcium hydroxide can be due to two reasons:

- *Chronically inflamed pulp* – There is no healing effect on inflamed pulp, and, in such situations, a full pulpectomy is indicated.
- *Extra-pulpal blood clot* – Such a blood clot prevents contact between the pulpal tissue and the cement and interferes with the wound healing process.

## Root Canal Filling Materials

The objectives of modern root canal therapy are:

- *To provide a clean canal* — The aim is to produce a reduction of bacteria to a non pathogenic level.
- *To provide an 'apical seal'* — This prevents the ingress of fluids which will provide nutrients for canal bacteria and also prevents irritants leaving the canal and entering the periapical tissues.

A wide variety of materials have been used in an attempt to produce a hermetic seal of the tooth root apex. The most widely used root canal sealing materials are a combination of root canal sealer cements and obturating points.

### *Obturating Points*

#### Gutta Percha

Gutta percha is a rubber that is tapped from the Taban tree. It was introduced into the UK in 1843 and has been used in endodontics for over a hundred years. Rubbers are polymers of

**Natural rubber (cis)**

**Gutta percha (trans)**

**128** The structure of isoprene rubbers. These are stereoisomers, which are compounds with the same order of connection between the atoms but with differing three-dimensional arrangements.

**Table 25** Composition of gutta percha points.

| Constituent | Amount (%) | Purpose |
|---|---|---|
| Gutta percha | 19–22 | Rubber |
| Zinc oxide | 59–75 | Filler |
| Heavy metal salts | 1–17 | Radio-opacifier |
| Wax or resin | 1–4 | Plasticiser |

**Table 26** Composition of a zinc oxide–eugenol cement based on Rickert's formulation.

| Powder | % | Liquid | % |
|---|---|---|---|
| Zinc oxide | 34–41 | Oil of cloves | 78–80 |
| Silver | 25–30 | Canada balsam | 20–22 |
| Oleoresin | 16–30 | | |
| Dithymoliodide | 11–13 | | |

isoprene (2-methyl-1,3-butadiene) and can take up two conformations as depicted in **128**. The *cis* arrangement is known as *natural rubber* and the *trans* arrangement as *gutta percha*.

These rubbers are soft and tacky unless they are hardened by *vulcanisation*, a process discovered by Charles Goodyear in 1839 (see section I.I). Vulcanisation involves heating the polymer with a few percent by weight of sulphur. The hardening occurs because *sulphur bridges* or *cross-links* form between the polymer chains, preventing the polymer molecules from slipping over one another.

Natural rubber is non-crystalline because of its *cis* double-bond geometry, whereas gutta percha is partially crystalline because its geometry allows the polymer chains to pack more closely together. Consequently, gutta percha is harder and more brittle than natural rubber.

The composition of commercially available gutta percha obturating points will vary from product to product, but typical values are shown in *Table 25*. The additional ingredients (listed in *Table 25*) are added to overcome the inherent brittleness of the rubber and to make it radio-opaque.

Gutta percha softens at 60–65°C and will melt at about 100°C, so it can not be heat-sterilised. If necessary, disinfection can be carried out in a solution of hypochlorite (5%). The use of solvents such as acetone or alcohol should be avoided, as these are absorbed by the gutta percha, causing it to swell. Eventually, the gutta percha will return to its unswollen state, thus compromising the apical seal. On exposure to light, gutta percha oxidises and becomes brittle. It is therefore important to check that the points have retained their flexibility before using them.

**Metal Points**

Metals, including gold, tin, lead, copper amalgam and silver, have long been used as root canal filling materials. It is suggested that silver is preferred because of its bactericidal effect.

Silver is a more rigid and unyielding material than gutta percha and is often used when access

**Table 27** Composition of Grossman's Sealer (Grossman).

| Powder | % | Liquid | % |
|---|---|---|---|
| Zinc oxide | 42 | Eugenol | 100 |
| Staybelite resin | 27 | | |
| Bismuth subcarbonate | 15 | | |
| Barium sulphate | 15 | | |
| Sodium borate | 1 | | |

**Table 28** Composition of Tubliseal (Kerr Mf.Co., USA).

| Base | % | Catalyst |
|---|---|---|
| Zinc oxide | 57–59 | Eugenol |
| Oleo resin | 18–21 | Polymerised resin |
| Bismuth trioxide | 7.5 | Annidalin |
| Thymol iodide | 3–5 | |
| Oils and waxes | 10 | |

and instrumentation is difficult due to a small cross-section or awkward anatomy. The rigidity of silver makes it impossible to adapt it closely to the canal wall and greater reliance is placed on the cements used to provide the seal. The other disadvantage with silver points is that they tend to corrode. This can give rise to apical discoloration of the soft tissues.

Corrosion can be limited by sealing the entire point within the root canal such that it is surrounded by the sealer cement.

Acrylic and titanium points are being used as alternatives to silver points in order to avoid the problems of corrosion.

# Root Canal Sealer Cements

It is well accepted that the sealing properties of conventionally applied and laterally condensed gutta percha or silver points are such that it is essential that they are used in conjunction with a root canal sealer cement.

The function of the cement is to fill the spaces between the obturating point and the wall of the root canal, producing an antibacterial seal.

Conversely, the use of root canal cements without obturating points is also contraindicated. When used in bulk, the cements are either too soluble or shrink excessively on setting. Additionally, it is difficult to gauge when, or if, the canal is adequately filled, and there is a danger that the cement may pass beyond the root apex into the surrounding tissues.

It is now well accepted that the current generation of root canal sealer cements are unable to provide a hermetic seal.

The root canal sealer cements fall into three groups:

- Zinc oxide–eugenol cements.
- Resin-based materials.
- Calcium hydroxide-based cements.

First, the composition of examples of the most widely used sealers will be described. Then, the characteristics which makes them suitable as sealers will be discussed, and finally the clinical data on their performance will be assessed.

## *Zinc Oxide–Eugenol-Based Cements*

There are many cements based on zinc oxide, used with eugenol, to which are added a variety of other substances to modify them for use as root canal sealers (see section II.IV). There are three major reasons for the additives in root canal sealers: to impart bacteriocidal properties, to increase their radio-opacity, and to improve the adhesion to the canal wall.

As with all zinc oxide–eugenol cements, the sealers consist of a powder which is mixed with a liquid. The complete list of ingredients of one widely used material (based on a formulation originally proposed by Rickert in 1931) is presented in *Table 26*. The powder is predominantly zinc oxide, to which silver is added to increase the radio-opacity. The resin acts as a plasticiser and the iodide as an antiseptic agent.

The problem with this formulation is that the silver is prone to causing discoloration of the dentine. This is problematical particularly in the coronal access cavity, and affects the appearance of the tooth.

Newer formulations such as Grossman's Sealer (*Table 27*) have replaced the silver with barium or bismuth compounds.

The particle size of the above preparations is fairly large and tends to produce a gritty texture to the resultant mix unless it is thoroughly spatulated. To overcome this, a new paste–paste system has been developed, and its constituents are presented in *Table 28*.

**Table 29** Composition of Sealapex (Kerr Mf. Co., USA).

| Base Paste | % | Catalyst Paste | % |
|---|---|---|---|
| Calcium hydroxide | 46 | Barium sulphate | 39 |
| Sulphonamide | 38 | Resin | 33 |
| Zinc oxide | 12 | Isobutyl salicylate | 17 |
| Zinc stearate | 2 | Colloidal silica | 6 |
| Colloidal silica | 2 | Titanium dioxide | 4 |
| | | Iron oxide | <1 |

## Resin-Based Cements

The attraction of resin systems is that these materials can readily be formulated in such a way that they have a rapid setting time and yet maintain a sufficiently long working time. Also, these products do not contain any coarse powders so they have a very smooth texture.

There are currently only two resin systems that have been around sufficiently long for some clinical data to have been gathered on them. These are an epoxy resin, AH26 (De Trey), and a polyvinyl resin, DIAKET (ESPE GMBH, West Germany). Both have very complex formulations, which will not be considered here. The main problem with these cements is the amount of shrinkage that takes place on setting, which compromises the apical seal.

## Calcium Hydroxide-Based Cements

Calcium hydroxide-based cements are relative newcomers. They are two-paste, polymeric calcium hydroxide root canal sealers, and consist of a resin similar to those used in the two paste resin composites, to which is added calcium hydroxide as a filler in place of the more usual glass fillers.

The composition of one of these materials is presented in *Table 29*. As yet, little is known about the clinical performance of this material

# Clinical Aspects Of Root Canal Materials

Root canal materials are in contact with living biological tissue that is not protected by any epithelial layer; therefore, their biocompatibility is of considerable importance. Their physical properties, relevant to the production of an apical seal, are also a major concern.

## Biocompatibility

In general, it is assumed that for a material to be biologically acceptable it must be as inert as possible. However, this is not always the case. In a sense, what is really desired is an interaction between the material and the biological environment that is beneficial to the biological environment and has no adverse effect on the material. This is very different from complete lack of interaction in the case of an inert material. The concern is over the form of the interaction.

When a sealer is placed at the apex of a root canal it will be in contact with vital tissue. It is important that the material does not elicit an inflammatory response in the tissues as this may induce irritation, pain or tissue necrosis. All of these responses are likely to lead to the loss of the tooth, which is just the opposite of the intended outcome.

A possibly beneficial response would be the formation of an intermediate layer of hard tissue that not only isolates the foreign material from the living tissue, but also helps to improve the quality of the apical seal.

A perennial problem in endodontic treatment is the likelihood of recurrent infection due to the presence of bacteria at the apex of the tooth. Thus, another feature one seeks in a root canal sealer is the ability to destroy bacteria.

As might be imagined, it is difficult to reconcile these two requirements as they would require a high degree of selectivity in the biological response. In general, materials that show antibacterial properties also induce some inflammatory response in the local tissues, while those that do not elicit an inflammatory response are at best bacteriostatic.

Given that a perfect seal *cannot* be achieved, the materials used must have sufficient antibacterial activity to prevent bacteria from infiltrating the canal space and proliferating. However, the antibacterial property of a material should not be achieved at the expense of its biocompatibility.

Gutta percha is a highly biocompatible material, having such a low cytotoxicity that it is the cements that are used with it that will determine the tissue response. This also applies to the silver points, as they too are non-irritant to the soft tissues. However, silver does corrode, and the corrosion products may be cytotoxic.

The zinc oxide–eugenol-based cements are all inclined to induce some inflammatory reaction in the tissues, probably due to the presence of free eugenol. It is therefore important that measures are taken to ensure that the cement does not leak beyond the apex and into the vital tissues. Some formulations must be avoided because they contain paraformaldehyde which may cause a severe inflammatory response, leading to tissue necrosis and bone resorption. Some cements have an incorporated steroid, and, again, their use is contraindicated.

The resin systems should have comparatively excellent biocompatibility, as none of them contain the eugenol that contributes to the poor biocompatibility of the zinc oxide cements. It has been reported, however, that AH26 is slightly toxic during the setting period but that once it has fully set any inflammation rapidly recedes. This moderate cytotoxic response of freshly prepared AH26 may be associated with the release of formaldehyde, which is produced as a by-product of the setting process. Since AH26 takes some time to set, a certain degree of sensitivity may be associated with the use of this sealer. In comparison, Diaket retains a degree of cytotoxicity even after it has set.

For the calcium hydroxide-containing resins (e.g. Sealapex) it is claimed that in addition to the excellent biocompatibility, the material promotes hard tissue formation, which is similar to that observed for the pulp capping agents based on calcium hydroxide.

## Sealing Properties

One of the difficulties in interpreting the information available on sealing properties is the lack of any standardised approach to the methods of measurement adopted, as this limits the value of the data available. This is particularly so for studies of the sealing properties, whether *in vivo* or *in vitro*, where so many methods have been used that direct comparison is unreliable, and only a general assessment is possible.

First, it is noticeable that there is no immediate distinction between the zinc oxide–eugenol cements and the resin-based materials. It would seem that some zinc oxide–eugenol cements are better than one or other resin system and that others are worse.

However, it should be appreciated that so much depends on the technique adopted that an acceptable result can most probably be obtained with any of them. As already noted, it is probably more important that an antibacterial seal is achieved than a physical seal, although both would be desirable. A physical seal by itself may not be good enough if the sealant does not provide an antibacterial barrier.

## Physical Properties

Since the results of endodontic treatment are so dependent upon the operator, it is important to choose a material which has the handling characteristics that most suit the particular individual. The working and setting times and flows of the cements determine their handling characteristics, while the film thickness, the solubility and the dimensional stability are important factors in determining their sealing ability.

Rickert's cement has a working time of some 15 minutes; it flows readily, but is inclined to have a thick film width due to the gritty nature of the powder. Grossman's sealer has a working time of one hour and also shows good flow; its solubility is lower than that of Rickert's cement. Tubli-seal is a two paste cement; it has a short working time (20 minutes), combined with good flow and a low film thickness.

The resin sealer Diaket has a very rapid set, and is sticky and viscous and difficult to manipulate. In comparison, AH26 has a much longer working time, a better flow and lower film thickness. Once set, both of these materials are virtually insoluble.

The calcium hydroxide filled resins are generally preferred from the point of view of their handling characteristics, but still require some clinical evaluation before they can be recommended for general use.

# Summary

The ideal of a hermetic seal of the root apex has been abandoned in favour of an antibacterial seal. Such an antibacterial seal can be achieved by the combined use of obturating points and root canal sealer cements. Amongst the obturating points, gutta percha is preferred over the silver points. There are many cements to choose from and the paste–paste system is the most popular.

It is perfectly possible to obtain an adequate antibacterial seal with currently available materials. Failure is more usually associated with problems of inadequate instrumentation, sterilisation or obturation, especially in inaccessible canals in multirooted teeth, and in unsealed lateral canals.

# Further Reading

Browne R. M. (1988) The *in vitro* assessment of the cytotoxicity of dental materials – does it have a role? Int. Endod. J. **21**, 50–58

Foreman P. C. & Barnes I. E. (1990) A review of calcium hydroxide. Int. Endod. J. **23**, 283–297

Ida K. *et al.* (1989) The pH values of pulp-capping agents. J. Endod. **15**, 365–368

Orstavik D. (1988) Antibacterial properties of endodontic materials. Int. Endod. J. **21**, 161–169

Pitt-Ford T. R. & Rowe A. H. R. (1989) A new root canal sealer based on calcium hydroxide. J Endod. **15**, 286–289

Tobia R. S. (1988) Antibacterial properties of dental restorative materials – a review. Int. Endod. J **21**, 155–160

Spangberg L. S. W. (1982) 'Endodontic filling materials' in *Biocompatibility of Dental Materials* vol. III, Smith D. C., Williams D. F. (Eds), Chapter 8, CRC Press, Boca Raton, USA

Zmener O. (1987) Evaluation of the apical seal obtained with two calcium hydroxide based endodontic sealers. Int. Endod. J. **20**, 87

# II.VII

# IMPRESSION MATERIALS

## Introduction

Impression materials are used to produce a detailed replica of the teeth and the tissues of the oral cavity. From this replica, or impression, a model can be made which is used in the construction of full dentures, partial dentures, crowns, bridges and inlays.

Over the years, a wide variety of impression materials and associated techniques have been developed, all striving to achieve the optimum in desirable characteristics. The impression materials can be classified in terms of rigid and elastic impression materials (*Table 30*).

The rigid impression materials can not engage undercuts that may be present on the teeth or the bone. Consequently, their use is restricted to edentulous patients without bony undercuts.

The elastic impression materials are subdivided into *hydrocolloid* and *elastomeric* impression materials. Both are able to engage undercuts and may be used in edentulous, partially dentate and fully dentate patients. The choice will depend upon the particular requirements of each individual case.

The choice of impression material may also be affected by the technique to be adopted, with a major consideration being the selection of a stock tray or special tray. These trays are needed to support the impression material (especially

when it is still fluid), so that it can be carried to the patient, inserted in the mouth, and removed once it is set. The trays also provide support when the model is poured from the impression.

The variety of applications and techniques used with the impression materials are presented in *Table 31*. The choice of impression tray is to some extent determined by the viscosity of the impression material.

An impression material that is very fluid when it is first mixed cannot be used with a stock tray, and a close fitting special tray needs to be produced. This can be done either by constructing an acrylic special tray from a preliminary model, or by using a high viscosity material which is placed in a stock tray, and, once this has set, a special tray is produced. Some impression

**Table 30** Categorisation of impression materials.

| Rigid | | |
|---|---|---|
| Plaster | | |
| Compo/zinc oxide–eugenol | | |
| **Elastic** | | |
| *Hydrocolloid* | Agar (reversible) | |
| | Alginate (irreversible) | |
| *Elastomeric* | Polysulphide | |
| | Polyether | |
| | Silicone (condensation-cured) | |
| | Silicone (addition-cured) | |

155

**Table 31** Indirect impression techniques.

| Application | Choice of Material | Impression Technique | Choice of Viscosity | Type of Tray |
|---|---|---|---|---|
| Full dentures | Plaster of Paris | Single stage | – | Stock/special tray |
| | Zinc oxide–eugenol | Single stage | – | Special |
| | Compo/zinc oxide–eugenol | Two stage | – | Stock |
| | Alginate | Single stage | – | Stock/special tray |
| Partial dentures | Alginate | Single | – | Stock/special tray |
| | Elastomers | Single | Medium | Special tray |
| Crowns, bridges | Compo | Copper ring | – | – |
| and inlays | Elastomer | Single | Medium | Special tray |
| | | Twin mix | Heavy/light | Special tray |
| | | | Putty/wash | Stock tray |
| | | Two stage | Heavy/light | Special tray |
| | | | Putty/wash | Stock tray |

materials are not available with a sufficiently high viscosity version for use in a stock tray, and these include zinc oxide–eugenol, polyether and polysulphide elastomers. Others, such as impression compound (compo) compo, plaster of Paris, alginate and the silicones are available in formulations that *can* be used with a stock tray.

The choice of impression material and the type of tray to use will depend upon the accuracy and the reproduction of the surface detail that is required.

For example, compo can be used in a stock tray, but the impression obtained does not give a very good reproduction of surface detail unless a zinc oxide–eugenol wash is used with it. Similarly, alginates, when used in a stock tray, do not always give the required degree of accuracy and are then better used in a special tray.

# Requirements Of An Impression Material

Some of the requirements of an impression material have already been touched upon in the above discussion and now need to be defined more explicitly. The important characteristics of impression materials can be identified from the point of view of the patient or the dentist (*Table 32*).

## Accurate Reproduction Of Surface Detail

The accuracy of the reproduction of the surface detail depends upon the viscosity of the mix and the ability of the impression material to adapt closely to both the soft and hard tissues. A low viscosity is therefore desirable, but it should not be so low that the material is not easily contained within the impression tray.

Some materials are hydrophobic (water repellent) and will be repelled by moisture on the surface. If this should happen in a critical area then important surface detail may be lost as a blow hole is formed on the impression surface. A dry field is essential for such materials. If this is not feasible, an alternative material must be used which is compatible with moisture and saliva.

There are instances in which the patient will have mobile soft tissues. (This occurs particularly with edentulous patients, who can present with a flabby ridge.) If the impression material is very stiff, it may displace such tissues and produce a distorted impression. When this is reproduced in the prosthesis, the soft tissues will need to adapt to the prosthesis rather than the other way round; this will cause discomfort to the patient. Such impression materials are classed as being muco-compressive.

Ideally, the impression material to be used should be sufficiently fluid upon placement to prevent displacement of the soft tissues, with

| Table 32 The requirements of an impression material. | |
| --- | --- |
| **The patient** | **The dentist** |
| Neutral taste and odour | Easily mixed |
| Short setting time | Short working time |
| Small tray | Easily removed |
| Easily removed | Good quality impression |
| Non-toxic | Low cost materials |
| | Easily disinfected |

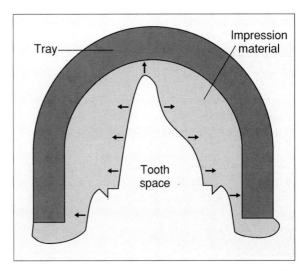

**129** Shrinkage of the impression material towards the tray resulting in the production of a model which is slightly larger than the original preparation.

such materials being considered to be mucostatic.

## *Dimensional Accuracy And Stability*

These are dependent upon :

### The Type Of Tray

If the tray is prone to distortion, then the resultant model poured from such a tray will also be distorted. Hence, highly flexible trays should be avoided. A good bond between the tray and the impression material is very important. If the impression material comes away from the tray, this will again distort the impression. Manufacturers of impression materials will supply a suitable adhesive for their material to ensure a good bond. It is important that the manufacturer's instructions are followed to the letter, otherwise failure of the adhesive bond may result. Additional retention may be achieved by the use of perforated trays.

### Shrinkage Of The Impression Material

Whether the impression material sets by a chemical reaction or some change in physical state, both usually result in some shrinkage of the impression material. Provided the impression material is firmly adhered to the tray, this increases the space previously occupied by the hard or soft tissues. In the case of a simple crown preparation, the result is a die which is slightly larger than the original tooth preparation (**129**). If the contraction of the impression material is excessive, this will result in a loosely fitting crown. Should the impression material expand on setting, then the opposite problem of a tightly fitting crown would result, with too little space for the cement that is needed to hold it in place.

In addition to the changes in dimensions on setting, there is also a slight thermal contraction of the impression material as it cools from mouth to room temperature. The coefficient of thermal expansion of both the tray and the impression material need to be small. Ideally, an impression material should show a very small contraction (<0.5%) as this will result in the production of a crown that is slightly larger than situation that it is designed for – this will provide the necessary space for the cement that is to be used.

### Permanent Set

When an impression is taken of a dentate patient, there will be undercuts due to the bulbous shapes of the tooth crowns. In this case, the impression material must be sufficiently flexible to allow removal from the undercut regions without causing distortion; rigid impression materials wouldtherefore be unsuitable. The elastic impression materials must be used, but, as most are actually viscoelastic materials (see section I.VII), there is a possibility of some permanent deformation.

### Storage Stability

There is usually a significant delay between the taking of an impression and its arrival in the dental laboratory where the model is poured. It is important that the impression material neither shrinks, expands nor distorts during this time period.

## Impression Technique

In the case of silicone impression materials particularly, there are a number of impression techniques that can be employed. It is important that the appropriate technique is used for each material. This will be dealt with later, in the discussion of the silicone impression materials.

Given that impression materials have to comply with a very wide range of requirements, it is perhaps not surprising that there are so many on the market. The rigid impression materials will be considered first, followed by the elastic impression materials.

# Rigid Impression Materials

## *Impression Compound (Compo)*

Impression compound is a thermoplastic material with a glass transition temperature of about 55–60°C. Above its glass transition temperature it becomes soft and will take up a new form. On cooling to mouth temperature, it hardens and can be removed, retaining an impression of the oral cavity. Thus, no chemical reaction is involved in the use of this material.

### Composition

The composition of impression compounds tends to vary from product to product and is usually a trade secret. They consist of a combination of resins and waxes, plasticisers and fillers, each having a specific function:

- *Resins and/or waxes* – Resins are amorphous organic substances which are insoluble in water. Typical, naturally occurring resins used in impression compound are shellac, dammar, rosin or sandarac. Some recent products use synthetic resins (e.g. coumerine-indene) to give greater control and consistency of the composition. Waxes are straight chain hydrocarbons of the general formula $CH_3(CH_2)_n CH_3$, where n is between 15 and 42. They are characteristically tasteless, odourless, colourless and greasy to the touch. Waxes used in impression compound include beeswax and colophany.

- *Plasticisers* – The waxes and resin, if used on their own, would tend to produce a brittle material with a tendency towards tackiness. The brittleness is overcome by the addition of plasticisers, such as gutta percha and now more commonly stearic acid.
- *Fillers* – To overcome the tackiness, to control the degree of flow and to minimise shrinkage due to thermal contraction, a filler is added. Commonly used fillers are calcium carbonate and limestone. The fillers also improve the rigidity of this impression material.

### Properties

*Impression compound* is muco-compressive, and is the most viscous of the impression materials used. This can present particular problems in those patients who have a flabby mandibular ridge.

Compo is rigid once cooled and therefore cannot be used to record undercuts. It has a high viscosity, so reproduction of surface detail is not very good.

However, the reproduction can be improved by reheating the surface of the impression material after taking the first impression and then reseating it in the patient's mouth. Even then, the surface detail is not as good as can be achieved with virtually all of the other impression materials. It is therefore better to use compo as a simple and quick means of producing a special tray, and then use a wash of zinc oxide–eugenol to provide the surface detail.

The coefficient of thermal expansion of resins and waxes is very high, as indicated in *Table 33*, and are highly non-linear within the temperature range of dental interest (**130**). Shrinkage is of the order of 1.5%, and is due to the thermal contraction from mouth to room temperature.

| **Table 33** Coefficient of expansion of waxes. | | | |
|---|---|---|---|
| Source | Name | Temperature range (°C) | Coef. of Exp. (ppm/°C) |
| Mineral | Paraffin | 20–28 | 307 |
| | | 28–34 | 1631 |
| Plant | Carnauba | 22–52 | 156 |
| Insect | Beeswax | 22–41 | 344 |
| | | 41–50 | 1048 |

The material has poor dimensional stability and the model must be poured as soon as possible after the impression is taken; this should take place within one hour.

The thermal conductivity of impression compound is very low, meaning that upon softening, the outside will always soften first. This can give the impression that the material is ready for use when the inside might still be quite hard.

Differential expansion gives rise to internal strains which relieve themselves in due course by distortion of the impression. Thus, the material must be placed in the water bath to allow sufficient time for it to achieve a uniform temperature. Even then, internal strains will inevitably build up during cooling, and will eventually give rise to distortion, which is why the model must be poured as soon as possible.

### Application

Its main application is for recording preliminary impressions of edentulous arches. This gives a model on which a special tray can be constructed, and which can subsequently be used with a low viscosity impression material (such as zinc oxide–eugenol) for recording the fine surface detail (see below). The material is used relatively little these days, as other impression materials are preferred.

## Zinc Oxide–Eugenol Paste

Whereas there are many zinc oxide–eugenol products that are presented as powder–liquid systems, the impression material is in the form of two pastes. There is typically a *base paste* consisting of zinc oxide, olive oil, linseed oil, zinc acetate and a trace of water, and a *reactor paste*, consisting of eugenol and fillers, such as kaolin and talc.

Zinc oxide and eugenol are the reactive components that take part in the setting reaction (see section II.IV). The water initiates the setting reaction, and the zinc acetate is present to speed up the setting process. The oils and fillers are inert substances which allow the material to be used in a paste–paste formulation, and help to provide the appropriate handling characteristics.

### Properties

The liquid is very fluid, i.e. muco-static, and, being a water-based system, readily adapts to

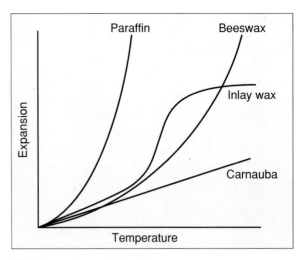

**130** Thermal expansion of waxes.

the soft tissues. It therefore provides a detailed reproduction of the soft tissues without causing displacement of the soft tissues, but is rigid once set and is thus unable to record undercuts. This limits its application to the edentulous mouth, where it is used with a special tray.

It has the advantage of being dimensionally stable and shows little shrinkage on setting. However, as it is used with a special tray, the tray may impose limitations on the dimensional stability of the whole impression.

Although the material is non-toxic, eugenol can cause a burning sensation in the patient's mouth and leave a persistent taste that the patient may find unpleasant. The paste tends to adhere to skin, so the skin around the lips should be protected with petroleum jelly.

## Impression Plaster

### Presentation And Composition

Impression plaster consists of a powder to which water is added to produce a smooth paste. The composition of the powder is similar to that of model materials discussed in more detail in section III.I, as is the setting process. The impression material consists typically of calcium sulphate β-hemihydrate $(CaSO_4)_2.H_2O$, potassium sulphate to reduce the expansion, borax to reduce the rate of setting, and starch to help disintegration of the impression on separation from the plaster/stone model.

### Properties

The impression plaster is easy to mix, but great care must be taken to avoid trapping air bubbles, as these will give rise to surface inaccuracies. The material has well-controlled working and setting characteristics, which are governed by the relative amounts of borax and potassium sulphate.

The amount of potassium sulphate is generally more than would be found in model plaster, since for impressions the expansion must be kept to a minimum.

Since the potassium sulphate also acts as an accelerator of the set, borax is needed to counteract it. The working time is of the order of 2–3 minutes as is the setting time.

The mixed material has a very low viscosity, and so is muco-static. It is hydrophilic and thus adapts readily to the soft tissues, recording their surface detail with great accuracy. The material is best used in a special tray, made of acrylic or shellac, to a thickness of 1.0–1.5mm. Alternatively, it can be used as a wash with a compo special tray.

The dimensional stability of impression plaster is very good, so a time delay in pouring the model is of no consequence, although extremes of temperature should be avoided. A separating medium (usually a solution of sodium alginate) must be used between the model plaster and the impression plaster.

The material is rigid once set and thus unable to record undercuts. This limits its application to the edentulous patient.

From the patient's point of view it is not an unpleasant material, although it tends to leave a sensation of dryness in the mouth for some time after the impression has been taken.

# Elastic Impression Materials

## *Colloids*

The word colloid is derived from the word *kola*, meaning glue, and *oid*, meaning like. Thus a colloid has a glue-like physical character.

The colloidal state represents a highly dispersed phase of fine particles within another phase, somewhere between a solution and a suspension:

- A solution is a homogeneous mixture consisting of a single phase.
- A suspension is a mixture of two distinct phases.
- A colloid is a heterogeneous mixture of two phases, where the two phases are not readily differentiated.

The difference between a colloid and a suspension is that in a colloid the dispersed phase is not readily detectable microscopically. Examples of colloids in dental use are:

- Colloidal silica in resin.
- Droplets of oil in water.
- Fillers in impression materials.

The size of the finely dispersed phase can not be defined accurately, but it is slightly greater than the simple molecular size, usually in the range of 1–500 nm.

The colloid can exist in the form of a viscous liquid, known as a *sol* or a solid, described as a *gel*. If the particles are suspended in water, then the suspoension is called a *hydrocolloid*, with the liquid being a *hydrosol* and the solid a *hydrogel*. In the case of the hydrogel there is an entanglement network of solid particles with the liquid trapped in the interstices. The solid particles are in the form of fibrils or chains of molecules.

The hydrocolloid impression materials come in two forms :

- Reversible, e.g. agar.
- Irreversible, e.g. alginate.

## *Agar*

Agar is a galactose sulphate which forms a colloid with water. It liquefies between 71°C and 100°C and sets to gel again between 30°C and 50°C. It is a long chain molecule, with a molecular weight of approximately 150 000. The structure of this polysaccharide is shown in **131**. The hydroxyl (OH) groups undergo hydrogen bonding, leading to the formation of a helical structure.

When heated, the hydrogen bonds are broken, the helix is uncoiled and the gel is turned into a viscous fluid. This process is therefore reversible in the manner shown below:

**131** The structure of a polysaccharide.

$$gel \xrightarrow[\text{heating}]{} sol \xrightarrow[\text{cooling}]{} gel$$

These materials are analogous to thermoplastics and have the advantage that they can be used repeatedly.

The agar is heated in a water bath until it becomes fluid. It is placed in a special metal tray through which water can be passed when it is placed in the patient's mouth. The water cools the agar, whereupon it resolidifies as a gel, having taken up the shape of the oral tissues.

**Composition**

The composition and purpose of the various ingredients of a typical agar impression material are as shown in *Table 34*. As can be seen from the composition, only a small amount of agar is needed to form a gel.

**Presentation And Application**

The material is provided in tube-like sachets for loading the tray, or in a syringe for easy adaptation to the teeth.

The agar content of the syringe-applied material is lower than that of the tray material, so it is more fluid and easy to eject from the syringe and inject around the teeth.

When immersed in a temperature-controlled water bath, both materials turns into a viscous liquid after approximately 8–12 minutes, and can be left for several hours.

It is important that the material is not over-heated, as this will cause breakdown of the polymer.

The water bath usually consists of three compartments, each held at a different temperature. One compartment contains water near its boiling point and is used for liquefying the agar. A second compartment is kept at 63–66°C for

**Table 34** Composition of an agar impression material.

| Component | Amount(%) | Purpose |
|---|---|---|
| Agar | 12.5 | Dispersed phase |
| Borax | 0.2 | Strengthens gel |
| Potassium Sulphate | 1.7 | Accelerator for model |
| Alkyl Benzoate | 0.1 | Prevents mould |
| Dyes and Flavouring | Trace | Appearance and taste |
| Water | 85.5 | Continuous phase |

storing the agar. The third compartment is kept at 46°C and is used for tempering the agar after it is placed in the special water cooled tray. This compartment is necessary to ensure that the agar is cooled to a temperature which the patient finds acceptable, and that will not burn the tissues. Due to the relatively small amount used, the syringe-applied material does not require tempering and can be kept in the storage compartment.

The contents of the tube are squeezed into an impression tray and placed in the tempering bath. Once the agar has cooled sufficiently, which takes about two minutes, the tray is placed in the patient's mouth. The water supply is connected only at this stage.

The temperature of the water for the water cooled tray should be around 13°C, so as to be comfortable for the patient; if it is too cold, the resultant thermal shock can cause considerable pain and discomfort. The water is allowed to circulate through the tray and after about five minutes the agar will have resolidified. The tray can now be removed from the patient's mouth and an accurate reproduction of the tissues obtained.

Should the material not be used, for whatever reason, it can be used again at a later date. The time required to reliquefy the material may be somewhat longer and can add up to four minutes to the process.

Each time the material is heated it will cause some breakdown of the polymer structure and the agar will become noticeably stiffer. Thus, it should not be reheated more than four times.

### Properties

As it is a highly fluid liquid when placed in the mouth and adapts readily to the contours of the hard and soft tissues because of its hydrophilic nature, this material provides very accurate reproductions. In addition to these advantages, the material closest to the water-cooled tray gels first, while the material in contact with the tissues stay liquid longest and can compensate for any inaccuracies due to shrinkage or unintentional movement of the tray.

The model should be poured from the impression immediately, and should this not be possible, the impression material should be kept at a relative humidity of 100% by wrapping it in a wet towel.

In any case, the model needs to be poured within one hour as the material suffers from two potential problems:

- *Syneresis* –This is a process whereby water is forced out onto the surface of the impression as the gel molecules are drawn closer together, with the main driving force being the relief of internal stresses. The water evaporates from the surface and causes the impression material to shrink.
- *Imbibition* – This is the uptake of water that occurs if the material has become dry, possibly due to inadequate storage technique. Distortion of the impression will result if this occurs, as the internal stresses that are always present are relieved during this process.

The material can readily be removed from undercuts, but great care must be exercised as the material tears very easily and does not bond to the stock tray. Although the tray is perforated, there is always the possibility that some separation occurs with severe undercuts.

The material is highly viscoelastic, so it is important that the tray is removed by a rapid snap-action so that a near elastic response results. This applies equally to many of the other polymer-based impression materials. It is necessary to have a reasonable thickness of the impression material to limit the extent of the deformation arising on the removal from an undercut.

The borax in the material, which is present to control the pH, has the adverse effect of reacting with the model material and thus slowing down its setting behaviour; this can result in a soft surface to the model. Potassium sulphate is added in order to avoid this.

The material is non-toxic and is non-irritant to the patient provided the recommended procedure is followed carefully. It is relatively cheap, and is used in some laboratories for making duplicate models as it can be recycled up to four times.

There are some disadvantages with the agar impression materials, in that one needs special equipment such as water-cooled trays and a temperature controlled bath, and there is an initial cost in providing this equipment. Also, the water-cooled tray is very bulky, which may cause some discomfort to the patient.

## *Alginates*

The alginates are based on alginic acid, which is derived from a marine plant. The structure of alginic acid is quite complex and is shown in **132**.

Some of the hydrogen molecules on the carboxyl groups are replaced by sodium, thus forming a water soluble salt, with a molecular weight of 20 000 to 200 000.

The composition of a typical alginate impression material is presented in *Table 35*.

### Setting Process

When mixed with water, a chemical reaction occurs that cross-links the polymer chain, so forming a three-dimensional network structure. This is an irreversible process, so the material can only be used once:

$$\text{sol} \quad \underset{\text{chemical reaction}}{\longrightarrow} \quad \text{gel}$$

### Setting Reaction

The calcium ions that are released from the calcium sulphate dihydrate, which is partially soluble, act as a cross-linking agent:

$$(CaSO_4).2H_2O \rightarrow 2Ca_2^+ + 2SO_4^{2-} + H_2O$$

**Table 35** Composition of an alginate impression material.

| Component | Amount (%) | Purpose |
|---|---|---|
| Sodium alginate | 18 | Hydrogel former |
| Calcium sulphate dihydrate | 14 | Provides calcium ions |
| Sodium phosphate | 2 | Controls working time |
| Potassium sulphate | 10 | Setting of model |
| Fillers (diatomeceous earth) | 56 | Controls consistency |
| Sodium silicofluoride | 4 | Controls pH |

Alginic acid

Sodium alginate

**132** Structure of sodium alginate with hydrogen ions in alginic acid replaced by sodium ions.

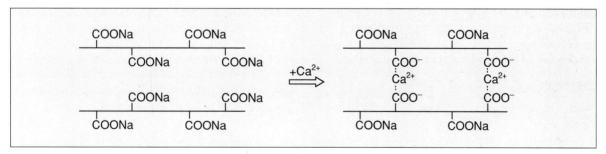

**133** Cross-linking reaction of sodium alginate in the presence of calcium ions.

The cross-linking mechanism is shown in **133** and can be described by the general reaction:

$$Na_nAlg + n/2\,CaSO_4 \rightarrow n/2\,Na_2SO_4 + Ca_{n/2}\,Alg$$

sodium + calcium → sodium + calcium
alginate sulphate dihydrate sulphate alginate gel

The working and setting times are determined by the release of calcium ions and their availability for cross-linking. Rapid dissolution of the calcium sulphate would give the material an inadequate working time, so, to overcome this, sodium phosphate is added to regulate the initial

| Table 36 A comparison of regular- and fast-set alginate. | | |
|---|---|---|
| | Regular-set | Fast-set |
| Mixing time (minutes) | 1 | 0.75 |
| Working time (minutes) | 3–4.5 | 1.25–2 |
| Setting time (minutes) | 1–4.5 | 1–2 |

burst of calcium ions. The sodium phosphate acts as a retarder, and the amount included can be varied to produce regular and fast setting versions of this impression material. Sodium ions are produced by the following reaction:

$$Na_3PO_4 \rightarrow 3Na^+ + PO_4^{3-}$$

The calcium ions will react preferentially with the phosphate ions to form an insoluble calcium phosphate:

$$3Ca^{2+} + 2PO_4^{3-} \rightarrow Ca_3(PO_4)_2$$

Thus, the first calcium ions that are released from the calcium sulphate dihydrate are not available for cross-linking as they react with the phosphate. Only when sufficient calcium ions have been released to react with the sodium phosphate that has been added will the subsequently released calcium ions be free to form cross-links.

There is a considerable pH change on setting, from a pH of 11 to one of about 7. This change in pH has been utilised in some formulations by the incorporation of pH indicators to allow a visual perception of the working and setting process.

**Properties**

These materials are now available as dust-free powders that overcome any potential irritation due to fine dust particles entering the atmosphere and being inhaled.

The powder should be mixed thoroughly before use to eliminate the segregation that may occur during storage, and to incorporate the surface layer which is often contaminated with moisture picked up from the atmosphere. The container must be resealed as soon as the required amount of powder has been removed. The correct proportioning of the powder and water is important, and the manufacturers supply a suitable measuring spoon. Mixing is most easily done in a rubber bowl with a spatula of the type used for mixing plaster and stone.

This material has a well-controlled working time, but it does vary from product to product. One can affect the working and setting times by using warm water, but it is better to choose a product with the times suited to your individual needs and use water at a temperature between 18°C and 24°C. Typical values for a regular- and fast-setting alginate impression material are shown in *Table 36*.

The clinical setting time can be detected by the loss of tackiness of the surface. The impression should be left in place for 2–3 minutes after the tackiness has gone from the surface.

The surface reproduction with these materials is not as good as that with agar or elastomers, and thus they are not recommended for crown and bridge work. However, they are very popular for full and partial denture work.

Alginates suffer from the same problems as agar in that they are susceptible to syneresis and imbibition. As with the agar, the model should be poured within one hour and kept wet in the meantime by placing a wet towel around the impression.

Like agar, alginate is highly viscoelastic and a snap-removal technique needs to be employed in order to get an elastic response. The amount of compression of the material may be of the order of 10% in areas of undercut. The permanent deformation in such circumstances may be of the order of 1.5%, which is just acceptable for the sort of applications in which these materials are used. The permanent deformation is somewhat higher than for agar impression materials, where, under the same conditions, the permanent set would be of the order of 1%.

The permanent deformation can be minimised by ensuring that there are no deep undercuts, as the deeper the undercut the greater the amount of compression. Using a snap removal will ensure that the time for which the material is under compression is as short as possible, which is an advantage because the longer the material is under compression, the higher the amount of permanent deformation due to the viscoelastic nature of the alginates. Some recovery of the deformation will occur once the impression is removed and the compressive load taken off.

$$\text{HS–(C}_2\text{H}_4\text{–O–CH}_2\text{–O–C}_2\text{H}_4\text{–S–S)}_x\text{–}\overset{\overset{\textstyle C_2H_5}{\textstyle |}}{\underset{\underset{\textstyle SH}{\textstyle |}}{C}}\text{–(S–S–C}_2\text{H}_4\text{–O–CH}_2\text{–OC}_2\text{H}_4\text{)}_y\text{–SH}$$

**134** A typical polysulphide.

However, although longer recovery times result in lower permanent sets, this advantage must be offset against the dimensional instability of the material.

The material has a very low tear strength, being less than that of the agar impression material. Fast loading rates, such as those that occur during snap removal will raise the tear strength, but even so it can not be used for crown and bridge work as excessive tearing will result on removal.

The impression must be rinsed after removal from the patient's mouth to remove any saliva as this will interfere with the setting of the gypsum model. Any surface water should be removed prior to pouring the model as residual water will dilute the model material and result in a soft surface which is easily damaged.

The alginate should not be left on the model for too long as it becomes difficult to separate if allowed to dry out. This would result in a poor surface finish as bits of the alginate are left on the surface of the model.

Patient acceptability is not a problem with these impression materials. The material is cheap but does have a limited shelf life, probably related to water contamination.

# Elastomeric Impression Materials

The impression materials discussed so far are not good enough generally for taking accurate impressions of the dentate patient. The alginates are inherently weak materials and provide a poor reproduction of surface detail; agar is dimensionally unstable and only suitable if laboratory facilities are close at hand; and the rigid impression materials can not be removed from deep undercuts. Thus, there is still a need for an impression material that is accurate, that shows a large recoverable deformation, and has adequate long-term dimensional stability. These goals can all be met with the elastomeric impression materials.

The elastomeric impression materials are characterised as polymers that are used at a temperature above their glass transition temperature, $T_g$. Such materials become more and more fluid as their temperature is raised above their glass-transition temperature.

The viscosities of the polymers that are used for impression materials are governed primarily by the molecular weight of the polymer (i.e. the length of the polymer chains) and by the presence of additives, such as fillers.

Thus, we have a material that is fluid at room temperature, but that can be turned into a solid by binding the long chain molecules together. This process of binding the chains to form a three-dimensional network is known as cross-linking, (as described in section I.V) and forms the basis of the liquid to solid transition of all the elastomeric impression materials.

There are essentially three main groups of elastomeric impression materials:

- Polysulphides.
- Polyethers.
- Silicones.

First, the chemistry of these impression materials will be described and then their relative merits will be considered.

## Polysulphides

The polysulphide polymer shown below has a molecular weight of 2000–4000, with terminal and pendant mercaptan groups (–SH) (see **134**).

The subscripts, x and y, in **134** denote different numbers of repeating units. These materials are also known as thiokol rubbers as they are derived from thiols, which are the sulphur

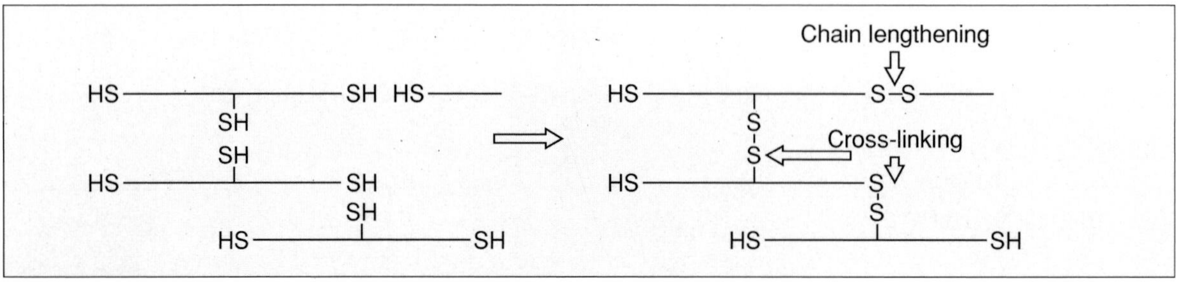

**135** Cross-linking and chain-lengthening of a polysulphide impression material.

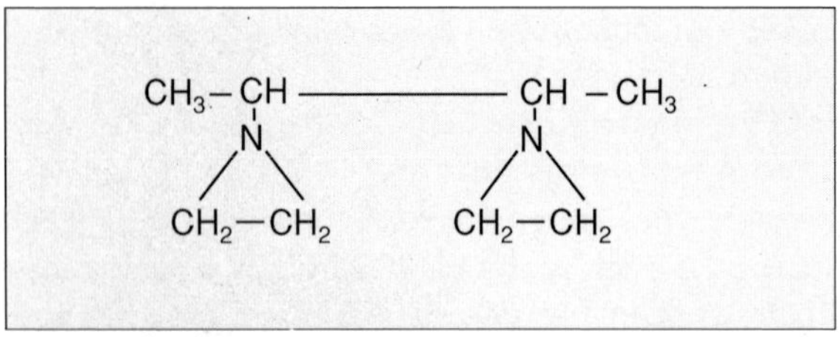

**136** Structure of a polyether.

analogues of the alcohols (e.g. ethanethiol, $CH_3CH_2SH$, rather than ethanol, $CH_3CH_2OH$).

The mercaptan groups are oxidised by an accelerator to bring about both chain lengthening and cross-linking, as shown in **135**. This reaction causes a rapid increase in the molecular weight of the polymer, which causes the paste to be converted into a rubber. Water is a by-product of the reaction.

The polymerisation reaction is exothermic, with a temperature rise of 3–4°C being typical, although this does depend upon the amount of polysulphide used.

**Presentation**

Polysulphides are presented as a base paste (containing polysulphide and an inert filler, such as titanium dioxide $TiO_2$ as 0.3 µm particles), and an activator paste (containing lead dioxide, which gives the distinctive brown colour, sulphur and dibutyl or dioctyl phthalate).

The viscosity of the base paste depends upon the amount of filler present, and heavy, medium and light bodied impression pastes forms are available. Note that there is no putty version of this impression material, so it must be used with a special tray, using either the medium-bodied material by itself or a combination of the heavy- and light-bodied materials.

## Polyethers

An interesting feature of the polyether based impression materials is that they were developed specifically with the dental profession in mind. They were introduced in the late 1960's. A simplified version of the polymer structure is shown in **136**.

The polymer is cured by a reaction with imine end groups. The setting reaction is shown in **137**. There is no by-product associated with this reaction, which is one reason why this material has good dimensional stability.

However, it *is* inclined to absorb water upon storage and must therefore be kept in a dry environment; certainly, one should never place the polymer in the same bag as an alginate impression.

**Presentation**

The polyethers come as two-paste systems: a base paste (consisting of polyether, a plasticiser such as glycoether or phthalate, and colloidal silica as an inert filler), and an activator paste (consisting of an aromatic sulphonate ester, a plasticiser, and an inert filler).

These materials are available only at a single viscosity. The idea is that it can be used in a special tray using a single viscosity mix. However, a thinner *is* available, and can be used to produce a low viscosity wash.

## Silicones

There are two important groups of silicone impression materials. One group is known as the condensation-cured silicones and the other as the addition-cured silicones. Both are based on the polydimethyl siloxane polymer but have different end groups giving rise to different curing mechanisms.

**137** Cross-linking reaction via the imine pendant groups of a polyether.

## Condensation-Cured Silicones

These materials are based on a polydimethyl siloxane polymer with hydroxyl terminal groups, as shown in **138**.

Cross-linking is achieved by the use of a tetra-ethyl silicate (TES), such that as many as three polymer chains can be linked together, as shown in **139**. (Three functional groups are needed to form a cross-linking network, as a functionality of two only gives rise to chain lengthening.)

The by-product of this reaction is an alcohol (R–OH).

## Presentation

The materials come as a base paste, containing silicone fluid and a filler, and an activator paste of tetra-ethyl silicate (the cross-linking agent).

A wide range of viscosities are available, varying from a putty, to a heavy, a medium and a light-bodied material. There are also some extra-fine materials of very low viscosity available. Thus, these materials can be used in a wide variety of impression techniques.

The difference in viscosity between the activator and base paste can present a problem in that it is difficult to obtain a uniform mix unless a good technique is employed.

It is also important that the amount of activator paste that is used is carefully controlled. Insufficient TES gives rise to an incomplete cure, leaving a material with poor mechanical characteristics, such as high permanent set. Conversely, an excess of TES also gives an incomplete cure, as in this case there are many unreacted ethyl end groups.

**138** Hydroxyl-terminated polydimethyl siloxane.

**139** Cross-linking reaction for a condensation-cured silicone impression material.

**140** Polydimethyl siloxane with vinyl end-groups.

## Addition-Cured Silicones

These materials are similar to the condensation-cured silicones in that they are also based on a polydimethyl siloxane polymer. However, in this case the terminal groups are vinyls, as shown in **140**.

**141** Cross-linking reaction for an addition-cured silicone impression material.

The setting reaction is via a platinum catalyst and a silanol as depicted in **141**. An important feature of this setting reaction is that there is no by-product.

### Presentation

The addition-cured silicones present as a base paste (of polyvinyl siloxane, silanol and a filler), and a catalyst paste (of polyvinyl siloxane, platinum catalyst and a filler).

As with the condensation-cured silicones, the material is available in a wide range of viscosities, varying from a putty, to a heavy, a medium and a light-bodied material.

Thus, these materials can also be used in a wide range of impression techniques. They have the advantage over the condensation-cured silicones in that the base paste and the catalyst paste for a given grade of material have the same consistencies, which makes them relatively easy to mix.

# Relative Merits Of The Elastomeric Impression Materials

## Handling Characteristics

The setting process of the polysulphide material is highly susceptible to changes in environmental conditions, such as temperature and humidity variation, and unless these are carefully controlled, the working and setting times can be very erratic.

Typically, the working time and setting time are 6 and 13 minutes respectively, which are quite long compared to some of the other impression materials. A high ambient temperature, combined with high humidity can give rise to much shorter working and setting times, and the converse is also true.

The condensation-cured silicones, too, can suffer from erratic setting behaviour, not only due to the possibility of a non-uniform mixing procedure, but also because the TES is susceptible to hydrolysis. If TES becomes contaminated with moisture it can become inactive, which could result in some embarrassing moments.

The setting behaviour of the polyether and addition-cured silicone impression materials is more consistent. However, it has been noticed that there is an inhibition of the setting of addition-cured silicone putties when the mixer is wearing latex gloves.

The mixing of the low viscosity addition-cured silicones has been made considerably easier with the introduction of gun delivery systems. These avoid both the potential for incomplete mixing and the introduction of air bubbles.

## Mechanical Properties

### Stiffness

The stiffness of the impression material once it has set can be a major consideration in the ease with which it is removed from undercuts. The relative stiffness of the set materials can be ranked as follows:

$$PS < CCS < ACS < PE$$

(excluding the putties and comparing similar viscosity materials). In the case of addition-cured silicones, problems have been experienced with the extremely stiff putties, where removal can be very difficult if the putty has been allowed to flow into large interdental spaces. Newer versions of the putties have been introduced which have a lower stiffness once set, the so-called *soft putties*.

### Permanent Set

Ideally, when the impression is removed from an undercut, the deformation that results should be totally and immediately recoverable.

All of the elastomeric impression materials are viscoelastic in behaviour, so it is important that they are removed from the mouth by a sharp tug. This will ensure that the impression material is strained for only a short time and that a near elastic response will be obtained. If the impression is removed slowly, the material will be given the opportunity to flow and not all of the induced strain may be relieved.

The silicones are particularly good at showing virtually no permanent deformation, while the polysulphides have a relatively high degree of viscous flow. The impression materials can be ranked as follows:

$$PS > PE > CCS > ACS$$

with the polysulphides most prone to permanent deformation, and the addition-cured silicones least prone.

### Tear Strength

The tear strength of the impression material is also important when an impression is taken of the dentate patient.

The polysulphides have the highest tear strength, followed a long way down by the polyethers and finally the silicones.

A high tear strength is nevertheless not necessarily a good thing, as too high a tear strength may give rise to difficulties in removing the impression from the mouth in cases where the impression material has flowed into the interdental spaces. Also, a considerable amount of deformation may occur for materials with a high tear strength before the impression material tears, and this deformation may not be totally recoverable.

Thus, the tear strength should be sufficient to prevent catastrophic failure, but not so high as to result in excessive deformation or difficulty in removal of the impression.

## Reproduction Of Surface Detail

All of the elastomeric impression materials are able to reproduce the details of the surface very accurately when a low viscosity material is employed. The ability to reproduce the surface detail is directly related to the viscosity of the impression material: the lower the viscosity, the better the reproduction. In fact, the reproduction is generally so good that the stone dies are unable to reproduce it.

Factors which give rise to inadequacies in the surface reproduction are generally related to poor technique. For example, great care must be exercised during the mixing of the two pastes to minimise the presence of air bubbles. Air bubbles are not a problem when they are within the bulk of the impression material, but they will present difficulties when close to or at the surface, as detail will be lost. Another problem which may manifest itself is the occurrence of areas where the impression material has not set properly and retains a tacky feel. This is usually due to improper mixing resulting in a non-homogeneous mix.

All of the elastomeric impression materials are hydrophobic, and, if the surface of the tooth has become contaminated with saliva, the impression material is unable to wet it – this can give rise to loss of surface detail. The ability of an impression material to wet a surface can be determined from contact angle measurements. The contact angles for water on the set materials have been measured, and are 49.3°, 82.1° and 98.2° for a polyether, polysulphide and an addition-cured silicone respectively. This shows that the silicones are particularly problematic, and that the polyethers are the easiest to work with from this point of view.

A number of so-called hydrophilic addition-cured silicones have recently come on the market. A surfactant has been added to these materials to alter the hydrophobicity of the surface and so reduce the contact angle to be closer to that of the polyether impression materials.

## Dimensional Stability And Accuracy

It is important that the model of the oral cavity is an accurate three-dimensional replica, since all of the laboratory work will be based on this model. Besides the problems of distortion, there are also the dangers of expansion and contraction of the impression.

With the advent of the addition-cured silicones and the polyethers, impression materials are most probably as accurate as they will ever need to be. Recently, attention has been paid to improving their handling characteristics; the dimensional stability of the addition-cured silicones can sometimes turn out to be somewhat of an embarrassment as discussed below.

## Other Factors

Factors which contribute to the production of an inaccurate model have already been discussed, but some deserve further comment in relation to specific impression materials.

### Polymerisation Shrinkage And Thermal Contraction

Polyether and addition-cured silicones have the lowest polymerisation shrinkage, followed by the polysulphides. The condensation-cured silicones have the highest degree of contraction due to polymerisation shrinkage. Thus, the impression materials can be ranked as follows in terms of their polymerisation shrinkage:

$$PE = ACS < PS < CCS.$$

The thermal contraction is important as the material is cooled from mouth temperature to room temperature. The polyethers have the highest thermal contraction (320 ppm/°C), followed by the polysulphides (270 ppm/°C) and then the silicones (200 ppm/°C). These can be ranked as follows:

$$CCS = ACS < PS < PE.$$

Of course, both the polymerisation shrinkage and the thermal contraction are affected by the amount of filler present, in that the higher the filler loading, the smaller the contraction. For this reason, the amount of light bodied material used should always be kept to a minimum.

### Storage Stability

The polysulphides are inclined to contract on storage, especially if they are kept in a low humidity environment, as the by-product of the setting reaction is water. Thus, the model will always be slightly larger than the tooth, leaving adequate space for the luting agent. Models should be poured very soon after the impression has been taken.

The polyethers are very stable on storage, unless they are placed in a high humidity environment upon when they will absorb water and expand. If this occurs, the resultant model is going to be smaller than the original tooth and a crown produced on such a model will not fit under any circumstances.

As this impression material absorbs water readily from alginate impression materials, the two should never be placed in direct contact.

The condensation-cured silicones show a considerable contraction with time. This has been ascribed to the loss of the alcohol by-product. So, as with the polysulphides, models should be prepared as soon as possible to avoid this problem.

The addition-cured silicones are extremely stable once set and show virtually no dimensional change on storage. Thus these materials are particularly good to use in situations where duplicate stone dies are needed.

## Impression Technique

The polysulphide and condensation-cured silicones display a measure of shrinkage, such that the model poured from the impression is invariably slightly larger than the tooth.

The amount of space thus created for the luting agent will depend upon the time that has elapsed between taking the impression and making the model. For the polyether impression material and the addition-cured silicones, the shrinkage is so small that there is very little space for the luting agent.

The high dimensional stability of the addition-cured silicones can cause problems if the wrong impression technique is used.

The wide variety of presentations of the silicone impression materials provides for the opportunity to use various impression-taking techniques. The most popular are putty/wash procedures which allow the use of a stock tray.

The consequences for the size of the model produced from the three impression techniques are shown graphically in **142**.

### Twin-Mix Technique

In this technique, the wash is mixed and placed in a syringe, and, while the impression material

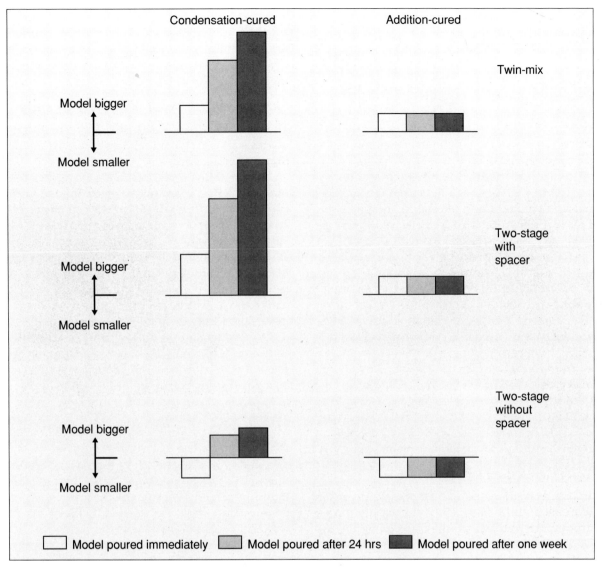

**142** Dimensional changes for an addition-cured and condensation-cured silicone impression material following different impression taking techniques.

is prepped around those teeth for which an accurate impression is needed, the putty is mixed and placed in the stock tray.

The loaded tray is then inserted in the patient's mouth, and the two impression materials allowed to set simultaneously. There will be some deformation of the impression material upon removal, most of which is recovered immediately by a recoil action.

If the model is poured virtually immediately, little or no shrinkage (due to cooling and storage contraction) will have taken place and the resultant model will be only slightly bigger than the tooth. Due to storage contraction (in the case of the condensation-cured silicone), the longer the delay before pouring the model, the larger the model will be. As the addition-cured silicones are extremely stable on storage, the model will be of the same size no matter when it is poured.

The potential problems with this technique are related to the removal of the addition-cured silicones. Although there are now some softer putties, removal can be difficult if the putty has flowed into the interdental spaces; the larger these are, the more difficult it will be to remove the impression. Another problem that may arise is that the putty may displace the wash in areas where surface accuracy is desirable.

### Two-Stage With Spacer Technique

This technique effectively involves the production of a special tray by using the putty first. A primary impression is taken either directly from the oral surfaces or sometimes with a thin cellophane sheet laid over the putty.

In the former situation, the poor quality impression of the teeth is then cut out, creating a channel for the wash material. After this, a second impression is produced using the wash which provides the necessary surface detail.

Generally, more of the wash material is required in this technique than in the twin-mix approach, and this means that there is more setting shrinkage as the wash has a much lower filler content. This is especially the case with the condensation-cured silicones which also show more shrinkage on storage.

The addition-cured silicones are relatively unaffected by such problems. The setting shrinkage is compensated for, to some degree, as the putty will have already set. This method is used with the addition-cured silicones, to avoid the need to remove a stiff putty material from undercuts.

### Two-Stage Without Spacer Technique

In this technique, the first impression is taken with the putty. Subsequently, the wash is placed around the teeth and in the tray containing the set putty, and is reseated in the mouth.

The process of reseating can in itself be quite problematic. As a certain amount of space is required by the wash, there will be some compression of the putty to accommodate this.

The excellent recovery of the silicone impression materials means that immediately after the material has set and is removed from the mouth, there will be a recoil action as the pressure on the putty is relieved.

If a model is poured virtually immediately, then for both impression materials the model is likely to be slightly smaller than the tooth. For the condensation-cured silicones, the shrinkage on storage will ensure that after a delay of 24 hours this situation will have reversed.

However, the addition-cured silicones are so dimensionally stable that the model will always be too small. This technique is doubly inappropriate for addition-cured silicones because the primary impression would be extremely difficult to remove from undercuts, once it has set, due to the high stiffness of the putty.

## Compatibility With Model Materials

The compatibility with the model materials does not present a problem for any of the elastomeric impression materials.

One limitation of the polysulphide impression material is that it can not be electroplated with copper to produce reinforced dies, as the polysulphide reacts with the electrolyte. The alternative process of silver plating is not readily available because of the dangers associated with the silver cyanide used in the plating process.

The susceptibility of the polyether impression materials to absorb water may give rise to some distortion during the plating process.

The condensation- and addition-cured silicones can be plated with either copper or silver. The only problem here is that the surface has to be made conductive, and it is difficult to apply a graphite coating because of the low surface tension of the silicones.

## Acceptability

The polysulphides have an unpleasant odour due to the mercapto groups. (Small amounts of thiols are added to natural gas to make it easier to detect and thiols are excreted by the skunk to ward off predators.) The polysulphides are also difficult to clean off clothing if spilled.

The polyether and silicone impression materials are highly acceptable and very clean to handle.

## Cost

The elastomers are considerably more expensive than the hydrocolloids and the rigid impression materials, with the addition-cured silicones being more expensive still.

# Disinfection Of Impression Materials

Particularly since the advent of AIDS there has been an increased awareness of the potential pathways for cross-infection when handling impression materials. Cross-infection may occur from the patient to the dentist, to the DSA and eventually to the laboratory technician.

There will come a time when dental laboratories will no longer accept impressions unless there is aguarantee from the dentist that they have been disinfected. This has presented the dentist with a serious problem, as the taking of accurate impressions is a difficult procedure at the best of times.

All the care and attention paid to the taking of a good quality impression could be totally undermined if the impression should distort during the disinfecting procedure.

It is up to the dentist to choose the most appropriate impression material and the associated disinfection procedure.

## Disinfectants

Disinfection of impressions can be carried out either by immersion in a disinfectant or by the use of sprays. There are a variety of solutions which may be used for spray or immersion disinfection of impression materials. These fall into the following main groups:

- *Chlorine solutions* –These tend to be harmful to skin, eyes etc., they bleach clothing, have an unpleasant odour and are highly corrosive to metals.
- *Aldehyde solutions* – These give off a suffocating odour and are irritating to the skin and eyes. Commercial products tend to be made from glutaraldehyde-based solutions rather than formaldehyde-based solutions. Glutaraldehyde-2% solutions are the preferred disinfectants.
- *Iodine solutions* (Iodophors 1%).
- *Phenols.*

## The Effects Of Disinfectants On The Accuracy Of Impression Materials

Over the last few years, a number of published articles have looked into the effects of disinfectants on the accuracy and dimensional stability of impression materials.

A summary is provided below of the current knowledge relating to the various classes of impression materials.

### Reversible Hydrocolloids

Agar impression materials should be avoided if impressions are to be disinfected by an immersion technique.

The guidelines presented by the American Dental Association, Council on Dental Materials, Instruments and Equipment (CDMEI, 1988), state that there is, as yet, insufficient information on the effects of disinfectants on reversible hydrocolloids.

Another potential hazard with agar is associated with the danger of cross-contamination from the conditioning baths.

*Reversible hydrocolloids must not be used in situations where disinfection is required.*

### Irreversible Hydrocolloids

A highly significant dimensional change occurs for alginate impression materials when immersed for 16 hours in glutaraldehyde, formaldehyde or sodium hypochlorite. Immersion for 15 minutes in neutral glutaraldehyde or Iodophor appears acceptable.

Sodium hypochlorite causes partial dissolution of alginates. However, alginate seems unaffected by immersion for 10 minutes in O-phenyl phenol, phenol, glutaraldehyde or sodium hypochlorite, but a significant change in dimensions occurs on storage for one hour in alkaline glutaraldehyde.

Silicone-modified alginates appear acceptable for up to one hour immersion in 2% buffered glutaraldehyde.

A new, antiseptic-containing alginate appears highly effective except that it still does not overcome the problem of how to disinfect the impression tray.

*Use a disinfectant spray and leave the impression in a sealed bag for the recommended disinfection time of 30 minutes.*

### Polysulphides

Studies using a wide range of disinfectants and periods of immersion varying from ten to thirty minutes indicate that no adverse effects are observed with polysulphide impression materials and that spray disinfectants are also acceptable.

*This impression material appears well suited to disinfection by immersion for up to 30 minutes.*

### Polyethers

Polyether impression materials are known to expand when exposed to moisture. It is not surprising then that immersion in a variety of disinfectants caused excessive swelling after 10 minutes. Dimensional changes become highly significant after four hours immersion in 10% aqueous succinic aldehyde, but are acceptable after 10 minutes immersion. Spray disinfectants are acceptable.

*Use a spray disinfectant or immersion in products with a short disinfection time (<10 minutes), such as chlorine compounds.*

### Condensation-Cured Silicones

Although condensation-cured silicones are chemically unaffected by prolonged immersion in a wide variety of disinfectants, the limiting factor with this impression material is its inherent dimensional instability.

*Almost all disinfection procedure are acceptable as long as the period of immersion does not exceed 30 minutes.*

### Addition-Cured Silicones

Many studies have been undertaken of the effects of disinfectants on the dimensional stability of addition-cured silicones. They conclude that no adverse effects result from even an extended exposure of addition-cured silicones to all varieties of disinfectants. The only drawback appears to be a reduced wettability of the model material on the set impression for the hydrophilic silicone impression materials.

*This impression material is ideal in those circumstances when disinfection is required, as it can be immersed in virtually any disinfectant for long periods.*

## *Disinfection Procedure*

Impressions should be rinsed in water immediately on removal from the patient's mouth to remove any obvious signs of saliva, blood and debris. Disinfection of the impression should be carried out before the model is cast or the impression is sent to an outside laboratory. It is the responsibility of the dentist to ensure that impressions are received by the dental laboratory without carrying contaminants. As can be seen from the above, the disinfection procedure to be adopted depends upon the type of impression material and the disinfectant used. It must be appreciated that the objective of the procedure is to disinfect and not to sterilise, the latter requiring extended immersion for an unacceptable period and in any case is not warranted.

The BDA Advisory Service (Advice Sheet A12) make the comment that certain types of impression materials can be disinfected with glutaraldehyde, but also note that there is as yet no universally applicable method for disinfecting all types of impression materials. They go on to recommend that disposable trays should be used and that technicians should wear gloves when handling impression materials and pouring models. The BDA therefore does not make a specific recommendation for the disinfection of impressions.

The American Dental Association CDMIE (1988) is less equivocal on specific procedures for disinfecting impressions. They suggest immersion for 30 minutes in a glutaraldehyde- based disinfectant for polysulphide, condensation- and addition-cured silicone impression materials and a chlorine compound spray disinfectant for irreversible hydrocolloid and polyether impression materials.

From the information available to date, the only impression materials that can be disinfected with virtually no adverse effects are the condensation- and addition-cured silicones and the polysulphides.

# Failures Of Impression Taking

As the quality of the prosthesis is directly dependent upon the quality of the impression, it is important that a poor quality impression is identified readily and is not passed to the dental laboratory for processing.

In many instances, the need for retakes can be avoided by being aware of the kinds of problems that might arise and how these may be avoided. The main failures are associated with poor reproduction of surface detail and poor fit of the prosthesis.

## *Poor Reproduction Of Surface Detail*

Factors that give rise to poor reproduction of surface detail are:

- *Rough or uneven surface on impression* – This may be due to incomplete setting (usually associated with premature removal), improper mixing or the presence of surface contaminants. A set that is too rapid will also give a poor surface reproduction and may be due to the wrong temperature, humidity or mix.
- *Bubbles* – These usually arise if the material is allowed to set too quickly or if bubbles have been introduced during the mixing process.
- *Irregular shaped voids* – These will appear due to moisture or debris on the surface.

## *Poor Fit Of Prosthesis*

Factors which give rise to poor fit are:

- *Distortion* – The use of excessively flexible trays will result in distortion of the impression as the tray is distorted during seating. If the working time of the impresion material is exceeded, the material will not flow properly and there is a temptation to use more pressure when taking the impression, causing distortion of the tray and permanent set of the impression material. Movement of the tray while the impression material is setting will also cause distortion. Adhesive failure between the tray and the impression material can occur if there is insufficient adhesive, if the wrong adhesive is used, or if insufficient time is allowed for the adhesive to become effective. An inappropriate disinfecting procedure will also give rise to distortion.
- *Castings too big or too small* – Although it would be difficult to distinguish between prostheses that fit poorly due to being the wrong size or being distorted, the most common causes of the wrong sized castings are: the use of inappropriate impression techniques, pouring the model at the wrong time, or the impression having been stored under unsuitable conditions of temperature and humidity.

# Further Reading

Bell J. W. & von Frauenhofer J. A. (1975) The handling of elastomeric impression materials: a review. J. Dent. **3**, 229–237

Brown D. (1981) An update on elastomeric impression materials. Brit. Dent. J. **151**, 35–41

CDMIE, (1988) Infection control recommendations for the dental office and the dental laboratory. J. Am. Dent. Assoc. **116**, 241–248

Jamani K. D., Harrington E. & Wilson H. J. (1989) Rigidity of impression materials. J. Oral. Rehab. **16**, 241–248

Johnson G. H., Drennon D. G. & Powell G. L. (1988) Accuracy of elastomeric impressions disinfected by immersion. J. Am. Dent. Assoc. **116**, 525–530

McCabe J. F. & Storer R. (1980) Elastomeric impression materials. The measurement of some properties relevant to clinical practice. Brit. Dent. J. **149**,73–79

McCabe J. F. & Wilson H. J. (1978) Addition curing silicone rubber impression materials. An appraisal of their physical properties. Brit. Dent. J. **145**, 17–20

Pamenius M. & Ohlsen N. G. (1987) The clinical relevance of mechanical properties of elastomers. Dent. Mater. **3**, 270

Pratten D. H. & Craig R. G. (1989) Wettability of a hydrophilic addition silicone impression material. J. Prosthet. Dent. **61**, 197–201

Rosen M., Touyz L. Z. G. & Becker P. J. (1989) The effect of latex gloves on setting time of vinyl polysiloxane putty impression materials. Brit. Dent. J. **166**, 374–375

Storer R. *et al.* (1981) An investigation of methods available for sterilising impressions. Brit. Dent. J. **151**, 217–219

Watkinson A. C. (1988) Disinfection of impressions in UK dental schools. Brit. Dent. J. **164**, 22

Wilson H. J. (1988) Impression materials Brit. Dent. J. **164**, 221

# III
# LABORATORY AND RELATED DENTAL MATERIALS

The materials described in this section are used mostly by the dental technician to construct prostheses. Although the clinician may not be involved fully in the various stages of construction, a thorough knowledge of the characteristics of the materials used is of paramount importance if the correct choice of material is to be made for a particular application. Additionally, the clinician will find that awareness of the various materials and procedures involved in the construction of a prosthesis greatly aids communication with the dental technician and avoids possible misunderstanding.

# GYPSUM PRODUCTS

## Introduction

Materials that are derived from gypsum are used in a variety of dental application. They include:

- Models and dies.
- Impression materials.
- Moulds.
- Investments.

A *model* is a replica of the fitting surfaces of the oral cavity; it is poured from an impression of the oral anatomy, and is then used to construct an appliance, such as a full or a partial denture. A *mould* is used for the construction of a denture. *Dies* are replicas of individual teeth, and are generally used in the construction of crowns and bridges. An *investment* is the gypsum-bonded ceramic that is used as the mould material for some of the gold casting alloys.

In this section we will deal only with the chemistry and properties of these materials.

## Chemistry Of Gypsum

### *Composition*

Gypsum is calcium sulphate dihydrate, $CaSO_4.2H_2O$. When this substance is heated to a temperature sufficiently high to drive off some of the water, it is converted into calcium sulphate hemihydrate, $(CaSO_4)_2.H_2O$.

The production of calcium sulphate hemihydrate can be undertaken in one of three ways, producing versions of gypsum with different properties and hence different applications.

It should be noted that the three versions are chemically identical, differing only in form and structural detail.

### Plaster

Calcium sulphate dihydrate is heated in an open vessel. Water is driven off, and the dihydrate is converted into hemihydrate, known as calcined calcium sulphate or $\beta$-hemihydrate.

The resultant material consists of large irregular porous particles. It needs to be mixed with a large amount of water to obtain a mix satisfactory for dental use, as much of the water is absorbed into the pores of the particles. The usual mix is 50 ml of water to 100 gm of powder.

### Dental stone

If the dihydrate is heated in an autoclave, the hemihydrate that is produced consists of small, regular shaped particles which are relatively non-porous. This autoclaved calcium sulphate is known as $\alpha$-hemihydrate. Due to the non-porous and regular structure of the particles, they can be packed more tightly together using less water. The mix is 20 ml water to 100 gm of powder.

### Densite (improved stone)

In the production of this form of calcium sulphate hemihydrate, the dihydrate is boiled in the presence of calcium chloride and magnesium chloride. These two chlorides act as deflocculants, helping to separate the individual particles that would otherwise tend to agglomerate. The hemihydrate particles that are produced are more compact and smoother than those of the dental stone. The densite is mixed in the ratio of 100 gm of powder to 20 ml of water.

## The Setting Process

Heating the hydrate to drive off some of the water produces a substance which is effectively dehydrated. As a consequence of this, the hemihydrate is able to react with water and revert back to calcium sulphate dihydrate as follows:

$$(CaSO_4)_2.H_2O + 3 H_2O \rightarrow 2 CaSO_4.2H_2O$$

The setting process for gypsum products is believed to occur in the following sequence:

- Some calcium sulphate hemihydrate dissolves in the water.
- The dissolved calcium sulphate hemihydrate reacts with the water and forms calcium sulphate dihydrate.
- The solubility of calcium sulphate dihydrate is very low and a supersaturated solution is formed.
- This supersaturated solution is unstable and calcium sulphate dihydrate crystals precipitates out as stable crystals.
- As the stable calcium sulphate dihydrate precipitates out of the solution, more calcium sulphate hemihydrate is dissolved and this continues until all the hemihydrate has dissolved.

## Working And Setting Times

The material must be mixed and poured before it reaches the end of its working time. The working times vary from product to product, and are chosen to suit the particular application.

For impression plaster, the working time is only 2–3 minutes, whereas it approaches 8 minutes for a gypsum-bonded investment. Short working times give rise to short setting times, as

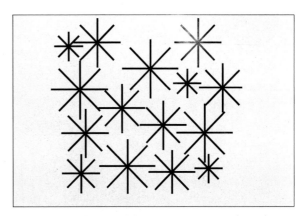

**143** Spherulitic structure of calcium sulphate dihydrate.

both are controlled by the speed of the reaction. Hence, for an impression plaster, the setting time is typically 2–3 minutes, whereas the setting time can vary from 20–45 minutes for gypsum-bonded investments.

The model materials have working times similar to those of impression plaster, but their setting times are somewhat longer. For plaster, the setting time is 5–10 minutes, while for stone it can be up to 20 minutes.

The handling characteristics are controlled by the inclusion of various additives. Additives which speed up to setting process are gypsum (<20%), potassium sulphate and sodium chloride. Those that slow down the setting rate are sodium chloride (>20%), potassium citrate and borax. These additives also affect the dimensional change on setting, as discussed later.

The manipulation of the powder–liquid system will also affect the setting characteristics. The operator can change the powder:liquid ratio, and, by adding more water, the setting time is extended. Increasing the spatulation time will result in a reduction of the setting time, as it has the effect of breaking up the crystals as they form, hence increasing the number of sites for crystallisation. A longer spatulation time will also tend to increase the setting expansion.

An increase in temperature has only a minimal effect, since the increased rate of dissolution is offset by the higher solubility of the calcium sulphate dihydrate in the water.

## Dimensional Changes On Setting

On setting, the crystals that are formed are spherulitic in appearance (**143**), not unlike snow

**Table 37** The change in molar volume that occurs as calcium sulphate hemihydrate is hydrated.

|  | $(CaSO_4)_2.H_2O$ + | $3 H_2O$ | → | $2 CaSO_4.2H_2O$ |
|---|---|---|---|---|
| Molecular weight | 290 | 54 |  | 344 |
| Density | 2.75 | 1.0 |  | 2.32 |
| Molar volume | 105 | 54 |  | 148 |
|  | Change in volume = (148 - 159) / 159 = - 7.1 % | | | |

flakes. These crystals impinge on one another as they grow, and try to push each other apart. The result of this action is that there is an apparent expansion on setting. The material in fact does shrink, in the sense that its molar volume is less, as shown in *Table 37*.

However, large empty spaces form between the crystals, leading to a high porosity. It is this that accounts for the apparent expansion.

The ability to expand on setting is a very important feature of this material, and it is the factor that makes it so useful for a large number of dental applications. In particular, models are best produced slightly larger than the oral anatomy. This is to ensure that crowns, bridges and dentures are not too tight a fit when placed in the mouth. The expansion is also made use of in investments, as it helps to compensate for the shrinkage of metallic casting on cooling from the melting temperature.

Although it is desirable generally that models produced from plaster or stone are slightly on the big side, the unchecked expansion of this material would be excessive. Thus there are various additives in gypsum products that are used to control the degree of expansion.

### Sodium Chloride

Sodium chloride provides additional sites for crystal formation. The higher density of crystals limits the growth of the crystals and hence reduces their ability to push each other apart. This results in a reduction of the apparent expansion.

The increased number of sites for nucleation of the dihydrate crystals has the effect of increasing the rate of setting of the material. The hemihydrate also dissolves more rapidly, which again increases the rate of reaction.

If present in high concentrations (>20%), the sodium chloride will deposit onto the surface of the crystal and prevent further growth. This reduces the reaction rate, rather than increasing it.

### Potassium Sulphate

Potassium sulphate ($K_2SO_4$) reacts with the water and hemihydrate to produce 'syngenite' ($K_2(CaSO_4)_2.H_2O$).

This compound crystallises very rapidly, and encourages the growth of more crystals. This has the effect of reducing the overall expansion and accelerating the setting reaction. When present as a 2% solution in water it will reduce the setting time from approximately 10 minutes to 4 minutes.

### Calcium Sulphate Dihydrate

The addition of a small amount of calcium sulphate dihydrate will provide additional sites for nucleation and act as an accelerator; it will reduce both the working and the setting times.

### Borax

The addition of borax ($Na_2B_4O_7.10H_2O$) is important because it counteracts the increased rate of setting due to the inclusion of the above additives. It is a *retarder* of the setting process. The addition of borax leads to the formation of calcium borate, which deposits on the dihydrate crystals and prevents further growth.

### Potassium Citrate

Potassium citrate acts as a retarder, and is sometimes added in addition to borax.

Thus, by carefully regulating the amount of the above additives, gypsum-based products can be produced with the correct degree of expansion and the correct working and setting times appropriate for various applications. Typically, the setting expansion for gypsum products is as shown in *Table 38*.

| Table 38 The setting expansions of some gypsum products. | |
| --- | --- |
| Plaster | 0.20–0.30 % |
| Stone | 0.08–0.10 % |
| Densite | 0.05–0.07 % |

| Table 39 The compressive strengths of some gypsum products. | |
| --- | --- |
| Plaster | 12 MPa |
| Stone | 30 MPa |
| Densite | 38 MPa |

The low setting expansion of stone and densite makes these materials ideal for the production of dies and models for both metal and ceramic work.

## Hygroscopic Expansion

The setting expansion can be increased substantially by immersing the material in water whilst it is setting. When it is in air, the surface tension of the free water tends to draw the crystals together, and this limits the ability of the crystals to grow.

However, when the crystals are immersed in water they can grow more freely, resulting in a greater degree of expansion. This process is called *hygroscopic expansion*, and is sometimes used with gypsum-bonded investments for the casting of alloys that have a high coefficient of thermal expansion or a high contraction on solidification.

## Dimensional Stability

Once the material has set, there is little or no dimensional change. The storage stability is excellent, although the material *is* slightly soluble in water. For this reason, washing the surface with hot water should be avoided.

# Properties

## Compressive Strength

The compressive strength is the mechanical property most commonly used for assessing the strength of gypsum products. These values are typically as shown in *Table 39*.

The compressive strength is affected considerably by the powder:liquid ratio that is used. It is clear from the above data that the reduction in the amount of water that is required to produce an acceptable mix gives a significant improvement in the compressive strength. Thus, the compressive strength of the set product is affected by straying from the recommended powder: liquid ratio.

The use of an excessive amount of water has the advantage that a smooth mix which can be readily poured is obtained. The air that is incorporated during the mixing process is more readily removed from such a mix for stone and densite by vibration, but the compressive strength after setting will be inferior. On the other hand, using less water than is recommended results in a thick mix from which incorporated air is more difficult to remove, leading to an increased porosity and a significantly reduced strength. There is also a danger that insufficient water will be present for the full reaction to take place.

Thus, using less water has the potential of increasing the compressive strength, but inferior properties are obtained if too little is used.

There is a marked difference in the wet and dry strength of plaster products. In general, the dry strength is about twice the wet strength.

## Tensile Strength

The wet tensile strength of plaster is very low (approximately 2 MPa). This is due to the brittle nature of the material, which has the disadvantage that teeth and margins on the model can be easily damaged if handled roughly. Dental stone has a tensile strength about twice that of plaster, and is therefore preferred for the production of crowns, bridge models and dies.

## Hardness And Abrasion Resistance

The surface hardness of gypsum products is very low, so the material is highly susceptible to scratching and loss through abrasion. Various methods of improving the surface hardness are available but these will not be discussed here.

| Table 40 The advantages and disadvantages of plaster for model making. | |
|---|---|
| Advantages | Disadvantages |
| Dimensionally accurate and stable | Low tensile strength, brittle |
| Cheap | Poor abrasion resistance |
| Good colour contrast | Poor surface detail |
| | Poor wetting of rubber impression materials |

### *Reproduction Of Surface Detail*

As the surface of gypsum products is slightly porous, minute surface detail at a microscopic level is not readily reproduced. However, macroscopic surface details are very accurately reproduced, although air bubbles (trapped between the plaster and the impression for example), can contribute to the loss of surface details.

## Summary

The advantages and disadvantages in the use of plaster for the production of models can be summarised as shown in *Table 40*.

## Further Reading

Combe E. C. & Smith D. C. (1964) Some properties of gypsum plasters. Brit. Dent. J. **117**, 237

Eames W. B., Edwares C. R. & Buck W. H. (1978) Scraping resistance of dental die materials: a comparison of brands. Oper. Dent. **3**, 66

Fan P. L., Powers J. M. & Reid B. C. (1981) Surface mechanical properties of stone, resin and metal dies. J. Am. Dent. Assoc. **103**, 408

# DENTURE BASE RESINS

## Introduction

Various materials have been used to construct dentures, including cellulose products, phenol-formaldehyde, vinyl resins and vulcanite. However, they have suffered from a variety of problems:

- Cellulose products suffered from warpage in the mouth, and from a taste of camphor due to its use as a plasticiser. This camphor leached out of the denture, causing blistering, staining and loss of colour within a few months.
- Phenol-formaldehyde (bakelite) proved to be too difficult to process and also lost its colour in the mouth.
- Vinyl resins were found to have a low resistance to fracture and failures were common, possibly due to fatigue.
- Vulcanite was the first material to be used for the mass production of dentures, but its aesthetic qualities are not very good and it has now been replaced by acrylic resins.

Acrylic resins are now the material of choice: they have the required aesthetic quality, and are cheap and easy to process. Even so, it is not ideal

**Table 41** The criteria for an ideal denture base material.

Natural appearance
Easy manipulation
High strength, stiffness, hardness and toughness
Low density
Dimensionally stable and providing accurate reproduction of surface detail
Absence of odour, taste or toxic products
Resistant to bacterial growth
Resistant to absorption of oral fluids
Good thermal conductivity
Good retention to other polymers, porcelain and metals
Radio-opaque
Easy to repair
Easy to clean
Good shelf life and inexpensive to use

in all respects. The ideal properties of a denture base material are shown in *Table 41*.

Acrylic resins are popular because they meet many of the criteria set out in *Table 41*. In particular, dentures made from acrylic resin are easy to process using inexpensive techniques, and are aesthetically pleasing.

# Composition And Structure Of Acrylic Resin

An acrylic resin denture is made by the process of free radical addition polymerisation to form polymethylmethacrylate (PMMA). The monomer is methylmethacrylate (MMA):

$$
\begin{array}{ccc}
H & & Me \\
| & & | \\
C & = & C \\
| & & | \\
H & & C = O \\
& & | \\
& & O \\
& & | \\
& & Me
\end{array}
$$

where Me stands for $CH_3$. The conversion of the monomer into a polymer involves the normal sequence of activation, initiation, propagation and termination as described in section I.VI.

The resins are available in either heat-cured or cold-cured forms. More recently, a light activated version has been introduced, but the chemistry of such materials is more akin to that of the composite restorative materials (see section II.II).

## *Heat-Cured Resins*

These materials consist of a powder and a liquid, which, upon mixing and subsequent heating, form a rigid solid. The constituents of the powder and liquid are shown in *Table 42*.

The reasons for the particular formulation of a powder/liquid system are twofold:

- Processing is possible by the dough technique.
- Polymerisation shrinkage is minimised.

The dough technique makes the processing of dentures a relatively straightforward process. By adapting the dough to the model and trimming off any excess, cold-cure varieties of the acrylics are easily manipulated (when in the doughy stage) to produce special trays.

The polymerisation shrinkage is reduced when compared to that of using a monomer, because most of the material that is being used

**Table 42** The constituents of a heat-cured resin.

| Powder: | Beads or granules of polymethyl methacrylate |
| --- | --- |
| | Initiator – benzoyl peroxide |
| | Pigments/dyes |
| | Opacifiers – titanium/zinc oxides |
| | Plasticiser – dibutyl phthalate |
| | Synthetic fibres – nylon/acrylic |
| Liquid: | Methyl methacrylate monomer |
| | Inhibitor – hydroquinone |
| | Cross-linking agent – ethylene glycol |
| | Dimethacrylate |

(i.e. the beads or granules) has already been polymerised.

Granules dissolve more readily in the monomer than beads and hence reduce the time taken to reach the doughy stage.

The monomer is extremely volatile and highly flammable, so the container must be kept sealed at all times and must be kept away from naked flames. The container is a dark glass bottle, which extend the shelf life of the monomer by avoiding spontaneous polymerisation from the action of light.

Hydroquinone also extends the shelf life of the monomer by reacting rapidly with any free radicals that may form spontaneously within the liquid and producing forms of stabilised free radicals that are not able to initiate the polymerisation process.

Contamination with the polymer beads or granules must be avoided, as these carry the benzoyl peroxide on their surface and only a tiny amount of the polymer is needed to start the polymerisation reaction.

The polymer powder is very stable and has a virtually indefinite shelf life.

A cross-linking agent such as diethylene glycol dimethacrylate is included in order to improve the mechanical properties (**144a**). These are incorporated at various points along the methylmethacrylate polymer chain and form cross-links with adjacent chains by virtue of their two double bond sites (**144b**).

Thus, although the polymethyl methacrylate (PMMA) is a thermoplastic resin, the inclusion of the cross-linking agent prevents post-processing.

(a)

Me
|
$CH_2=C$

Me
|
$C=CH_2$   or   N–N

|
$C–OOCH_2–CH_2OO–C$

(b)

R - M - M - M - M - N - M - M - R
|
R - M - N - M - N - M - M - M - R
|
R - M - M - N - M - M - M - N - M - R
|
- M - N - M - M - etc

**144** Diethylene glycol dimethacrylate (a), and its formation of cross-links (b).

## Cold-Cure Resins

The chemistry of these resins is identical to that of the heat-cured resins, except that the cure is initiated by a tertiary amine (e.g. dimethyl-P-toluidine or sulfinic acid) rather than heat.

This method of curing is not as efficient as the heat curing process, and tends to result in a lower molecular weight material. This has an adverse effect on the strength properties of the material and also raises the amount of uncured residual monomer in the resin. The colour stability is not as good as for the heat-cured material, and the cold-cured resins are more prone to yellowing.

The size of the polymer beads is somewhat smaller than in the heat-cured resin (which has a bead size of 150 µm) to ease dissolution in the monomer to produce a dough. The doughy stage has to be reached before the addition curing reaction begins to affect the viscosity of the mix and prevents the adaptation of the mix to the mould walls.

The lower molecular weight also results in a lowering of the glass transition temperature, with $T_g$ being typically 75–80°C. Whilst one might think that this makes the material more inclined to warpage, as no external heat source is used to cure the resin there is a lower build up of internal strain. Nevertheless, the material is highly susceptible to creep, and this can contribute significantly to the eventual distortion of the denture when in use.

## Pour-And-Cure Resins

These are cold-cure resins that are sufficiently liquid when mixed that they can be poured into a mould made of a hydrocolloid. They give excellent reproduction of surface detail but are inferior to both the heat- and cold-cured acrylics in so many other respects that they are not much used.

## Visible-Light Cured Resins

This is a relatively recent innovation and still awaits full evaluation of the clinical efficacy. The material has more in common with a composite restorative material than with the denture base resins considered above. It is composed of a matrix of urethane dimethacrylate that contains a small amount of colloidal silica to control the rheology. The filler consists of acrylic beads that become part of an interpenetrating polymer network structure when it is cured.

# Aspects of manipulation

## Powder:Liquid Ratio

It is important to use the correct powder:liquid ratio (2.0:1.0 wt%; 1.6:1.0 vol%). Too much powder could result in under-wetting of the polymer beads by the monomer, resulting in a weak material. Too much monomer will produce excessive polymerisation shrinkage and a loss of quality of fit to the denture bearing surface.

The additives tend to settle out at the bottom of the container and it is important that the container is shaken before use to ensure an even distribution of the powder ingredients.

## Control Of Colour

The colouring pigment is usually incorporated in the polymer powder, but in some cases it may simply be on the surface of the polymer beads and may be washed off by too rapid a contact of the monomer. In this case, the polymer should be added to the monomer slowly. Too little powder will produce too light a shade.

## Mould Lining

There is a danger that the resin may penetrate the relatively rough surface of the plaster mould and adhere to it. To prevent this, a separating medium must be employed. Nowadays, the separating medium is usually a solution of sodium alginate, although some still recommend the use of tin foil.

## Processing

There are two problems in particular to watch out for in the processing of acrylics for dentures: one is their porosity and the second is the presence of processing strains.

### Porosity

The problem one is most likely to experience with acrylic resin dentures is the occurrence of porosity during the processing stage. There are two major causes of porosity: polymerisation shrinkage, termed *contraction porosity*, and volatilisation of the monomer, termed *gaseous porosity*.

Contraction porosity occurs because the monomer contracts by some 20% of its volume during processing. By using the powder/liquid system, this contraction is minimised and should be in the region of 5–8%. However, this is not translated into a high linear shrinkage, which, on the basis of the volumetric shrinkage, should be of the order of 1.5–2%, but is in fact somewhere in the region of 0.2–0.5%. It is believed that this is because the observed contraction is due to thermal contraction in the change from curing temperature to room temperature and not to the curing contraction.

At the curing temperature, the resin is able to flow into the spaces created by the curing contraction. The driving force for this flow is provided by pressure that is exerted during the processing; packing a slight excess of denture base material into the mould ensures that the material is under pressure when the mould is closed. This pressure is maintained throughout the processing cycle.

The resin only becomes rigid once it gets below its glass transition temperature, at which point the curing contraction will have been completed. From this point on, it is the thermal contraction that contributes to the observed changes in dimensions of the denture base. Cold-cure resins should give a better fit for the denture, as the processing temperature is considerably lower (around 60°C, compared to 100°C for the heat-cured resin). However, the fit is normally compromised due to the increased likelihood of creep from the lower $T_g$.

It is therefore important that sufficient dough is packed in the mould to ensure that the material is under pressure during processing. This will cause any voids present in the mix to collapse, and should also help to compensate for the curing contraction. Thus, the packing of the mould should only be carried out when the mix has reached the doughy stage, as, prior to this, the high flow causes a rapid loss of pressure. If there is evidence of localised porosity, it may be due to poor mixing of the components or to packing the mould before the doughy stage is reached. The associated differential contraction can lead to distortion of the denture.

On polymerisation, there is an exothermic reaction which could cause the temperature of the resin to rise above its boiling temperature, which is just above 100°C. If this temperature is exceeded before the polymerisation process is completed, gaseous monomer will be formed – this is the cause of gaseous porosity. The amount of heat generated depends upon the volume of resin present, the proportion of monomer and the rapidity with which the external heat reaches the resin. The occurrence of gaseous porosity can be avoided by allowing the temperature to be raised in a slow and controlled fashion.

Thus, it can be seen that polymerisation must be carried out *slowly* (to prevent gaseous porosity) and *under pressure* (to avoid contraction porosity).

### Processing Strains

The restriction imposed upon the dimensional change of the resin will inevitably give rise to internal strains. If such strains were allowed to relax, the result would be warpage, crazing, or distortion of the denture base. Although many of the strains generated during the curing contraction can be relieved by the flow that occurs above the glass transition temperature, some strain that is due to thermal contraction will remain. The level of the internal strain can be minimised by using acrylic rather than porcelain teeth (so that there is no differential shrinkage on cooling) and by allowing the flask to cool slowly.

The relief of internal strain can produce tiny surface cracks in the resin. These are known as *crazes*, and can be identified by a hazy or foggy appearance to the surface of the denture base. Sometimes the cracks may be visible with the naked eye.

The crazes may be formed in response to heat (due to polishing, for example), differential contraction around porcelain teeth, or attack by solvents such as alcohol. The introduction of cross-links in the polymer chains has been found to reduce the potential for craze formation.

# Properties

## *Biocompatibility*

In general, PMMA is highly biocompatible and patients suffer few problems. Nevertheless, some patients will show an allergic reaction. This is most probably associated with the various leachable components in the denture, such as any residual monomer.

The allergic reaction tends to be virtually immediate, and is more likely to occur with cold-cured resin dentures because of their higher residual monomer content. Sometimes it may be possible to overcome this problem by subjecting the denture to an additional curing cycle, but there is a danger that this will cause the denture to distort as internal processing stresses are relieved.

Alternative denture base materials, such as polycarbonates, may have to be considered.

## *Dimensional Stability And Accuracy*

Given that the denture is placed on an adaptable cushion of soft tissues, one may wonder why it is so important that the denture does not change its shape. In fact, it is a matter of great concern to the *retention* of the denture, where retention can be defined as the resistance to forces that tend to displace the denture in an occlusal direction. This is distinct from *stability*, which is the resistance to movement in a horizontal direction.

The factors that determine the retention of dentures in the mouth are essentially physical in nature. Anatomical factors such as undercuts are a nuisance rather than an advantage, as the denture is rigid and can not engage them. In some instances preprosthetic surgery may be required to remove the undercut.

The most appropriate explanation of the factors that govern the retention of a denture is the viscous flow model (as discussed in section I.X), which is based on the relationship

$$F = \frac{3\pi\eta R^4}{2h^3} \frac{\delta h}{\delta t}$$

for a disc with radius, R, and a thickness of saliva, h.

Adhesion of the denture to the mucosa is provided by saliva, and the greater the surface area the better the adhesive bond (i.e. R should be as large as possible).

At the same time, it is important that the cohesion of the saliva film is not destroyed and this is best guarded against by having as thin a film of saliva between the mucosa and denture as is possible (i.e. h should be small), so the denture should fit as accurately as possible.

The establishment of a peripheral seal around the edge of the denture is very important for retention. The tighter the seal, the more difficult it is for additional saliva to enter the space between the denture and the mucosa, and this means that more force needs to be applied to separate the denture from the mucosa.

Anything that may upset the peripheral seal, such as over-extension, interferences (e.g. a frenal notch) and occlusal imbalance, will impair the retention of the denture.

As patients get older, the rate of production and the consistency of their saliva may change. The saliva becomes less adhesive to the denture, due to poor wetting of the surface by an inadequate supply of saliva, and it also becomes less viscous. Denture retention can then become a particular problem, and denture fixatives may have to be employed.

Thus, for a denture to have the optimum retention it should:

- Cover the maximum area of mucosa compatible with the functional muscular activity.
- Be a close fit, so as to minimise the thickness of the saliva film and retain a good peripheral seal.

## Mechanical Properties

The tensile strength of acrylic resins is typically no more than 50 MPa. The elastic modulus is low, and the flexural modulus being in the region of 2200–2500 MPa. When this is combined with a lack of fracture toughness, it is perhaps not surprising that dentures are prone to fracture.

Most fractures are associated with some traumatic incident to the denture, although this may not be easily recognised. If dropped on the floor a denture does not necessarily break instantly, but the chances are that a crack will have formed that will continue to grow until the denture fails suddenly and catastrophically.

Some fractures may be associated with poor quality processing. Lack of bonding between the resin and the acrylic teeth is such a possibility, and gives rise to a weak interface from which a fracture is likely to be initiated.

For those patients who fracture their dentures on a regular basis, it is possible to consider a high-impact-resistant denture base resin. These resins are formulated with a rubber toughening agent, such as a fine dispersion of butadiene styrene. The rubbery inclusions cause a lowering of the flexural modulus but also stop cracks developing, showing a higher degree of resistance to fracture as a consequence.

Creep is a problem with acrylic resins (particularly the cold-cured resins) as they are viscoelastic materials. The addition of a cross-linking agent reduces the amount of creep, but it cannot be totally eliminated.

## Physical Properties

### Thermal Conductivity

The thermal conductivity of PMMA is approximately $6 \times 10^{-4}$ cal.gm$^{-1}$.cm$^{-2}$. This is very low, and can present problems during denture processing as the heat produced cannot escape, leading to a temperature rise.

From the patient's point of view, the problem with a low coefficient of thermal conductivity is that the denture isolates the oral soft tissues from any sensation of temperature. This can lead to a patient consuming a drink that is far too hot without realising it, which may lead to the back of the throat and possibly even the oesophagus being scalded.

### Coefficient Of Thermal Expansion

The coefficient of thermal expansion is approximately 80 ppm/°C. This is quite high, as one might expect from a resin. In general, this does not present a problem, except that there is a possibility that porcelain teeth set in denture base resin may gradually loosen and be lost due the differential expansion and contraction.

### Water Sorption And Solubility

Due to the polar nature of the resin molecules, PMMA will absorb water. This water sorption is typically of the order of 1.0–2.0% by weight.

In practice, this helps to compensate for the slight processing shrinkage. However, given the low rate of diffusion of water through the resin, it would take the denture some weeks of continuous immersion in water to reach a stable weight.

Although PMMA is soluble in most solvents (e.g. chloroform), it is virtually insoluble in most of the fluids that it may come into contact with in the mouth. However, some weight loss *will* occur, due to leaching of the monomer in particular, and possibly some of the pigments and dyes.

## Summary

The advantages of the use of polymethylmethacrylate are that it:

- Has excellent aesthetics.
- Is easy and cheap to process.
- Has a low density.

The disadvantages are that the material:

- Has barely adequate strength characteristics.
- Is susceptible to distortion.
- Has a low thermal conductivity.
- Is radiolucent.

# Denture Lining Materials

The denture lining materials fall essentially into three groups, namely:

- Hard relining materials.
- Soft liners.
- Tissue conditioners.

| Table 43 The two types of cold-cured resin. | | |
|---|---|---|
| | Type I | Type II |
| Powder | Polymethyl methacrylate | Polyethyl methacrylate |
| | Benzoyl peroxide | Benzoyl peroxide |
| | Pigments | Pigments |
| Liquid | Methyl methacrylate monomer | Butyl methacrylate |
| | Di-n-butylphthalate | Amine |
| | Amine | |

## Hard Reline Materials

If the fitting surface of a denture needs to be replaced to improve the fit of the denture, a *hard reline* material can be employed. This can be achieved either with a cold-cure acrylic resin at the chair-side, or the denture is sent to a dental laboratory for relining with a heat-cured acrylic.

The heat-cured acrylics used by laboratories are identical to those used for the construction of dentures. The cold-cured resins come in two types, with constituents as listed in *Table 43*.

The reason for the second type of reline material is that methylmethacrylate (MMA) can be very irritant to soft tissues and can sensitise the patient.

The polyethylmethacrylate (PEMA) and butylmethacrylate are less irritant to the patient, but have the disadvantage that they cause a reduction in the $T_g$, and this increases the possibility of dimensional instability.

One of the most serious drawbacks with attempting a chair-side reline is that there is little control over the amount of denture material removed and the thickness of the reline material that replaces it. At best, it should be considered only as a temporary expedient, with laboratory relines being much preferred.

## Soft Liners

Occasionally, a patient will complain of persistent pain and discomfort from a denture, even though the denture would appear totally satisfactory in all other respects.

This problem is seen most commonly in the lower jaw, where there is a smaller surface area over which to distribute the load, and where patients may have a sharp, thin or heavily resorbed alveolar ridge. In such cases, the patient has difficulty in tolerating a hard denture. If the pain persists when all possible measures have been taken to minimise the occusal load, the

| Table 44 Glass transition temperatures for polymethacrylate esters. | |
|---|---|
| Group | Transition Temperature (°C) |
| Methyl | 125 |
| Ethyl | 65 |
| Propyl | 38 |
| Butyl | 33 |

denture may be made more comfortable by the use of a soft liner. This provides a means of absorbing some of the energy involved in mastication, by interposing a highly resilient material between the denture and the mucosa.

Polymers with a glass transition temperature just above the temperature in the mouth will have a rubbery behaviour and are highly resilient.

Some polymers have a naturally low glass transition temperature (e.g. silicone polymers) and others (e.g. polymethylmethacrylate) can be modified by the inclusion of plasticisers to reduce their glass transition temperature (see *Table 44*).

The plasticiser acts as a lubricant for the polymer chains, making it easier for them to slide past one another, allowing the material to deform more easily and giving it a lower elastic modulus. In fact, soft liners are usually constructed from these two materials.

### Silicone Rubber

The silicone rubber consists of a polydimethylsiloxane polymer to which filler is added to give it the correct consistency. The material solidifies by a cross-linking process rather than by a polymerisation process, as the material is already a polymer. This cross-linking can be achieved either by heat, using benzoyl peroxide, or at room temperature, using tetraethylsilicate.

Silicone rubber does not bond readily to the acrylic resin of the denture, so an adhesive needs

**Table 45** Relative merits of soft liners.

| Silicone Rubber | Acrylic |
|---|---|
| Highly resilient | Less resilient |
| Retain softness | Go hard with time |
| Requires bonding agent | Self adhesive |
| Susceptible to growth of *Candida albicans* | More resistant to bacteria |
| Weak bond | Permanent bond |
| Poor tear strength | Acceptable tear strength |
| No permanent deformation | Susceptible to creep |

to be employed. This adhesion can be achieved using silicone polymer dissolved in a solvent, or by the use of an alkyl–silane coupling agent.

In both cases the bond is very weak, and usually fails within a relatively short time. Another drawback is that this material tends to support the growth of *Candida albicans*, which leads to denture stomatitis.

### Acrylic Soft Liners

These soft liners have the advantage that they bond well to the PMMA denture. They can be subdivided into those which contain leachable plasticisers and those which contain polymerisable plasticisers.

### Leachable Plasticiser Systems

Polyethylmethacrylate (PEMA) has a glass transition temperature of only 66°C, compared with 100°C for PMMA. A combination of these two polymers, with a small amount of plasticiser (such as dibutylphthalate) is highly resilient. Thus, the powder is a mixture of PEMA and PMMA and the liquid is MMA, containing 25–50% plasticiser.

Unfortunately, the plasticiser gradually leaches out, and the liner becomes stiff as it looses its resilience. How rapidly this transition takes place depends to some extent on the patient's regime for cleaning the denture. In general, high temperatures and strong bleaching agents should be avoided.

### Polymerisable Plasticiser Systems

New plasticisers have been developed that polymerise, and thus resist dissolution, but which maintain their lubricating effect .

Exact formulations of this new material are not known, but some use alkyl-maleate or alkyl-itaconate, while for one experimental system the liquid component is known to be a mixture of tridecylmethacrylate, 2-diethylhexyl maleate and ethylene glycol dimethacrylate. The liquid is mixed with either PEMA or copolymers of n-butyl and ethylmethacrylate.

The material is fairly hard at room temperature, which makes it easy to finish, and softens when taken up to mouth temperature.

## Relative Merits Of Soft Liners

The relative merits of the silicone and acrylic soft liners are outlined in *Table 45*.

## Tissue Conditioners

In some instances, the denture can give rise to inflammation or ulceration of the load-bearing soft tissues.

A simple solution would be for the patient to stop wearing the denture until the inflammation has subsided. This is not generally acceptable to the patient, and a tissue conditioner can be employed to overcome the problem.

A tissue conditioner is a soft material that is applied temporarily to the fitting surface of the denture for the purpose of allowing a more even stress distribution. This permits the mucosal tissue to return to its normal shape, and to resolve any inflammation of the denture bearing tissues. Once the inflammation has receded and the tissue has recovered, an impression can be taken for a new denture.

Such a material must be exceptionally soft, yet not so soft as to squeeze out from between the denture and the mucosa. These materials consist of a powder of PEMA, which, when mixed with a solvent such as ethyl alcohol and an aromatic ester such as a plasticiser (e.g. butyl phthalyl-butylglycolate), produces a gel-like substance.

The alcohol and plasticiser will leach out quickly, and, therefore, the tissue conditioner needs to be replaced every few days if the traumatised tissue is to revert to a healthy state as soon as possible.

These tissue conditioners are sensitive to denture cleansers, and are best cleaned with plain soap and water.

# Further Reading

Abou-Tabl Z. M., Tidy D. C., Combe E. C. & Grant A. A. (1983) The development of modified denture base materials. J. Biomed. Mat. Res. **17**, 885

Lamb D. J., Ellis B. & Priestley D. (1983) The effects of processing variables on levels of residual monomer in autopolymerizing dental acrylic resin. J. Dent. **11**, 1

Huggett R., John G., Jagger R. G. & Bates J. F. (1982) Strength of the acrylic denture base tooth bond. Brit. Dent. J. **153**, 187

McCabe J. F. & Basker R. M. (1976) Tissue sensitivity to acrylic resin. Brit. Dent. J. **140**, 347

Stafford G. D., Huggett R., MacGregor A. R. & Graham J. (1986) The use of nylon as a denture-base material. J. Dent. **14**, 18

Turrell A. J. W. (1966) Allergy to denture base material – fallacy or reality? Brit. Dent. J. **120**, 415

Wright P. S. (1976) Soft lining materials: their status and prospects. J. Dent. **4**, 247

# III.III

## CASTING ALLOYS FOR METALLIC RESTORATIONS

## Introduction

The production of metallic restorations, such as crowns, bridges, inlays, cast posts and cores and partial dentures in the dental laboratory is carried out by the *lost wax casting* technique. This method of casting has been around for a considerable time, and is much used by craftsmen to produce intricate jewellery and ornaments. Its history can be traced back beyond 3000 B.C., but it was not used in dentistry until the 1890s.

The basic principles are simple. A wax model is produced of the desired shape, and this model is invested in a material resistant to high temperatures. The wax is then removed by melting and burning, leaving behind a cavity of the desired shape. This can now be filled with molten metal, so that the metal assumes the shape of the original wax carving. The stages in the production of a dental casting are therefore as follows:

- Preparation of the dentition.
- Production of an impression.
- Pouring of a model.
- Waxing of the desired shape.
- Investing the wax pattern.
- Burn-out and heating.
- Melting and casting the alloy.
- Finishing and polishing.
- Heat treatments.

Thus, it can be seen that many different materials are involved in the production of a metal casting. These include impression materials, model and die materials, waxes, investment materials and casting alloys. Some of these have already been discussed already in previous sections.

A detailed account of the various practical stages involved in the production of a metal casting will not be provided here as this process is the prerogative of the dental technician. Instead, attention will be focused on the alloys that are used and the requirements that are placed upon them for their applications in restorative dentistry.

It is the responsibility of the dentist to request the most suitable alloy for a particular application when instructing a dental laboratory to produce a prosthesis. This choice should not be left to the dental technician. After all, it is the dentist who will be placing these materials in the patient's mouth and therefore it is the dentist who needs to know what they are providing their patient with. This requires a knowledge of the types of alloys available, their composition and properties.

The main alloys that are employed in dentistry are gold alloys, palladium alloys, and various non-noble metal alloys such as Co–Cr or Ni–Cr.

**Table 46** Composition of high-gold alloys.

| Type | Description | Au% | Ag% | Cu% | Pt% | Pd% | Zn% |
|------|-------------|------|-------|-------|-----|-----|-----|
| I | Soft | 80–90 | 3–12 | 2–5 | – | – | – |
| II | Medium | 75–78 | 12–15 | 7–10 | 0–1 | 1–4 | 0–1 |
| III | Hard | 62–78 | 8–26 | 8–11 | 0–3 | 2–4 | 0–1 |
| IV | Extra hard | 60–70 | 4–20 | 11–16 | 0–4 | 0–5 | 1–2 |

# Desirable Properties

The choice of alloy is governed by a number of factors. Cost is a serious consideration due to the increased price of gold today. Other considerations are the biocompatibility of the alloy and its resistance to corrosion and tarnish. It is these factors that particularly limit the range of alloys available for dental applications.

Suitability for a specific application, be it a low-stress bearing inlay or a posterior bridge, is determined primarily by the mechanical properties of the alloy, such as its stiffness, strength, ductility, and hardness.

Stiffness is a consequence both of design and of the elastic modulus of the alloy. The higher the elastic modulus, the stiffer the structure will be for the same shape. This is an important consideration, especially for long-span bridges, cast posts, partial dentures and denture clasps. These restorations are also likely to be subjected to fairly high loads and therefore need to be resistant to permanent deformation. This requires the alloy to have a high yield stress or proof stress.

However, for such things as clasps, high strength needs to be balanced against ductility, since it is important that the alloy is not so brittle as to fracture when small adjustments are made.

In the case of inlays, where marginal adaptation is usually improved by burnishing, ductility is even more important. Alloys for these applications need to be very ductile and soft if they are not to fracture during this procedure.

Thus, alloys with a wide range of properties are needed to satisfy these varied requirements.

Another important consideration is the quality of fit of the restoration. This is governed by the ease of casting of the alloy. The dental technician will want to know what the melting range and casting temperature is for the alloy, as, in general, the higher these are, the more problems the alloy presents in handling.

The density of the alloy is also important. Most castings are carried out in a centrifugal force-casting machine, and the higher the density of the alloy, the easier it is to force the air out of the mould space and to fill the space completely with alloy.

Casting shrinkage and cooling contraction are other considerations. These have to be accounted for if the casting is not to be too small. The higher the shrinkage, the more of a problem this becomes.

Thus, it is important to have a close working relationship with the dental laboratory, and to take into account their views when choosing an alloy.

# High-Gold Alloys

This is a group of alloys that have been around for some considerable time and that can be distinguished from other alloys used in dentistry by their high noble metal content, which must not be less than 75%. The noble metal content is usually made up of gold, silver, platinum and palladium. These alloys can be classified into four distinct groups as indicated in *Table 46*.

The amount of gold in an alloy is defined in one of two ways:

- *Carat* – Pure gold has a carat value of 24, and an alloy's carat is expressed in terms of the number of 24th parts of gold within it. Thus, an alloy with 50% gold would be designated as a 12 carat gold alloy. Much jewellery is 9 carat gold (37.5%) or 18 carat gold (75%).
- *Fineness* – Pure gold has a fineness rating of 1000, so that 18 carat gold is 750 fine, and 9 carat gold is 375 fine.

Thus, the dental gold alloys in *Table 46* vary from 21.6–14.4 carat, or 900–600 fine.

## Alloying Elements In Dental Gold Alloys

The largest fraction by far of these alloys is gold, with lower amounts of silver and copper. Some formulations also contain very small amounts of platinum, palladium and zinc.

The silver has a slight strengthening effect and counteracts the reddish tint of the copper.

The copper is a very important component as it increases the strength, particularly of the Type III and IV gold alloys, and reduces the melting temperature. The limit to the amount of copper that can be added is 16%, as amounts in excess of this tend to cause the alloy to tarnish.

Platinum increases both the strength and the melting temperature. Palladium has the same effect as platinum, but is considerably cheaper.

Zinc acts as a *scavenger* during casting, preventing oxidation, and improves the castability.

A variety of other elements, such as iridium, ruthenium and rhenium (<0.5%) may be present. These have very high melting temperature and act as nucleating sites during solidification, thus helping to produce a fine grain size.

## Strengthening Mechanism

Although all of the alloying elements give rise to some increase in the yield strength of the gold alloy by forming a solid solution, the most effective strengthening mechanism is the addition of copper, in what is known as *order-hardening*.

This hardening heat treatment is carried out after the homogenising anneal at approximately 700°C, which is carried out to ensure a uniform composition throughout the casting. It involves reheating the alloy to 400°C and holding it at that temperature for approximately 30 minutes. Rather than being randomly distributed the copper atoms arrange themselves in little ordered clusters.

This ordered structure prevents slippage of the atomic layers, which has the effect of raising the yield stress and the hardness of the alloy. There must be at least 11% copper in the gold alloy for order hardening to occur, so it can not occur in Type I and Type II gold alloys. Type III gold alloys have just enough copper, and a small improvement in strength is observed. For Type IV gold alloys, the improvement in strength is quite significant.

The effect of this strengthening process is shown in *Table 47*. The addition of copper, combined with the hardening heat treatment can result in a ten-fold increase in the yield strength. The importance of the hardening heat treatment for the Type III and IV gold alloys is also indicated. However, there is a price to pay in terms of a reduction in the ductility of the alloy, as shown by the lower percentage elongation at which failure occurs. Thus, excessive bending may give rise to brittle fracture, a problem that may arise when producing partial denture clasp arms out of a Type IV gold alloy.

For some alloys, the hardening process is to allow the alloy to cool slowly on the bench rather than quenching it immediately on casting. This technique is commonly known as *self-hardening*.

The disadvantage with this approach is that it is not as well-controlled as when the alloy is first given a homogenising anneal and then a hardening heat treatment. It is important that the dentist stipulates to the dental technician that a hardening heat treatment is to be carried out if a Type III or IV gold alloy is chosen, unless a self hardening alloy has been selected in which case it should be allowed to cool slowly on the bench and should not be quenched.

## Other Features

As the alloying elements form a solid solution readily with the gold, the difference between the liquidus and the solidus is small. This makes these alloys relatively easy to cast and produces a reasonably homogeneous result. The addition of platinum and palladium gives a larger gap between the liquidus and the solidus, and makes a homogenising anneal more desirable for the Type III and IV gold alloys.

Due to their low casting temperature, the casting shrinkage is readily compensated for by the use of a gypsum-bonded investment.

The low Vickers hardness values (VHN) make these alloys easy to polish to a smooth surface finish, although in the case of the heat-hardening alloys this is better done in the as-cast condition.

In general, it can be said that the use of these alloys does not present a major problem to the dental technician, and good quality, well fitting castings can be produced. Their corrosion and tarnish resistance is excellent, as is their biocompatibility.

**Table 47** Range of mechanical properties of high-gold alloys.

| Type | Condition | $\sigma_y$ (MPa) | UTS (MPa) | Elongation (%) | VHN |
|------|-----------|--------|-----------|----------------|-----|
| I | As cast | 60-140 | 200-310 | 20-35 | 40-70 |
| II | As cast | 140-250 | 310-380 | 20-35 | 70-100 |
| III | As cast | 180-260 | 330-390 | 20-25 | 90-130 |
|  | Hardened | 280-350 | 410-560 | 6-20 | 115-170 |
| IV | As cast | 300-390 | 410-520 | 4-25 | 130-160 |
|  | Hardened | 550-680 | 690-830 | 1-6 | 200-240 |

**Table 48** Composition of medium- and low-gold alloys.

| Alloy | Type | Colour | Au (%) | Pd (%) | Ag (%) | Cu (%) | In (%) |
|-------|------|--------|--------|--------|--------|--------|--------|
| Solaro 3 (Metalor) | Medium-gold | Yellow | 56 | 5 | 25 | 11.8 | – |
| Stabilor G (Degussa) | Medium-gold | Yellow | 58 | 5.5 | 23.3 | 12.0 | – |
| Mattident E (Johnson Matthey) | Medium-gold | Yellow | 55 | 8.0 | 24.0 | 11.5 | – |
| Palaginor 2 (Metalor) | Low-gold | White | 12.5 | 18.9 | 53.7 | 14.2 | – |
| Palliag MJ (Degussa) | Low-gold | White | 12.5 | 20.9 | 55.0 | 8.5 | – |
| Mattident B (Johnson Matthey) | Low-gold | White | 11.0 | 20.0 | 54.5 | 12.5 | – |
| Realor (Degussa) | Low-gold copper-free | Yellow | 20.0 | 20.0 | 39.0 | – | 16.0 |
| Selector 3 (Metalor) | Low-gold copper-free | Yellow | 20.0 | 21.0 | 38.7 | – | 16.5 |
| Mattieco J (Johnson Matthey) | Low-gold copper-free | Yellow | 20.0 | 20.0 | 40.1 | – | 17.8 |

## *Applications*

Given their different mechanical properties, the recommended applications for the use of these alloys is as follows:

- *Type I alloys* – These are best used for inlays in low stress situations. As they are relatively soft and easily deformed they need plenty of support to prevent deformation under occlusal loading. The low yield stress of these alloys allows the margins to be burnished easily. Given the high ductility, they are unlikely to fracture.
- *Type II alloys* – These can be used for most inlays. However, those with thin sections should be avoided as deformation is still a possibility.
- *Type III alloys* – These can be used for all inlays, onlays, full coverage crowns and short-span bridges, cast posts and cores because of their greater strength than Type I and Type II alloys. However, they will be more difficult to burnish, and have a higher potential for localised fracture if they are burnished excessively.
- Type IV alloys – these are used for cast posts and cores, long-span bridges and in partial denture construction, particularly clasp arms. Clasp arms can be adjusted in the as-cast state, and then heat hardened. Of course, this will not be possible when using a self hardening alloy. The low elastic modulus and high yield strength of the gold alloy provide a high degree of flexibility to clasp arms, which allows them to be withdrawn over quite severe undercuts without danger of permanent deformation. These alloys can not be burnished in their hardened state, and are therefore unsuitable for inlays.

# Medium- And Low-Gold Alloys

The rapid rise in the prices of noble metals in the 1970s has stimulated manufacturers to produce many new alloys with reduced gold contents. Compositions of a few representative commercial examples are presented in *Table 48*. Some of these may be classed as medium-gold alloys, with the gold content varying from 40–60%.

These medium-gold alloys were introduced in the early 1970s, and have become very popular in recent years. The palladium and silver contents were increased to compensate for the reduced gold content, while the copper content is in the range of 10–15%. Palladium is added to counteract the tendency of silver to tarnish.

The palladium, silver and copper readily form substitutional solid solutions, with the gold producing a single phase structure throughout the entire compositional range. The presence of copper allows order hardening, just as with the Type III and IV gold alloys.

There are also a number of low-gold alloys which have gold contents typically of the order of 15–20%. The other elements are silver (40–60%) and palladium (up to 40%); these alloys could thus be described as Ag–Pd alloys, but we will leave that description for those alloys containing minor amounts of gold (<2%) or no gold at all.

Due to the reduced gold content, these alloys are white in appearance; they are less attractive to the patient who prefers the appearance of the yellow gold alloys. In order to overcome this disadvantage, there are also a number of copper-free low-gold alloys which contain high levels of indium. These have a two-phase structure consisting of a FCC matrix with islands of a BCC phase due to the high indium content.

The matrix phase is essentially a Ag–Au solid solution with minor additions of palladium, indium and zinc. The BCC phase consists of Pd–In with substantial amounts of gold, silver and zinc, giving the alloy its yellow colour. Thus, the colour seems to be related to the presence of the indium rather than the absence of copper.

### Properties And Applications

Some of the properties of these alloys are compared in *Table 49*. The medium-gold alloys are recommended for the same applications as Type III and IV gold alloys. Their ductility tends to be lower than that of the Type IV gold alloys and their high yield stress makes them difficult to burnish. There is even a danger of fracture on burnishing, due to the localised work-hardening that occurs and further reduces their ductility. However, they are very suitable for long-span prostheses and may be used for implant-supported prostheses and posts and cores.

The low-gold content alloys tend to have lower mechanical properties than the medium-gold alloys, and are recommended as an alternative to Type III gold alloys. However, their white colour makes them less popular than they might otherwise be. These alloys are extensively used for posts and cores, where the white colour does not present a problem as the casting will be covered with another material.

The removal of the copper and the addition of the indium again produces alloys with properties similar to those of the Type III gold alloys, but with the advantage of the yellow colour. However, the gap between the solidus and the liquidus is greater, which can result in a less homogeneous structure, and their melting temperature is considerably higher, making the casting process more difficult.

Although, in general, the medium-gold alloys are a suitable alternative to the Type IV gold alloys, and the low-gold alloys for Type III gold alloys, one problem with these alloys is that their properties are more variable from alloy to alloy than for the four types of high-gold alloys. This requires the dentist to examine carefully the properties of each alloy, and, if necessary, to seek advice from the dental laboratory in order to determine the suitability of an alloy for a particular clinical application (*Table 49*).

The biocompatibility of these alloys appears to be excellent, and corrosion does not seem to be a problem, even with the two-phase low-gold copper-free alloys.

# Silver–Palladium Alloys

As the name implies, Ag–Pd alloys contain predominantly silver with significant amounts of palladium.

The palladium improves the resistance to corrosion and helps to prevent tarnish, which is usually associated with the silver. These alloys were introduced in the 1960s as an alternative to the high-gold alloys, and are commonly called 'white golds'.

The composition and the properties of some representative alloys after their heat hardening treatment are presented in *Table 50*. Although there is some self-hardening with these alloys if they are left to bench cool, the properties are generally inferior when compared to a carefully controlled hardening heat treatment.

**Table 49** Comparison of some properties of medium- and low-gold casting alloys compared to a Type IV gold alloy.

| Alloy | Type | Vickers Harness Number | Elastic Modulus (GPa) | 0.2% Proof Stress (MPa) | Elongation (%) | Solidus–Liquidus Temperature (°C) | Casting Temperature (°C) |
|---|---|---|---|---|---|---|---|
| Aurofluid 3 | Type IV | 255 | 80 | 480 | 10 | 885–920 | 1070 |
| Solaro 3 | Medium-gold | 285 | 90.5 | 600 | 10 | 870–920 | 1070 |
| Stabilor G | Medium-gold | 275 | – | 830 | 6 | – | 1000–1100 |
| Mattident E | Medium-gold | 269 | – | 685 | 7 | 885–945 | 1045–1145 |
| Palaginor 2 | Low-gold | 170 | 82 | 340 | 12 | 875–970 | 1200 |
| Palliag MJ | Low-gold | 265 | – | 630 | 4 | 940–1010 | 1100–1200 |
| Mattident B | Low-gold | 256 | – | 645 | 3.5 | 945–1000 | 1100–1200 |
| Realor | Low-gold Cu-free | 185 | – | 405 | 6 | 860–1035 | 1200 |
| Selector 3 | Low-gold Cu-free | 180 | 75 | 370 | 8 | 875–1035 | 1200 |
| Mattieco J | Low-gold Cu-free | 200 | – | 740 | 5 | 870–940 | 1080–1150 |

*Data taken from the manufacturers' data sheets

**Table 50** Composition and properties of silver/palladium alloys.

| Alloy | Ag (%) | Pd (%) | Cu (%) | Zn (%) | VHN | 0.2% Proof Stress (MPa) | Elongation (%) | Solidus-Liquidus Temperature(°C) | Casting Temperature (°C) |
|---|---|---|---|---|---|---|---|---|---|
| Palliag W (Degussa) | 70.0 | 27.5 | – | – | 55 | 80 | 33 | 1080–1180 | – |
| Mattico 25 (Johnson Matthey) | 68.5 | 25.0 | – | 3.0 | 199 | 500 | 31 | 1050–1110 | 1210–1290 |
| Palliag M (Degussa) | 58.5 | 27.4 | 10.5 | – | 310 | 940 | 3 | 950–1040 | 1100–1200 |
| Palliag NF IV (Degussa) | 52.0 | 39.9 | – | 4.0 | 270 | 595 | 6 | 1070–1145 | 1200–1250 |
| Mattident P (Johnson Matthey) | 46.6 | 33.4 | 19.0 | – | 290 | 780 | 3 | 1005–1040 | 1140–1240 |

* Data taken from manufacturers' data sheets.

There are two notable features of the data presented in *Table 48*. First, there is the wide range of properties in the different alloys, which again highlights the need to select the alloy for the application in mind very carefully. The low strength and hardness and the high ductility of one of the alloys shown (Palliag W) suggests that this alloy is suitable only for low stress-bearing inlays. The other alloy with a similar composition (Mattieco 25) has superior mechanical properties, being more comparable to a Type III gold alloy, and could be used for crowns, short-span bridges and post and cores.

However, those alloys with reduced silver content and increased palladium content have properties similar to those of the Type IV gold alloys. Their use for long-span prostheses is generally contraindicated. This may be associated with the high casting temperatures for these alloys which is the second most notable feature of these materials.

These high casting temperatures require the use of phosphate-bonded investments and high temperature casting techniques, and it is well recognised that accurate casting at high temperatures is a problem for the dental technician.

**Table 51** Properties of some Co–Cr alloys.

| Alloy | Co (%) | Cr (%) | Mo (%) | Vickers Hardness Number | 0.2% Proof Stress (MPa) | Elongation (%) | Solidus-Liquidus Temperature (°C) | Casting Temperature (°C) |
|---|---|---|---|---|---|---|---|---|
| Biosil H (Degussa) | 65.7 | 28.5 | 4.5 | 360 | 600 | 8 | 1320-1380 | 1500 |
| Vitallium (Nobelparma) | 60.6 | 31.5 | 6.0 | 428 | 616 | 3 | 1300-1370 | 1550 |
| Wisil (Krupp) | 65 | 28 | 5 | 390 | 580 | 7 | 1355-1375 | 1535 |
| *Data taken from manufacturers' data sheets | | | | | | | | |

The alloys have a tendency to work-harden rapidly, which precludes excessive adjustment and any burnishing. Although they are highly biocompatible, tarnishing does occur with these alloys. These disadvantages have resulted in this group of alloys being considerably less popular than the medium- and low-gold alloys.

# Cobalt–Chromium Alloys

Co–Cr alloys were first introduced to the dental profession in the 1930s, and since then have effectively replaced the Type IV gold alloys for the construction of partial denture frameworks, primarily due to their relatively low cost, which is a significant factor with these large castings.

## Composition

The alloy consists of cobalt (55–65%) with up to 30% chromium. Other major alloying elements are molybdenum (4–5%) and in at least one case titanium (5%) (see *Table 51*).

The cobalt and chromium form a solid solution for up to 30% chromium, which is the limit of solubility of chromium in cobalt; additional chromium would produce a highly brittle second phase.

In general, the higher the chromium content, the better the corrosion resistance of the alloy. Therefore, the manufacturers try to maximise the amount of chromium without introducing the brittle second phase. Molybdenum is present in order to refine the grain size by providing more sites for crystal nucleation during the solid-ification process. It has the added benefit that it produces a significant solid solution hardening effect, an effect shared by the addition of iron. Nevertheless, the grains are very large, although grain boundaries are difficult to identify due to the coarse dendritic structure of the alloy.

Carbon, which is present only in small quantities, is nevertheless an extremely important constituent of the alloy, as small changes in the carbon content can significantly alter the strength, hardness and ductility of the alloy.

Carbon can combine with any of the other alloying elements to form carbides. The fine precipitation of these can dramatically raise the strength and hardness of the alloy. However, too much carbon will result in excessive brittleness. This presents a problem for the dental technician who needs to ensure that no excess carbon is absorbed by the alloy during melting and casting.

The distribution of the carbides also depends upon the casting temperature and the cooling rate, with discontinuous carbide formation at the grain boundaries being preferable to continuous carbide formation.

The commercially available alloys do not usually contain nickel or beryllium. Nickel is a well known human allergen, and its use in the mouth may trigger an allergic reaction. Therefore, for patients known to have a propensity for allergic reactions, it is advisable to use a nickel-free Co–Cr alloy. Beryllium is not so much a problem for the patient as for the dental technician. The mechanical grinding and polishing process causes the release of beryllium, which is a known carcinogen.

## *Properties*

For the dental technician, these alloys are considerably more difficult to handle than the gold alloys, because they must be heated to high temperatures before they can be cast.

This problem has largely been overcome with the introduction of induction casting equipment. Accuracy is compromised at these high temperatures, which effectively limits the use of these alloys to partial dentures.

The high hardness of these alloys makes them difficult to polish mechanically. Electrolytic polishing is used for the fitting surfaces, so as not to compromise the quality of fit, but non-fitting surfaces are still mechanically polished. The benefit is that the highly polished surface is retained for a very long time, which is a distinct advantage with a removable prosthesis.

The lack of ductility, so easily exacerbated by carbon contamination, *does* present problems, especially as these alloys are also prone to casting porosity. These limitations combine to give rise to a common problem with partial dentures: clasp fractures. This problem becomes even more pronounced when an attempt is made to adjust a clasp arm, and excessive or frequent adjustments will invariably lead to a clasp-arm fracture.

Nevertheless, there are some features of these alloys that make them ideally suited to the construction of partial denture frameworks. The modulus of elasticity of a Co–Cr alloy is typically 250 GPa, whereas for the alloys previously discussed the modulus is in the range 70–100 GPa. This high modulus of elasticity has the advantage that the denture, and particularly the clasp arms, can be made thinner in cross-section whilst maintaining adequate rigidity. When this is combined with a density of about half that of the gold alloys, it means that the castings are considerably lighter. This is of great benefit to the comfort of the patient.

The addition of chromium makes this a highly corrosion resistant alloy, as can be emphasised by the fact that the alloy also forms the basis of many surgically implanted prostheses, such as hip and knee joints. It can be said, therefore, that these alloys have an excellent history of biocompatibility.

## Summary

A rapidly growing number of casting alloys are used in dentistry. In order to make a rational choice from the current spectrum of high-gold alloys and their alternatives, the dentist needs to have more knowledge about their appearances and their physical and mechanical properties than ever before.

To make this choice, it is important that the dentist liaises closely with the dental laboratory and finds out which alloys are regularly used by them, and what their recommendations are. This becomes all the more important when the dentist should wish to use alternative alloys such as medium- or low-gold alloys rather than the high-gold alloys, because of the wide range of properties that are obtainable.

Although the cost of the alloy is an important consideration, one generally finds that the cost savings on the prostheses are less than might be expected. This is because the lower cost of the alloy is often offset by the increased cost of production.

Also, in general, it can be said that the higher the gold content of the alloy, the better the quality of fit of the restoration.

At the end of the day, the ultimate responsibility for the materials used in the patient's mouth rests with the dentist, and not the dental technician.

## Further Reading

Asgar K. (1988) Casting metals in dentistry: Past – Present – Future. Advances in Dental Research **2**, 33

Bates J. F. (1965) Studies related to the fracture of partial dentures. Brit. Dent. J. **118**, 532

CDMIE (1985) Report on base metal alloys for crown and bridge applications: benefits and risks. J. Am. Dent. Assoc. **111**, 479

Cruickshank-Boyd D. W. (1981) Alternatives to gold 1: Non-porcelain alloys. Dental Update **8**, 17

Cunningham D. M. (1973) Comparison of base metal alloys and Type IV gold alloys for removable partial denture frameworks. Dent. Clin. N. Am. **17**, 719

Huget E. F. (1978) Base metal alloys in *An Outline Of Dental Materials And Their Selection* O'Brien and Ryge (Eds) Chap. 23, p. 284, W. B. Saunders Co.

Landesman H. M., de Gennaro G. G. & Martinoff J. T. (1981) An 18-month clinical evaluation of semi-precious and nonprecious alloy restorations. J. Prosthet. Dent. **46**, 161

Mezger P. R., Stols A. L. H., Vrijhoef M. M. A. & Greener E. H. (1989) Metallurgical aspects and corrosion behaviour of yellow low-gold alloys. Dent. Mater. **5**, 350

van Noort R. & Lamb D. J. (1984) A scanning electron microscope study of Co-Cr partial dentures fractured in service. J. Dent. **12**, 122

# III.IV

## DENTAL CERAMICS

## Introduction

It could be said that the ceramic material known as porcelain holds a special place in dentistry because, notwithstanding the many advances made in composites and glass–ionomers, it is still considered to produce aesthetically the most pleasing result. Its colour, translucency and vitality can not as yet be matched by any materials except other ceramics.

Its traditional use is in the construction of artificial teeth for dentures, crowns and bridges. More recently, the use of ceramics has been extended to include veneers and inlays/onlays. The construction of such restorations is usually undertaken in dental laboratories by technicians skilled in the art of fusing ceramics.

As people retain their teeth for much longer than in the past, the need for aesthetically acceptable restorations is continuing to increase. This is reflected in the growing use by dentists of restorative procedures using ceramics.

In the UK, the demand for porcelain jacket crowns has been increasing at the rate of 50% every four years. Therefore, ceramics will continue to be important restorative materials for many years to come.

## Historical Perspective

### *Pottery In Europe Up To 1700 A.D.*

The achievement of making usable pottery was a considerable feat, and involved many trials and tribulations for the early potters. The raw material used for pottery is clay, and this presented the potter with two major problems.

The first problem the primitive potter met, was how to get the clay into a form that provided the best consistency for manipulation and firing. Clay is usually too sticky to handle when simply mixed with water, and this problem was overcome by the addition of sand and ground seashells. In addition, clay shrinks as it dries out and hardens. If this shrinkage is non-uniform, either in rate or in overall amount, the pots will crack even before they have been fired. Again, the addition of a coarse-grained filler went some way towards overcoming this problem.

It was during the firing of the pots that the problems really began to be serious. Gases present in the mixture, whether air bubbles or gases formed during heating (such as water vapour and $CO_2$), create voids in the clay and may even cause the clay to fracture during firing. Early potters overcame this problem by beating the

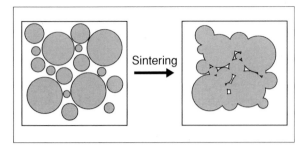

**145** Sintering of ceramic particles.

clay prior to moulding to get rid of the air. (*Wedging* is the term often used by the craftsmen to describe this process.) Another development was the technique of raising the temperature very gradually during the firing process, as then, the steam and gases could diffuse out of the clay slowly, rather than bursting out and causing the pot to crack.

The most serious obstacle during this phase in the development of ceramic technology was the temperature at which the pottery could be fired. The conversion of clay from a mass of individual particles loosely held together by a water binder to a coherent solid relies on a process known as *sintering*. In this process, the points at which the individual particles are in contact fuse at sufficiently high temperatures (**145**).

The process relies on diffusion, which is greatly accelerated by elevated temperatures. The demand for high, uniform temperatures could not be met by the traditional open fires, and this led to the invention of the *kiln*. The earliest of these was the *up-draught kiln*, in which higher temperatures and greater uniformity of temperature were obtained by drawing air through the fire and putting the pots in the rising hot gases.

Early kilns were able to reach temperatures of up to 900°C, and pottery fired at this temperature is called *earthenware*. The resultant pottery is porous, as the sintering process has only just managed to fuse the particles of clay where they touch. Such pots were suitable for the storage of solid foods but could not hold any liquids. This problem was overcome eventually by fusing a thin layer of a glassy material, i.e. a glaze, over the surface of the pot. This technology was used as far back as 5500 B.C. in various places, including Turkey.

Gradual progress was made towards higher kiln temperatures, so that many more clays could be partially melted. The liquid phase would invariably solidify as a glass, resulting in impervious pottery that is generally known as *stoneware*. Stoneware appeared in Europe in the 15–16th centuries A.D.

## Chinese Porcelain

In contrast to what was happening in Europe, stoneware had been produced in China by 100 B.C., and, by the 10th century A.D., ceramic technology in China had advanced to such a stage that they were able to produce:

'A ceramic so white that it was comparable only to snow, so strong that vessels needed walls only 2–3 mm thick and consequently light could shine through it. So continuous was the internal structure that a dish, if lightly struck would ring like a bell.'

### This is porcelain!

As trade with the Far-East grew, this infinitely superior material came to Europe from China during the 17th century. Until then, there had been a distinct lack of interest in tableware. The majority of the population ate off wooden plates, and the nobility were satisfied with eating off metal plates. For special occasions, gold and silver tableware would be used.

This all changed with the introduction of Chinese porcelain, which stimulated demand for high quality ceramic tableware. There was no way in which the trade with the Far-East could possibly satisfy this demand, so strenuous efforts were made by the European pottery industry to imitate the Chinese porcelain.

Passable imitations were made by using tin oxide as a glaze (producing the white appearance of porcelain), but it was found impossible to reproduce the translucency of Chinese porcelain.

For example, Meissen in Germany in 1708 managed to produce what they called 'white porcelain', but their product more closely resembled northern Chinese stoneware. Many other manufacturers, now well established names, were unable to produce genuine porcelain but still made a name for themselves with high quality stoneware, such as Majolica from Italy, Wedgwood from England and Delft's Blue from Holland.

In the up-draught-kiln they had the technology to produce high temperatures, although the Chinese down-draught kiln was somewhat superior at controlling the temperature. The problem of reproducing Chinese porcelain was essentially one of selecting the material and the method of processing. Many, such as John Dwight of Fulham who was granted a patent by Charles II in 1671, claimed to have discovered the secret of Chinese porcelain, but really only managed to make white stoneware.

In order to produce porcelain, the material has to remain or to become white on firing, and must be so strong that vessels with walls less than 3 mm thick can be produced. If the product needs to be made with walls thicker than 3 mm, even porcelain appears opaque.

So, the major differences between stoneware and porcelain are that porcelain is white and can be made in such thin sections that it appears translucent. Stoneware could be made to look white, but had to be use in such a thickness that it was invariably opaque.

This situation prevailed for some time, until, in 1717, the secret was leaked from China by a Jesuit missionary, Father d'Entrecolles. He performed his missionary work in a place called King-te-Tching, which, at that time, was the porcelain centre of China. Going amongst the people in their place of work he managed to acquire samples of the materials used. He sent the samples to a French friend of his, together with a detailed account of how the porcelain was manufactured. The samples and the description were passed on to M. de Reamur, a scientist, who was able to identify the components used by the Chinese as kaolin, silica and feldspar.

Kaolin, known as china clay, is a hydrated aluminium silicate. The silica is in the form of quartz, and remains as a fine dispersion after firing, and the feldspar is a mixture of sodium and potassium-aluminium silicates.

In a way, it is a little surprising that it took so long before the composition of the Chinese porcelain was unravelled. The art of making porcelain involves no complex chemistry, since the process is one of taking three rather common minerals (kaolin, feldspar and flint) and firing them at high temperatures.

Once the mystery had been unravelled however, it did not take long for new porcelains to be developed in Europe. Soon it was possible to make it in any shade or tint, and its translucency gave such a depth of colour that it was not long before the dental potential of this material was recognised.

The dental application of porcelain dates from 1774, when a French apothecary named Alexis Duchateau considered the possibility of replacing his ivory dentures with porcelain.

Ivory, being porous, soaks up oral fluids and eventually becomes badly stained, as well as being highly unhygenic. Duchateau, with the assistance of porcelain manufacturers at the Guerhard factory in Saint Germain-en Laye, succeeded in making himself the first porcelain denture. This was quite a feat, since the porcelain shrinks considerably on firing. This shrinkage had to be taken into account if the denture was going to fit at all well in the mouth.

Since then, other materials such as vulcanite and more recently polymethylmethacrylate have helped to replace porcelain for denture applications.

Porcelain teeth, in conjunction with an acrylic denture base are still extensively used. However, the most important application of dental porcelain is in the construction of crowns and bridges, where the aesthetic qualities of the porcelain are still superior to that of any other substitute for enamel and dentine.

Many new materials have appeared on the market over recent years that are described as porcelains, but are in fact very different forms of ceramic when compared with the early porcelains. Thus, it is now more appropriate to use the more general description of *dental ceramics*, within which the *dental porcelains* are but one group of materials. These were the first materials used in the construction of the porcelain jacket crown

# Construction Of A Porcelain Jacket Crown (PJC)

The production of a porcelain jacket crown involves three technical stages:

- Compaction.
- Firing.
- Glazing.

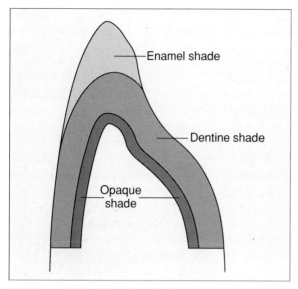

**146** Porcelain build-up for a jacket crown.

## Compaction

In the construction of a porcelain jacket crown, the porcelain powder is mixed with water and made into a paste. This paste is applied to the die, which has been coated beforehand with a very thin platinum foil, to allow the porcelain crown to be separated from the die and transported to the furnace.

A porcelain jacket crown is made from a number of porcelain powders because it is impossible to recreate all of the aesthetic features of a tooth by the use of a single porcelain. Conventionally, three basic types of porcelain powder are used. These are an opaque shade to mask the colour of the underlying structure, which may be an amalgam or silver-cermet core or a metal post and core construction. Then a dentine shade is applied and finally an enamel shade. The exact enamel shade is selected from a guide that is used to compare with the shade of the natural tooth. The final construction is as shown in **146**.

The powder is mixed with water and a binder to form a slurry which can be applied to the die in a number of ways, such as spatulation, brush application, whipping or vibrating, all of which are aimed at compacting the powder. The object of these condensation techniques is to remove as much water as possible, resulting in a more compact arrangement with a high density of particles that minimises the firing shrinkage. The particle size and shape are extremely important, as they affect the handling characteristics of the powder and have an effect on the amount of shrinkage on firing. The binder helps to hold the particles together as the material is extremely fragile in this so-called *green state*.

## Firing

Initially, the crown is heated slowly in the open entrance to the furnace. This is carried out in order to drive off excess water before it has a chance to form steam. If the water in the mix was allowed to turn into steam, it would cause the fragile powder-compact to crack as the steam tried to escape to the surface. Once the compact has been dried, it is placed in the furnace and the binders are burnt out. Some contraction occurs during this stage.

As the porcelain begins to fuse, continuity is only achieved at points of contact between the powder particles. The material is still porous, and is usually referred to as being at the *low bisque stage*.

As the exposure to the elevated temperature continues, more fusion takes place as the molten glass flows between the particles, drawing them closer together and filling the voids. A large contraction takes place during this phase, and the resultant material is non-porous. The cause of the high shrinkage of porcelain on firing is therefore the fusion of the particles during sintering, as the powder particles are brought into close contact.

The firing of the porcelain must be carried out exactly according to the manufacturers' instructions. If the crown should remain in the furnace for too long it will lose form due to *pyroplastic flow* (flow of the molten glass) and will become highly glazed.

A very slow cooling rate is essential in order to avoid the possibility of cracking or crazing. The furnaces available offer usually a considerable degree of automation, and can be used for air- or vacuum-firing. Vacuum-firing produces a denser porcelain than air-firing, as air is withdrawn during the firing process. Fewer voids are formed, resulting in a stronger crown with a more predictable shade. Areas of porosity in air-fired porcelain alter the translucency of the crown, as they cause light to scatter. An additional problem is that air voids will become exposed if grinding of the superficial layer

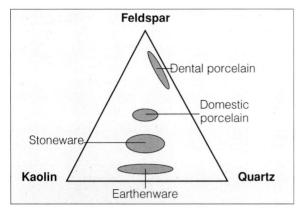

**147** Relative composition of ceramic products based on feldspar, kaolin and quartz.

**Table 52** Compositions of household and dental porcelains.

| Porcelain | % Kaolin | % Quartz | % Feldspar |
|-----------|----------|----------|------------|
| Household | 50 | 20–25 | 25–30 |
| Dental | 0 | 25 | 65 |

should be necessary, giving rise to an unsightly appearance and a rough surface finish.

## *Glazing*

There will always be some porosity in the porcelain, with small air voids being exposed at the surface. These will allow the ingress of bacteria, oral fluids and act as potential sites for the build-up of plaque. To avoid this, the surface is glazed to produce a smooth, shiny and impervious outer layer. There are two ways in which this can be achieved:

- Glasses that fuse at low temperatures are applied to the crown after construction, and a short period at a relatively low temperature is sufficient to fuse the glaze.
- Final firing of the crown under carefully controlled conditions fuses the superficial layer to an impervious surface glaze.

# Dental Porcelain

## *Composition Of Dental Porcelain*

The earliest dental porcelains were mixtures of kaolin, feldspar and quartz, and were quite different for earthenware, stoneware and domestic porcelain, as indicated in **147**.

**Table 53** Typical oxide composition of a dental porcelain.

| Material | wt% |
|----------|-----|
| Silica | 63 |
| Alumina | 17 |
| Boric oxide | 7 |
| Potash ($K_2O$) | 7 |
| Soda ($Na_2O$) | 4 |
| Other oxides | 2 |

It was not until 1838 that Elias Wildman produced dental porcelain with the translucency and shades that reasonably matched those of the natural teeth. The compositions for domestic and dental porcelain are shown in *Table 52*.

Kaolin is a hydrated aluminium silicate ($Al_2O.2SiO_2.2H_2O$) and acts as a binder, increasing the mouldability of the unfired porcelain. It is opaque however, and when present,even in very small quantities it meant that the earliest dental porcelains lacked adequate translucency.

The quartz remains unchanged during the firing process and acts as a strengthening agent. It is present as a fine crystalline dispersion throughout the glassy phase that is produced by the melting of the kaolin and the feldspar. The feldspar fuses when it melts, forming a glass matrix. Modern dental porcelain does not contain kaolin and can thus be considered to be a feldspathic glass with crystalline inclusions of silica.

The feldspars are mixtures of potassium aluminium silicate ($K_2O.Al_2O_3.6SiO_2$) and sodium aluminium silicate, also known as albite ($Na_2O.Al_2O_3.6SiO_2$). Feldspars are naturally occurring substances, so the ratio between the potash ($K_2O$) and the soda ($Na_2O$) will vary somewhat. This affects the properties of the feldspar, in that the soda tends to lower the fusion temperature and the potash increases the viscosity of the molten glass.

During the firing of porcelain there is always the danger of excessive pyroplastic flow that may result in rounding of the edges and loss of tooth form. It is important that the right amount of potash is present to prevent this. These alkalis are present either as a part of the feldspars, or they may be added as carbonates to ensure the correct ratio. The typical oxide composition of a dental porcelain is presented in *Table 53*.

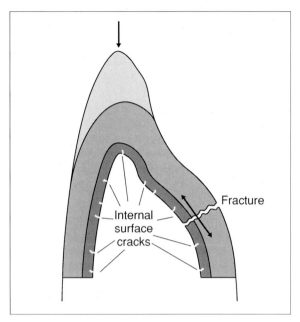

**148** Palatal fracture of a porcelain jacket crown initiated from an internal surface flaw.

The porcelain powder that is used by the dental technician is not a simple mixture of the ingredients in *Table 53*. These powders have been fired once already. The manufacturer mixes the components, adds additional metal oxides, fuses them and then quenches the molten mass in water. The resultant product is known as a *frit*, and the process is known as *fritting*. A consequence of the rapid cooling is that large internal stresses build up in the glass, resulting in extensive cracking. This material can be ground very easily to produce a fine powder for use by the dental technician.

Thus, during the firing of a porcelain jacket crown for example, there is no chemical reaction taking place; the glass is simply melted and cooled down again. All that has happened is that the individual particles have fused together by sintering to produce a coherent solid.

The particle size distribution is critical in ensuring that the particles pack together as tightly as possible, in order that the shrinkage on firing is minimised. The average particle size is generally in the region of 25 µm, with a wide distribution of other particle sizes such that the smaller particles fill in the spaces in between the larger particles. Some porcelain powders have a multimodal particle size distribution to increase the packing density.

A number of other ingredients will be present in the dental porcelain powders. These include metal oxides, which provide the wide variety of colours of the porcelain.

Iron acts as a brown pigment, copper oxide as a green pigment, titanium oxide as a yellowish-brown, and cobalt oxide imparts a blue colour. A binder, consisting of starch and sugar, may also be present to help in the manipulation of the powders.

## The Properties Of Dental Porcelain

Porcelain is chemically very stable, and provides excellent aesthetics that do not deteriorate with time.

The thermal conductivity and the coefficient of thermal expansion are similar to those of enamel and dentine, so, in the presence of a good marginal seal, marginal percolation is less likely to be a problem.

Although the compressive strength of dental porcelain is high (350–550 MPa), its tensile strength is very low (20–40 MPa). The material, being a glass, lacks any fracture toughness. The maximum strain that a glass can withstand is less than 0.1%. They are extremely sensitive to the presence of *surface microcracks*, and this represents one of the major drawbacks in the use of porcelain.

On cooling from the furnace temperature, the outside of the porcelain will cool more rapidly than the interior, particularly as the porcelain has a low thermal conductivity. The outside surface contracts more than the inside initially, resulting in a compressive load on the outside and a residual tensile stress on the inside as the interior is being prevented from shrinking by the outside skin.

If the differential dimensional change is sufficiently high, the internal surface layer that is under tension will rupture to relieve the stresses. This will result in the internal surface containing a large number of minute cracks, and it is these that will ultimately cause the crown to fracture catastrophically (**148**).

The application of a glaze with a slightly lower coefficient of expansion would potentially fill in the cracks and also place the surface under compression. Unfortunately, this is not possible on the fitting surface of the crown, as it may result in the crown not seating properly.

# High Strength Ceramics

The feldspathic porcelains are not strong enough to be used for the manufacture of multi-unit bridges, and problems even arise for porcelain jacket crowns, especially when they are in situations of heavy occlusion. The tiny surface flaws in the interior of the crown act as initiating sites for catastrophic failure. The inherently low tensile strength of feldspathic porcelains (20–40 MPa) would restrict their use to low stress-bearing applications.

In order to extend the use of porcelain, ceramics with improved tensile strength are needed. Since all ceramics tend to fail at the same critical strain of 0.1%, one means of achieving this is to increase the elastic modulus of the material. If, at the same time, the propagation of cracks is made more difficult, a higher strength ceramic will result.

A number of new ceramic systems have been introduced in recent years which show a marked improvement in their resistance to fracture. The flexural strengths of a number of ceramics are shown in *Table 54*.

As the tensile strength is a difficult property to measure (giving rise to a wide degree of scatter in the data), it is common practice to determine the flexural strength. Although the silicon nitrides and carbides and the zirconia are attractive from the viewpoint of strength, they are not suitable because of the difficulties associated with the manufacture of individual crowns, the colour differences and the mismatch in the coefficient of thermal expansion.

The three major developments that are worthy of further consideration are the aluminous porcelains, the cast-glass ceramics and the high expansion porcelains.

## *Aluminous Porcelains*

The aluminous porcelains were introduced in the early 1960s; they consist of a core porcelain containing 40–50% alumina. The alumina particles are far stronger than the glass, and are more effective at preventing crack propagation.

Whereas the flexural strength of feldspathic porcelain is approximately 60 MPa, this is raised to 120–180 MPa for the aluminous porcelains, which represents a two- to three-fold increase in the strength of a porcelain jacket crown.

| Type of ceramic | Flexural Strength (MPa) |
|---|---|
| Hot-pressed silicon nitride | 800–900 |
| Hot-pressed silicon carbide | 400–750 |
| Partially stabilised zirconia | 640 |
| Alumina 98% pure | 420–520 |
| Dicor* castable glass ceramic | 140–150 |
| Aluminous core porcelain | 125–150 |
| High expansion core porcelain | 120–130 |

**Table 54** Typical strength values for high strength ceramics.

* Dentsply International Inc, York, Pa

Commonly nowadays, the opaque shade shown in **146** is an aluminous porcelain. It is still necessary to use the weaker dentine and enamel shades of the feldspathic porcelains because it is not possible to produce aluminous porcelains with the required translucency; the alumina causes the porcelain to appear dull and opaque. Although the improvement in strength is considerable, it is still insufficient to allow the construction of even a two-unit bridge.

Even if the crown or bridge could be made out of high density alumina which has a flexural strength of 420–560 MPa, this is only just approaching that of the metals such as gold and Ni–Cr alloys.

A recent variant on the aluminous porcelain is a core porcelain, produced by Vita Zahnfabrik, (Bad Säckingen, FRG) under the name of Hi-Ceram. The core material is different from the conventional porcelain core materials in that it has a very high alumina content. This raises its flexural strength, which is reported to be greater than that of Vita Dur aluminous core porcelain. When this core material is fired directly on the refractory model a naturally rough surface finish is obtained which contributes to the retention of the restoration.

It has been noted that too high a temperature or too long a firing cycle can cause the porcelain to fuse to the refractory. This would suggest that excessive flow of the glass phase has taken place, resulting in too close an adaptation to the refractory.

The addition of alumina to the feldspathic glass during the prefritting process limits the

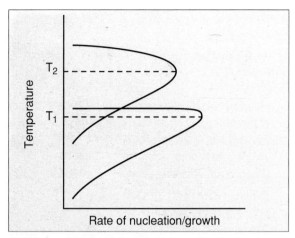

**149** Rate of nucleation ($T_1$) and growth ($T_2$) of crystals in a glass ceramic.

amount of alumina that can be incorporated. An alternative approach has been adopted in a new system called In-Ceram (Vita Zahnfabrik, Bad Säckingen, FRG). A ceramic core is formed onto a refractory die from a fine slurry of alumina powder and is lightly sintered. The highly porous structure is then infiltrated with molten glass, producing a dense ceramic. Very high flexural strength values have been claimed for this ceramic.

## Castable Glass Ceramics

In order to surmount the problems of the poor aesthetics and the inherent inaccuracies of the fit of the aluminous porcelains, attention has recently been paid to the possibility of using glass ceramics (e.g. DICOR), which employ a casting process for the manufacture of crowns, veneers and inlays.

The concept of producing porcelain restorations using a casting technique is by no means new, and was first attempted in the 1920s. It is only with the recent introduction of the cast glass ceramics that this has become possible.

The technique uses the same principles as for the lost-wax casting process of metallic restorations. The restoration is waxed up on a die, using conventional materials. The pattern is removed from the die and invested in a special phosphate-bonded investment. Then an ingot of the castable ceramic material is placed in a special crucible and centrifugally cast at a temperature of 1380°C. The casting then requires a further heat

treatment to develop the strength. The desired shade is achieved by firing self-glazing shading porcelains on the surface.

Their flexural strength is comparable to that of the aluminous porcelain, but they have the advantage that they can be made with the required translucency. In addition, they offer the advantage of allowing the production of a single casting of complex design and high accuracy, which would otherwise require great skill and time on the part of the dental technician to produce.

The first glass ceramics were developed by Corning Glass Works in the late 1950s. In principle, an article is formed while liquid, and a metastable glass results on cooling. During a subsequent heat treatment, controlled crystallisation occurs, with the nucleation and growth of internal crystals. This conversion process from a glass to a partially crystalline glass is called *ceraming*, and is accompanied by a small but controlled volume change.

Thus, a glass ceramic is a multiphase solid containing a residual glass phase with a finely dispersed crystalline phase. The controlled crystallisation of the glass results in the formation of tiny crystals that are evenly distributed throughout the glass. The number of crystals, their growth rate and thus their size is regulated by the time and temperature of the ceraming heat treatment.

There are two important aspects to the formation of the crystalline phase: crystal nucleation and crystal growth. The schematic in **149** shows that the rate of crystal nucleation and the rate of crystal growth are at a maximum at different temperatures.

The ceraming process consequently involves a two-stage heat treatment. The first heat treatment is carried out at the temperature for maximum nucleation of crystals, so as to maximise the number of crystals formed. The material temperature is then raised, after a suitable period of time, to the higher temperature to allow crystal growth. It is held at the higher temperature until the optimum crystal size is formed.

To ensure a high strength for the glass ceramic it is important that the crystals are numerous and are uniformly distributed throughout the glassy phase. The crystalline phase will grow during ceraming, and can eventually occupy from 50% to nearly 100% of the material.

## Composition And Optical Quality Of Dental Glass Ceramics

Most glass ceramics are opaque or cloudy and would not be suitable for dental use. The first glass ceramic employed in dentistry was introduced by MacCulloch in 1968 for the construction of denture teeth, and was based on the $Li_2O.ZnO.SiO_2$ system. At the time, the use of acrylic denture teeth was becoming popular, and the idea of glass ceramics was not exploited further.

The exploration of glass ceramics for dental use was taken up by other researchers, and has resulted in at least two commercially available products.

Fluoromicas are products such as Dicor (Dentsply DeTrey). Dicor is based on the composition $SiO_2.K_2O.MgO.Al_2O_3.ZrO_2$, with the addition of some fluorides to impart fluorescence in the prostheses, in a way similar to that encountered in the natural dentition.

For this composition, the ceraming process results in the nucleation and the growth of tetrasilicate mica crystals within the glass. Mica has an unusual microstructure in that it consists of many small interlocking plate-like crystals that are randomly oriented. This is ideal from the point of view of strength. The mica readily cleaves along its long axis, causing cracks to deflect, branch or blunt. Thus, the propagation of cracks through this material is arrested by the mica crystals, providing a substantial increase in the flexural strength.

The passage of light through the material is affected by the crystal size and the difference in the refractive indices of the glass phase and the crystalline phase. If the crystals are smaller than the wavelength of visible light ($0.4–0.7\mu m$) the glass will appear transparent. The refractive index of the small mica crystals is closely matched to that of the surrounding glass phase such that the tendency for light to scatter is lower than for the aluminous porcelains. This produces a translucency close to that of enamel.

Apatite glass ceramic is based upon a $CaO.MgO.P_2O_5.SiO_2$ system. The crystalline phase formed on ceraming is a hydroxyapatite $[Ca_{10}(PO_4)_6.2OH]$, which is the same basic constituent from which enamel is made. Thus, it represents a material which, at least in composi-

tion, is the closest match to enamel that has been achieved so far. It has been suggested that these materials can readily be bonded to tooth tissues with the glass–ionomer cements.

The glass–ionomer cements are believed to bond primarily to the apatite component of the enamel and dentine, and thus should also bond to the apatite phase within the glass ceramic. To enhance this possibility, a special etchant has been made available which preferentially removes the glassy phase from the surface of the glass ceramic thus exposing the apatite phase. The glass–ionomer cement can then bond to this apatite phase as well as providing some micromechanical interlocking.

The high degree of translucency of the glass ceramics prior to the ceraming process has the added advantage that the glass casting can be checked for any internal defects. The characterisation is obtained by firing feldspathic porcelains of appropriate shade and translucency onto the surface.

## Magnesia-Core Porcelains

In the USA in particular, the use of all porcelain crowns is not as widespread as in the UK. Thus, the majority of dental laboratories tend only to stock the porcelains used in metal-bonded restorations.

These have relatively high coefficients of expansion (13–14 ppm/°C) in order to match those of the metals used. The coefficient of expansion of an aluminous porcelain is typically in the region of 6–8 ppm/°C. Thus, the aluminous core materials can not be used in conjunction with these porcelains because of the large mismatch in the coefficients of expansion.

Thus the laboratory would need to have experience of the use of two different sets of dentine and enamel porcelains, and would need to keep duplicate stocks. One way of overcoming this problem is to develop a core porcelain of high strength which also has a high coefficient of expansion. Such a core material has been developed using magnesium oxide which has a high coefficient of expansion. The flexural strength matches that of the aluminous porcelains due to fine dispersion of crystalline magnesium oxide.

A marked increase in the flexural strength is achieved when the internal fitting surface is glazed. The internal surface of the magnesium

209

oxide porcelain is quite porous, and the glaze can penetrate into these pores. An improvement in flexural strength from 130 MPa to 270 MPa may be achievable.

Firstly, the surface microcracks are much reduced in size, and, secondly, by using a glaze porcelain with a lower coefficient of expansion, the surface is placed under a compressive stress.

Although one might expect a similar improvement in the flexural strength of aluminous porcelain upon glazing, this appears not to be the case and may be related to the smooth fitting surface of aluminous porcelain.

# Mechanical Properties Of High Strength Ceramics

The mechanical properties are believed to be greatly influenced by:

- Particle size of the crystalline phase.
- Volume fraction of the crystalline phase.
- Interfacial bond strength between phases.
- Differences in elastic moduli.
- Differences in thermal expansion.

Fracture in brittle solids is nearly always initiated at a small internal or surface defect, such as a microcrack, that acts as a stress raiser.

If the crystalline phase is relatively strong, then the cracks will form in the glassy phase. The dimension of these microcracks canthus be limited to the distance between the crystalline particles. Therefore, the critical parameter is the mean free path, in the glassy phase, $L_s$, which is given by:

$$L_s = \frac{d(1 - V_f)}{V_f}$$

where d is the crystal diameter and $V_f$ is the volume fraction of the crystalline phase.

Thus, the smaller the crystals and the larger the volume fraction of the crystals, the shorter the mean free path will be, and, consequently the greater the strength of the material. A feature of glass ceramics is that the size and the amount of the crystalline phase can be carefully controlled during the ceraming process.

As yet, the strength of the high-strength ceramics would not be considered sufficiently high to enable them to be used for extensive bridge construction, but if the strength can be improved such that even simple bridges are possible, then this would represent an exciting new development. Particularly, the aesthetics could be far better than the metal-bonded system, as it would not be necessary to mask out the metal coping.

A number of additional strengthening mechanisms are open to exploration with the ceramics. These strengthening mechanisms rely on the formation of a compressive surface layer.

## Ion Exchange

The surface of the material can be placed under compression by replacing some of the ions in the surface with larger ions via an ion-exchange mechanism. This process is carried out in a fused salt bath of the appropriate composition at a temperature of approximately 850°C.

An example of this is a glass ceramic placed in a solid solution of beta-spodumene, where the exchange of lithium ions for the larger sodium ions leads to the formation of a surface compression layer during cooling, with a three-fold increase in the flexural strength.

## Heat Treatment

A compressive surface layer can be formed during the heat treatment of glass ceramics that is used to control crystallisation in the bulk of the material.

An example is the addition of fluoride to glass ceramics that are based on $Na_2O.K_2O.SiO_2$. A glassy surface layer is formed that has a thermal expansion lower than that of the material that is crystallised in the bulk phase. Alternatively, a crystalline surface layer can form with a lower thermal expansion than the bulk phase, due to the slower transformation on the surface than in the bulk of the material.

## Surface Glazes

If a surface glaze with a lower thermal expansion than the bulk ceramic is fired onto the surface, a thin layer over the surface will be under compression once the material has cooled.

At this stage, the experience with these new materials is very limited, and more information

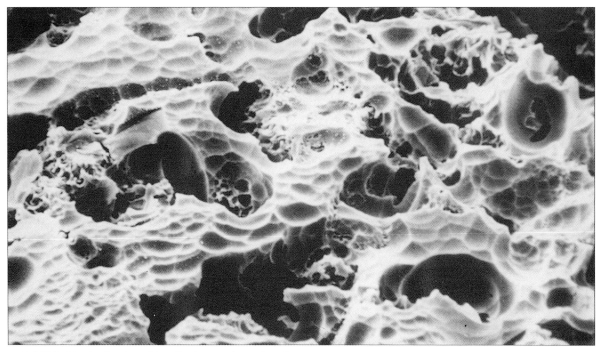

**150** SEM of hydrofluoric acid etched ceramic surface.

is needed to assess whether the cast glass ceramics and high expansion porcelains are a viable alternative to the aluminous porcelain crown.

The relatively low cost of the aluminous porcelain and the good aesthetic qualities engendered over many years of experience will make it difficult for other ceramics to replace them, particularly in those countries where the porcelain jacket crown is extensively used.

# Resin-Bonded Ceramic Crowns, Veneers And Inlays

One way in which the traditional approach is being challenged is the development of new adhesive techniques. These have extended the use of ceramics to areas not previously thought possible.

The combination of adhesion and improved strength characteristics has produced restorations with excellent mechanical integrity. In fact, the adhesive bond has the effect of eliminating the internal surface flaws and thus reduces the potential for fracture. This has led to a growth in the use of ceramics for crowns, veneers and inlays.

The concept of using ceramics as veneers is not new, and can be traced back to Dr Charles Pincus of Beverley Hills, who, in 1928, described the use of porcelain veneers with actors in Hollywood. The porcelain veneers were baked on platinum foil and retained on the teeth by denture powder.

However, the veneers broke frequently because the thin porcelain was brittle and they were frequently removed from the teeth. When acrylic resin was introduced in 1937, he used this material for the acting profession. This developed into the use of composites for the production of veneers.

The use of porcelain was reintroduced in 1983 by Dr Horn in America. He fabricated the veneers on a foil backing and discovered that the fitting surface could be etched with hydrofluoric acid, thus improving the micromechanical retention (**150**). Using the acid-etch technique he was able to bond the veneers permanently to the teeth with a resin based composite.

Porcelain veneers are considered superior to composites because of their superior aesthetics, colour stability, surface finish, abrasion resistance and tissue compatibility. They are also chemically very stable and have a coefficient of expansion similar to that of enamel.

The finishing of porcelain veneers is more difficult than that of composites due to their high hardness. The thin feathered margins are more easily damaged than the margins of crowns, both in the laboratory and in the surgery.

However, they have the distinct advantages over crowns that improved aesthetics can be achieved with minimal tooth reduction, and the palatal surface of the tooth is unchanged so that incisal guidance is maintained.

Veneers are relatively new and are still not clinically proven to the same degree as porcelain jacket crown restorations. They also incur higher laboratory costs and placement is more time consuming than for a porcelain jacket crown.

## Construction Of Veneers And Inlays

In effect, there are four methods for the construction of veneers and/or inlays.

### The Foil Technique (Veneers Only)

There are two forms for this technique:

- *Type 1 – no core shade* – The etched bonded veneering system consists of dentine and enamel shade porcelains which are fired on to a 25 µm thick platinum foil matrix. After shaping and glazing, it is etched with hydrofluoric acid to obtain a rough surface finish. These veneers are extremely thin and show a high degree of translucency.
- *Type 2 – core shade* – When veneers are required to mask discoloration, it is possible to incorporate an opaque layer by firing a layer of aluminous core porcelain before placing the dentine and enamel shades.

This technique has two advantages. Firstly, providing the foil is kept in place, the veneer can be tried in the mouth prior to glazing. This allows adjustment of contour and check of occlusion. Secondly, there is a choice between opaque and translucent veneers.

The disadvantages are that on firing, the resultant shrinkage can distort the platinum foil and pull the margins away from the model, and that, for multiple veneers, more tooth structure must be removed so as to separate the contact points. This allows the stone dies to be separated and pinned.

### Refractory Die Technique

In this system, the dentine and enamel shades are placed and fired directly on a refractory die material which is designed to withstand the high firing temperature. It is important that the ceramic and the refractory are closely matched in expansion characteristics in order to prevent cracking of the restoration on cooling.

A high surface roughness is obtained after removal of the refractory die by grit blasting. A core material can be applied to mask discoloration.

The advantages are that no costly platinum foil is required, that there is a reduced possibility of distortion during firing, that the veneer is more easily finished to a knife edge, allowing minimal tooth reduction, and that contact points need not be separated, as multiple units can be fired on the same model.

The disadvantages are the need to remove the refractory die material from the fitting surface by grit blasting (which can lead to damaged margins), and that the use of a core material requires some degree of tooth reduction to avoid over-contouring.

### Ceraming Technique

In principle, the veneer or inlay is cast from a glass using the lost-wax casting technique. The glass that is formed is metastable, and, during a subsequent *ceraming heat treatment*, controlled crystallisation occurs. The fine dispersion of the crystalline phase in the glassy phase produces a material with a high strength and high translucency.

The advantages are the superior aesthetics, the high strength, and the control over the opacity. The disadvantages are the difficulty of using the technique because of the thin sections of wax, and that the characterisation is obtained by surface glazes which can wear away.

### CAD–CAM (inlays only)

The CAD–CAM technique involves the use of a computer controlled milling machine for the construction of the inlay. This technique is very much in its infancy and insufficient data are available at the time of writing to judge its performance.

## Ceramic Bonding

The fitting surface of ceramics that are constructed on a refractory die is inherently rough due to the grit blasting process used to remove the refractory.

The application of hydrofluoric acid to the fitting surface of these ceramics enhances the surface roughness even more, due to the preferential removal of either the crystalline phase or the glassy phase. Thus, a micromechanical bond can be created by the use of a composite luting cement.

The composite luting cements are, in effect, lightly filled composites with small sized filler particles to ensure thin film thickness. Whereas the first cements were visible light activated, the tendency is now towards the use of light and optional dual-cure cements. This makes the cements suitable for both veneers and inlays.

The concern is that visible light curing cements may not cure properly when they are used to cement large inlays, as the light would be unable to penetrate to the full depth of the inlay.

Similarly, the move towards the use of resin-bonded crowns requires the use of a dual-cure cement in order to ensure that complete polymerisation of the composite luting cement occurs.

Many of these cements are now provided with a silane coupling agent that can be applied directly to the clean fitting surfaces of veneers or inlays as they are received from the dental laboratory, or that can be used for the repair of fractured ceramic restorations. The silane coupling agents work in exactly the same way as described in section I.X for the resin to glass filler bond in composites.

A thorough cleaning of the ceramic surfaces with isopropyl alcohol, acetone or phosphoric acid is needed after the veneer or inlay has been checked for satisfactory fit and prior to applying the silane. This is necessary in order to remove any surface contaminants, such as grease or saliva, that would interfere with the application of the silane coupling agent.

For some products, it is recommended that a phosphoric acid solution is added to the silane coupling agent to hydrolyse the silane prior to applying it to the fitting surface. Others are made up of a dilute solution of the activated silane in ethyl alcohol. In this case, the addition of phosphoric acid solution is therefore not necessary because the silane is already hydrolysed, although this will limit the shelf life of the silane coupling agent.

In the case of repairs, the surface of the porcelain must first be etched *in situ* with hydrofluoric acid solution to create a micromechanically retentive surface. Acidulated phosphate fluoride gels can also be used, but the etching time of 20 minutes is prohibitive.

Phosphoric acid is ineffectual as an etchant since the ceramic is totally resistant to attack from this acid. A fractured surface, even if roughened by a diamond bur, will not be as effective at providing micromechanical retention as an etched surface.

### General Problems With Hydrofluoric Acid Etching

There are three main problems:

- If the hydrofluoric acid is not neutralised completely, it may leach out and cause tissue damage at a later date.
- The hydrofluoric acid gel tends to slump, such that the lateral borders of the veneer (in particular), may not be fully etched. This may cause marginal leakage.
- Damage to the labial gingival margin of the veneer or inlay by the etchant can lead to plaque retention, inflammatory gingival response and secondary caries.

## Failures Of Veneers

There are four main causes for the failure of a veneer:

- *Aesthetic failures* – Colour matching is difficult when only one tooth is discoloured. If the shade cannot be corrected by tints and coloured composite luting cements, a remake is necessary.
- *Polymerisation failure* – A curing time of at least 60 seconds is essential. If a small tipped curing unit is used, each area under the tip must be cured for 60 seconds. Incomplete cure of the resin will result in fracture of the veneer.

- *Marginal failure* – This may be due to inadequate luting cement and a healthy excess is necessary. Poor etching and bonding technique can also give rise to this problem. Care must be taken to avoid 'suck back' of air, which can cause the formation of voids underneath the restoration.
- *Fracture of veneers* – The most common cause of fracture is incorrect occlusion. It is essential to check the occlusion carefully with articulating paper and identify any interferences. It is also best to ensure that the opposing tooth is never in contact with the ceramic–enamel junction.

# Further Reading

Banks R. G. (1990) Conservative posterior ceramic restorations: a review of the literature. J. Prosthet. Dent. 63, 619

Christensen G. (1985) Veneering of teeth. Dent. Clin. N Am. 29, 373

Clyde G. (1988) Porcelain veneers: a preliminary review. Brit. Dent. J. 164, 9

Duret F., Blouin J-L. & Duret B. (1988) CAD-CAM in dentistry. J. Am. Dent. Assoc. 117, 715

Grossman D. G. (1985) Cast glass ceramics. Dent. Clin. N. Am. 29, 725

Horn H. (1983) Porcelain laminate veneers bonded to etched enamel. Dent. Clin. N. Am. 27, 671

MacCulloch (1968) Advances in dental ceramics. Brit. Dent. J. 142, 361

Piddock V. & Qualtrough A. J. E. (1990) Dental ceramics – an update. J. Dent. 18, 227

Toh C. G., Setcos J. C. & Weinstein A. R. (1987) Indirect laminate veneers: an overview. J. Dent. 15, 117

# III.V

## METAL-BONDED CERAMICS

## Introduction

One approach to the development of stronger and stronger ceramics is the elimination of microcracks.

In the case of ceramic crowns, the multitude of microcracks on the internal fitting surface is the major source of weakness, and their removal would significantly improve the crown. Glazing the internal fitting surface is one possibility. Another possibility is bonding the ceramic to a metal substrate such that these microscopic cracks are effectively eliminated, with the consequence that the structure is considerably stronger. This is the basic premise behind the metal-bonded system (**151**).

It has been shown that metal-bonded ceramic crowns are up to three times stronger than ceramic crowns. The crown consists of a cast metal coping onto which is fired a ceramic veneer. If a proper bond is created then the internal cracks are eliminated as the metal presents a barrier to the propagation of cracks by virtue of its high fracture toughness. One of the most likely modes of failure with this system is the separation of the ceramic from the metal due to an interfacial breakdown. Thus, the success of the system depends upon the quality of the bond.

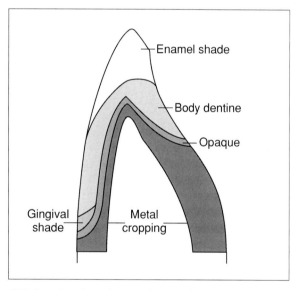

**151** Construction of a metal–ceramic crown.

Another concern for metal-bonded ceramic restorations is the potential for a mismatch between the coefficients of expansion of the ceramic and the metal. If the mismatch is too great then stresses will build up during the cooling process after firing. These stresses can be sufficient to result in crazing or cracking of the ceramic. The issues of the bond and the coefficients of expansion both require careful consideration.

# The Bond

The nature of the bond between the metal coping and the ceramic has been extensively studied and it is agreed generally that there are three mechanisms involved:

- Mechanical retention.
- Compression.
- Chemical bonding.

Mechanical retention occurs as the ceramic flows into the microscopic spaces in the surface of the metal. The roughness of the surface is enhanced often by applying an alumina–air abrasive or by grinding, so that the amount of interlocking is increased. This has the added benefit of producing a very clean surface that aids the wetting of the ceramic onto the metal.

Good bonding relies on an intimate contact between the ceramic and the metal coping and any contaminants will jeopardise the quality of the bond. Before the ceramic is applied to the surface of the coping, the coping is subjected to a degassing cycle in the furnace which burns off any remaining impurities and reduces the formation of bubbles due to trapped gasses at the interface. The various stages in the surface preparation of the metal coping are described in more detail at a later stage.

On cooling, the metal will try to contract more than the ceramicdue to its higher coefficient of expansion. This leaves the ceramic in a state of compression, which is highly beneficial for this brittle material. It is important that the mismatch in the coefficients of thermal expansion is only small, otherwise the internal stresses created during cooling could cause the ceramic to fracture, with the most likely place for failure being the interface between the metal and the ceramic.

There is now considerable evidence that a strong chemical bond is created between the ceramic and the oxide coating on the metal. During firing, the ceramic is taken above its glass transition temperature such that it can flow and fuse with the oxides on the metal surface by migration of the oxides into the ceramic. In the case of gold alloy copings, small amounts of oxide-forming elements are added to the alloy because gold does not naturally form an oxide.

As a consequence, the strength of the bond between the metal and the ceramic is increased manifold. This shows the importance of the presence of the surface oxides.

# Preparation Of The Metal Surface

In order to obtain a good bond between the metal coping and the ceramic veneer it is important that the metal surface is carefully prepared. This involves a number of technical stages that warrant closer examination. The main reasons for the surface preparation of the metal are to ensure the removal of any contaminants and to produce a surface oxide layer of the correct composition and character for the ceramic to fuse to. The various stages can be identified as:

- Surface grinding.
- Heating under partial vacuum.
- Acid pickling.
- Heating in air.

## Surface Grinding

When the metal casting is removed from the investment there is always residual investment bonded to the surface of the casting. The surface is also contaminated with unwanted oxides, small porosities and fine projections, especially if the investment is susceptible to fracture of the surface layer.

The grinding process is carried out to remove all of these imperfections, and the increased surface roughness is believed to aid the retention of the ceramic by micromechanical interlocking.

However, the grinding process can itself suffer from the problem of debris such as oils, waxes, bits of skin tissue or gasses becoming trapped in undercuts. Even though the ceramic may be very effective in wetting the surface of the metal, it cannot always penetrate deep fissures.

The presence of trapped air and contaminants that may decompose upon firing results in the presence of gas bubbles at the interface between the metal and the ceramic, causing a marked degradation in the bond strength and the aesthetics of the prosthesis.

In general, methods of grinding that do not result in the formation of deep fissures, porosities or undercuts are preferred, and to this end, the use of fissure burs or carbide burs appear to be the recommended procedures.

Cleaning the casting in an organic solvent (e.g. carbon tetrachloride) in a sealed ultrasonic bath will remove surface contamination that has arisen during the handling of the casting.

## Heating Under Partial Vacuum

In the as-cast condition, the metal will not have the ideal oxide coating on its surface. (Gold alloys will have virtually no oxide coating given the noble nature of this metal.)

An oxide film can be formed by heating the casting at a temperature near to the firing temperature of the ceramic. This has the effect of allowing the metallic elements that are incorporated in the alloy to migrate to the surface and form an oxide surface layer.

Great care must be taken to ensure that the correct heating cycle is used. Too brief a heat treatment could result in the formation of a thin or partial oxide coating, providing a poor substrate for the ceramic to fuse to. An excessively long heating cycle could result in the depletion of the oxidising elements from the surface layer of the gold alloy.

No bond will form if all of the oxide formed is removed during the subsequent acid pickling process and none of the oxidising elements are left sufficiently close to the surface to allow the formation of additional oxides.

Carrying out the heat treatment under reduced pressure aids the removal of gasses that have been absorbed by the metal in great amounts during the casting process. The removal of these gasses helps to prevent the formation of interfacial bubbles.

In the case of base metal alloys, where nickel and chromium are commonly used, the metals oxidise very readily and the problem is generally the opposite of that for the gold alloys, in that too much of the oxide is formed.

Although oxides will naturally form during the firing of the ceramic it has been found that it is better to preform the oxide coating, as this improves the wetting of the ceramic on the metal surface.

## Acid Pickling

The heat treatment of gold alloys will produce not only tin oxide but various other oxides on the surface as well.

The acid pickling procedure seeks to remove the unwanted oxides in preference to the tin oxide. There is the added advantage that the dark surface of the alloy is lightened from grey to white due to increased concentration of tin oxide on the alloy surface. Commonly used acids are 50% hydrofluoric acid or 30% hydrochloric acid, with the latter preferred because of the hazards associated with the use of hydrofluoric acid. Niether this, nor the following procedure are generally required for base metal alloys.

## Heating In Air

A further heat treatment in air is frequently carried out in order to form an oxide coating of the correct thickness and quality.

The optimal oxide film on precious metal alloys should have a mat, greyish white appearance, being composed mainly of tin oxide. If the surface has a glossy appearance, this indicates a lack of oxide film and is usually the consequence of too many repeated surface treatments.

# The Importance Of Thermal Expansion

The composition of the ceramic for metal–ceramic restorations needs to be different from that of the ceramic used in porcelain jacket crowns.

The coefficient of thermal expansion, $\alpha$, of the latter, at 8 ppm/°C, is far too low when compared to that of the alloys, which is typically in the region of 12 ppm/°C. This mismatch would give rise to serious problems due to excessive differential shrinkage on cooling. Depending upon their composition, the coefficient of thermal expansion of the alloys can differ quite considerably, and, for this reason, *it is extremely important that the correct combination of metal and ceramic is used.*

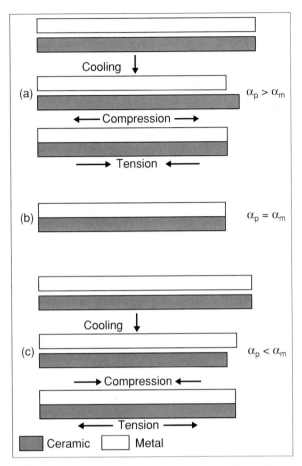

152 The effect of thermal mismatch on residual stress in the metal and the ceramic.

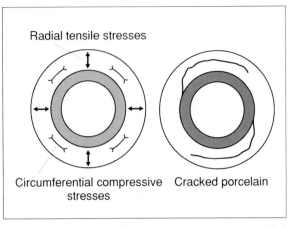

153 Cracking of metal-bonded-ceramic due to radial tensile stresses when $\alpha_p \ll \alpha_m$

## Thermally Induced Stresses

The ceramic loses its thermoplastic fluidity once it is cooled below its glass transition temperature, which is in the range 600–700°C. From this point on, any difference in the coefficients of expansion will produce stresses in the ceramic as the ceramic attempts to shrink more or less than the metal substructure, depending upon the type of mismatch. There are three possible scenarios which can be considered, namely:

$$\alpha_p > \alpha_m$$
$$\alpha_p = \alpha_m$$
$$\alpha_p < \alpha_m$$

The stresses that result from each of the above conditions are shown in 152.

When $\alpha_p > \alpha_m$, the ceramic will attempt to contract more than the metal (152a). As the metal prevents this from happening, the ceramic will be under a state of tension when it is cooled to room temperature, with the metal being in a state of compression. The surface tensile stresses cause the formation of surface cracks and a crazed surface.

When $\alpha_p = \alpha_m$, the two materials will shrink at the same rate and no differential stresses are generated (152b)

When $\alpha_p < \alpha_m$, the metal will attempt to shrink more than the ceramic and this places the ceramic in a state of compression (152c). This substantially reduces the potential for the ceramic to crack, since these compressive stresses have to be overcome before the ceramic is placed under tension. The metal will be in a state of tension, but, since the tensile strength of the alloys used is quite high (500–1000 MPa) there is no danger of the metal failing. Thus it would appear that the best situation is that when the coefficient of expansion of the metal is greater than that of the ceramic.

Whereas it would appear from the above discussion that the greater the mismatch the better (as the ceramic will be under a higher compressive stress); this is in fact not the case. The mismatch should not be too great, as the stresses generated in the system may cause crazing or fracture of the ceramic, or debonding from the metal surface.

The reason for this is best explained by considering ceramic that is fused to a circular metal structure, especially as this is more akin to the real situation, and is shown in 153. When the metal attempts to shrink more than the ceramic, radial tensile stresses and a circumferential compressive stress are generated. The latter are advantageous, but the former can be sufficient to cause debonding between the ceramic and the metal. If the mismatch is very large, the radial tensile stresses can cause the ceramic itself to fracture, with the fracture appearing circumferentially. Thus, the best situation is one where the coefficient of expansion of the ceramic is only slightly lower than that of the metal.

### The Effect of Composition of the Ceramic

The mismatch in the coefficient of expansion between the ceramics used in the manufacture of porcelain jacket crowns and the metals available for ceramic bonding is normally far too great. To overcome this problem, the alkali content of the ceramic is increased, as indicated in *Table 55*. Both soda ($Na_2O$) and potash ($K_2O$) are added to push up the coefficient of expansion to be in the region of 12 ppm/°C.

The addition of these oxides results in the formation of a crystalline phase in the glassy matrix. This crystalline phase is known as *leucite* and has a high coefficient of thermal expansion.

The amount of precipitated leucite is carefully controlled to provide the ceramic with the correct coefficient of expansion for a particular alloy, and can be 30–40% of the volume of the material. The reduction in firing temperature has the benefit of reducing the potential for distortion due to creep of the alloy.

After the ceramic frit is prepared by the manufacturer, it is held at an elevated temperature for a specific time to allow the formation of leucite crystals. Thus, this is a process very akin to the ceraming of the glass ceramics, so these materials are perhaps best described as leucite-reinforced glass ceramics.

An increase in the number and size of the leucite crystals will occur on firing the ceramic onto the metal. In the case of multiple firings, this will increase the coefficient of expansion of the ceramic. Such an increase can compromise the compatibility of the metal and the ceramic. Thus, excessive multiple firing of the metal-ceramic system is contraindicated. Slow cooling can also have the same effect as repeated firing, as can post-soldering, and the temperature

**Table 55** Typical compositions of metal-bonded ceramics as compared with a PJC porcelain.

|  | PJC Porcelain | Metal-Bonded Ceramic | |
|---|---|---|---|
| SiO$_2$ (%) | 66.5 | 66.4 | 59.2 |
| Al$_2$O$_3$ (%) | 13.5 | 14.5 | 18.5 |
| Na$_2$O (%) | 4.2 | 6.2 | 4.8 |
| K$_2$O (%) | 7.1 | 10.2 | 11.8 |
| Firing Temp. (°C) | 960 | 940 | 900 |

should be raised and lowered as quickly as possible without giving rise to thermal shock effects.

The opaque shade of the ceramic when it is first laid down on the metal coping tends to contain larger amounts of metallic oxides that help to mask the colour of the coping.

Great care must be exercised during the firing process, since the ceramic has a tendency to devitrify by a process of recrystallisation. This results in cloudiness of the ceramic as the small crystals that are formed act as scattering sites for light.

## Choice Of Metal–Ceramic Alloys

The requirements for alloys used in the metal-bonded ceramic system are somewhat different from those for the all-metal constructions. As it is necessary to fire ceramic onto the surface of the metal at high temperatures, the metal must have a high melting temperature.

If the melting temperature of the metal is too close to the firing temperature of the ceramic, partial melting of thin sections of the coping may occur, or the coping may deform. Especially in the construction of long-span bridges, the metal must have a high elastic modulus and high yield stress. The resultant high stiffness of the bridge structure will prevent the occurrence of excessively high strains (that the ceramic cannot cope with) on occlusal loading. In addition, a low stiffness of the metal framework can result in distortion due to the differential contraction stresses that are generated on cooling after porcelain firing.

**Table 56** Typical compositions of metal-ceramic alloys.

| Type | Au % | Ag % | Pd % | Pt % | Ni % | Cr % | Mo % | In, Cu, Zn, Ga % |
|------|------|------|------|------|------|------|------|------------------|
| High-gold | 88 | 1 | 6 | 4 | – | – | – | Balance |
| Au–Pd | 50 | 10 | 38 | – | – | – | – | Balance |
| High-palladium | – | – | 80 | – | – | – | – | Balance |
| Pd–Ag | – | 30 | 60 | – | – | – | – | Balance |
| Ni–Cr | – | – | – | – | 70 | 20 | 10 | – |

At one time, only high-gold alloys were available, but, with the rising cost of gold, a variety of alternative alloys have been developed, which may be classified as shown in *Table 56*.

## High-Gold Alloys

For the high-gold alloys, the melting temperature is raised by the addition of platinum and palladium, both of which have a high melting temperature.

An immediately obvious difference between the non-ceramic gold alloy and the ceramic–gold alloy is the omission of copper in the latter. This is done because copper reduces the melting temperature and also will react with the ceramic, producing a green discoloration. This is another feature of the alloys: they must not react with the ceramic, as this may spoil the aesthetics of the restoration.

The high-gold alloys have the advantage that they have been around for some considerable time and clinical experience has shown that they are extremely successful. In particular, the bond between the ceramic and the metal is very strong and highly reliable.

The main disadvantages of high-gold alloys are their relatively low melting temperatures, their susceptibility to creep at high temperatures and their low elastic moduli. A minimum coping thickness of 0.5 mm is required with their use.

In situations of limited biological width, this can give rise to aesthetic problems and often results in over-contouring to mask the metal colour. In this respect, the Pd–Ag and base metal alloys are more attractive.

## Gold–Palladium Alloys

One reason for the introduction of the Au–Pd alloys in the early 1970s was the rapidly rising cost of gold. Their performance is comparable to that of the high-gold alloys in terms of castability, accuracy of fit and corrosion resistance.

However, there are some alloy–porcelain combinations that should be avoided due to a mismatch in thermal expansion characteristics.

## High-Palladium Alloys

These alloys are primarily palladium, with small additions of other elements, such as copper, gallium and tin.

The copper, which can be present in amounts up to 15%, may be a surprising addition since this might have been thought to cause porcelain discoloration. However, unlike gold alloys, the inclusion of copper in palladium alloys does not seem to have this effect.

Their sag resistance can be poor, and, as such, these alloys are contraindicated for long-span bridges where this may present a particular problem.

Although clinical experience with these alloys is limited, they are rapidly gaining in popularity.

## Palladium–Silver Alloys

The Pd–Ag alloys have the most favourable elastic modulus of all of the precious metal alloys, producing castings with low flexibility and a reduced tendency to sag on porcelain firing. The alloys are somewhat less forgiving in terms of castability and fit, but as long as appropriate procedures are followed, results can be as good as with the gold alloys.

Due to the presence of high amounts of silver, there is concern that porcelain discoloration may occur. This problem appears to be more severe with certain alloy–porcelain combinations than others, and can be minimised by careful selection of the metal–porcelain combination.

Mutiple firings should be kept to a minimum, and overheating of the alloy avoided.

## Nickel–Chromium Alloys

The Ni–Cr alloys are very stiff as, their elastic modulus can be some 2.5 times higher than that of the high-gold alloys. This has the advantage that the coping thickness can be reduced from 0.5 mm to 0.3 mm, which lessens the problem of over-contouring.

They would be better for the construction of long-span bridges, as they provide greater rigidity, and, because of the high melting temperature, there is less potential for sag during firing.

The disadvantage with these alloys is that casting is more difficult, and the higher casting shrinkage can give rise to problems of poor fit. Also, clinical experience would indicate that the ceramic to metal bond is not as reliable as for the other alloys.

However, as more experience is gained with these alloys, so their performance may well improve. The low cost of the alloy is certainly very attractive.

# Resin-Bonded Bridges

In 1973, Rochette first reported the use of metal structures that were bonded by resins to acid-etched enamel. He used thin, perforated metal castings, bonded with cold-cure acrylic resins, to splint mobile lower incisors that were affected by advanced bone loss.

Following the successful retention of these devices, he had occassion to extract one of the incisors, and it was then that the idea of adding a pontic to the splint was first conceived. As resin technology improved, so the concept was explored in greater detail by other workers.

One weakness of the Rochette bridge design was the use of small perforations for retention. These exposed the resin to wear and meant that the attachment was to a relatively small area of the metal retainer.

This problem was overcome in the early 1980s when electro-etching of Ni–Cr alloys was developed. This technique provides a highly retentive surface that adheres strongly to the composite luting resins due to the high degree of micromechanical interlocking introduced. It bonds the entire area of the retainer to the etched

enamel and protects the underlying resin. This is the basis of the *Maryland bridge*, now in widespread use. Later developments relied on the bonding of chemically adhesive composite luting resins to roughened oxidised retainer surfaces.

The main advantages of resin-bonded bridges are that the minimal enamel preparation does not require local anaesthetics, that it leaves the teeth largely intact, such that traditional treatment options can still be used in the future, and that it prevents possible irritation of the pulp as there is no exposure of dentine.

Disadvantages include a high debonding rate for the retainers, and colour changes in anterior abutment teeth due to the metal retainer shining through. The latter can be overcome to some degree by using opaque composite luting resins. The former requires a careful consideration of design of the retainers.

Since the prosthesis relies on the presence of enamel for its attachment, sufficient enamel is required on which to bond the retainers. Short crowns, extensive restorations, congenital defects and tooth surface loss would prevent the use of these resin retained castings.

Also, for unsightly abutment teeth, conventional bridges would be a better proposition.

## Retention Systems

The composite luting resins are essentially very similar to composite restorative materials, except that they are invariably two-paste chemically-cured systems as the access of light is restricted by the metal retainers.

The filler loading may be slightly lower in order to ensure a low film thickness.

These resins do not adhere well to untreated metal surfaces, relying primarily on weak physical attraction and mechanical adhesion. In order to improve the adhesive bond of composite luting resins to the metal surface, two techniques are now commonly used.

### Micromechanical Adhesion

With this method, the entire fitting surface of the retainer is rendered micromechanically retentive by either electrolytic or acid-gel etching.

This technique is only applicable to Ni–Cr or Co–Cr alloys, which have a eutectic microstructure as shown on **154**. The etching process preferentially removes one of the phases, which

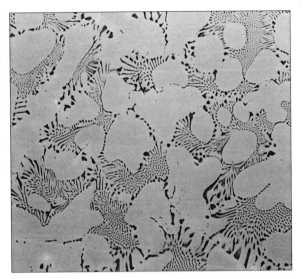

**154** Eutectic microstructure of a Ni–Cr alloy as it appears under the scanning electron microscope using back scattered electron imaging.

results in a pitted and grooved surface appearance as shown in **155**. The main alloys used are Ni–Cr alloys rather than Co-Cr alloys because of greater difficulty of fusing ceramic to the latter. The gold- and palladium-based alloys cannot be used, as these do not have the requisite microstructure. This means that they do not etch in the same way, and provide no enhanced micromechanical retention.

Retainers can be made to a minimum thickness of 0.3 mm, and can be waxed directly onto investment models, resulting in a good accuracy of fit.

Since electro-etching requires a high degree of skill and specialist equipment, the gel-etching process has become the more popular of the two. The gel is a high concentration solution of hydrofluoric acid, which is highly toxic and needs to be handled with great care.

### Grit Blasting

A variety of composite luting resins are available in which the resin component has the ability to bond chemically to suitably prepared metal surfaces.

In one system, the active constituent is the resin 4-META (4-methacryloxyethyl trimellitate anhydride), and, in another, a resin incorporating a phosphate group is used.

Grit blasting of base metal alloys with 50 μm alumina grit produces some surface roughening

for mechanical adhesion, as shown in **156**, but the main bond is obtained by a chemical interaction between the resin and the metal oxide on the surface.

Unlike the etched retainer, there is no need for special laboratory equipment or the use of dangerous chemical reagents. The Bis-GMA or UDMA based composite luting resins may also be used on grit-blasted surfaces, but only if the metal surface is first treated with a metal primer such as phosphinic acid. The direct bond to a grit-blasted metal surface is not sufficiently strong for these luting resins.

There is a reluctance on the part of some clinicians to use Ni–Cr alloys, as nickel is a known allergen. Some of the alloys also contain beryllium, which is highly toxic in its free state. (When alloyed with other elements it does not usually present a problem; this behaviour is not unlike mercury's.)

However, beryllium may be released during grinding and polishing of the castings, and therefore dental technicians are more at risk than either the dentist or the patient. Beryllium is usually present in order to improve the castability of the Ni–Cr alloy and to provide a superior eutectic microstructure.

The chemically adhesive luting resins can now be used with gold or palladium alloys by first plating the alloy with a thin layer of tin oxide or silica. A major disadvanatage in the use of these alloys as opposed to Ni–Cr alloys is that the retainers will be less rigid, due to their lower elastic modulus, and, the more flexible the retainer, the more likely it is that debonding will occur. The way to overcome this is to make the retainers thicker, but this creates problems if it leads to occlusal interferences.

## Recementing Debonded Bridges

Resin-bonded bridges may fail by total or partial debonding.

The most common mode of failure is cohesive fracture of the luting cement close to the cement–metal interface, with large amounts of the luting cement remaining on the tooth surface and relatively smaller amounts on the metal surface. Although the reasons for this have not been resolved, it is probable that the retainer is too flexible and the luting cement too brittle. On loading, tensile stresses are generated in the

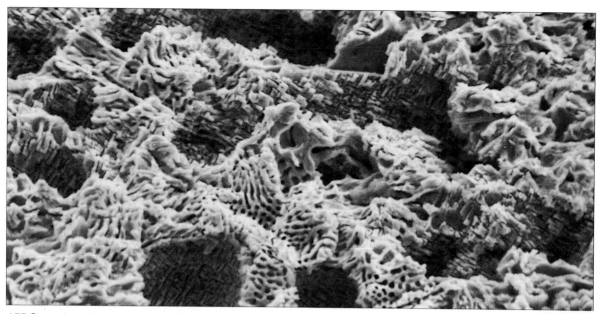

**155** Scanning electron micrsocope view of the surface of a Ni–Cr alloy after having been etched with a gel etchant.

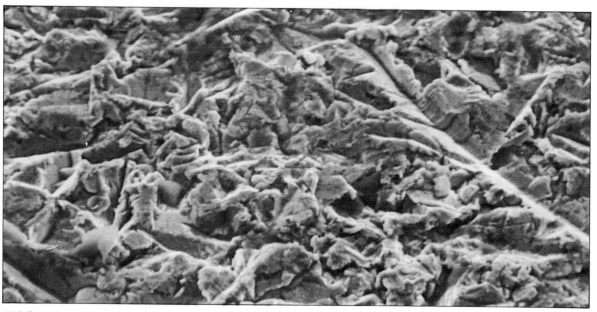

**156** Scanning elctron micrsoscope view of the surface of a Ni–Cr alloy after grit blasting with alumina.

adhesive layer which it is unable to bear. This situation is probably exacerbated by fatigue, which will help to increase the rate of fracture initiation and growth. If the failure occurs at the enamel–resin interface, then this indicates contamination or inadequate etching of the enamel surface.

If complete debonding has occurred, then the resin can be burnt off the retainer and this can be followed by ultrasonic cleaning. It should not be necessary to re-etch the metal surface. Alternatively, the surface of the metal may simply be grit blasted, which can now be done at the chairside with an intra-oral grit blaster. This will roughen the surface sufficiently for use with one of the chemically adhesive cements.

Any composite luting cement remaining on the tooth surface will need to be removed, with care being taken to avoid damaging the enamel; this can be extremly difficult when tooth coloured luting resins have been used. The enamel will need to be re-etched.

It should be said that the survival rate with rebonded resin-bonded bridges is generally not as good as that first time around. This may be because the design of the bridge is such that it is prone to debonding and a more conventional bridge design might be required.

# Summary

The main advantage of the metal–ceramic restoration over the all-ceramic restoration is its resistance to fracture. Bridges cannot as yet be made out of ceramics, and metal-bonded ceramic is the only option available.

The introduction of the resin-bonded ceramic crowns, veneers and inlays is challenging many of the situations where traditionally a metal–ceramic crown would have been used. This is because the latter are more conservative in the use of tooth tissue and provide superior aesthetics, especially at the margins of the restoration. However, the metal–ceramic crown has provided sterling service for many years, whereas the ceramic restorations are relative newcomers.

Whatever the advantages and disadvantages of the different systems, the following recommendations should be followed:

- *The responsibility for the choice of alloy rests with the dentist and should not be delegated to the dental laboratory technician.*
- *Ensure that the correct metal–ceramic combination is used.*

# Further Reading

Anusavice K. J. (1985) Noble Metal Alloys for Metal-Ceramic Restorations. Dent. Clin. N. Am. **29**, 789

Bagby M., Marshall S. J. & Marshall G. W. (1990) Metal ceramic compatibility: a review of the literature. J. Prosthet. Dent. **63**, 21

Betolotti R. L. (1984) Selection of alloys for today's crowns and fixed partial denture restorations. J. Am. Dent. Assoc. **108**, 959

Clyde C. S. & Boyd T. (1988) The etched cast metal resin-bonded (Maryland) bridge: a clinical review. J. Dent. **16**, 22

CDMIE (1981) Porcelain-metal alloy compatibility: criteria and test methods. J.Amer.Dent.Assoc. **102**, 71

Creugers N. H. J. & Käyser A. F. (1992) An analysis of multiple failures of resin-bonded bridges J. Dent. **20**, 348

Lawson J. R. (1991) Alternative alloys for resin-bonded retainers. J. Prosthet. Dent. **65**, 97

Livaditis G. J. & Thompson V. P. (1982) Etched castings: an improved retentive mechanism for resin-bonded retainers. J. Prosthet. Dent. **47**, 52

Murakami I. & Schulman A. (1987) Aspects of Metal-Ceramic Bonding Dent. Clin. N. Amer. **31**, 333

Rochette A. L. (1973) Attachment of a splint to enamel of lower anterior teeth. J. Prosthet. Dent. **30**, 418

Saunders W. P. (1989) Resin-bonded bridgework: a review. J. Dent. **17**, 255

Wood M. (1985) Etched Castings – an alternative approach to treatment Dent. Clin. N. Am. **29**, 393

# III.VI

# STAINLESS STEEL

## Introduction

Most of us are familiar with stainless steel as a widely used quality product for both domestic and industrial applications.

However, it is also extensively used in medical and dental applications, such as for the production of dental instruments, e.g. scalpel blades and forceps, orthodontic wires, denture bases and partial denture clasps. The material has generally been heavily worked to get it into the desired shape and is therefore defined as a *wrought alloy*. A wrought alloy distinguishes itself from the many casting alloys used for the construction of crowns and bridges in that it is: *a cast alloy which has been formed by mechanical processing such as rolling, extrusion or drawing to give it a new desired shape.*

Many alloys are available in wrought form besides stainless steel, such as gold alloys, Ni–Ti alloys, Co–Cr–Ni alloys and pure titanium, and are mainly used in the construction of orthodontic appliances. Only stainless steel will be considered in detail in this chapter.

Steels are available in a wide variety of compositions, with each having very specific properties that are carefully tailored to suit their particular application. One feature of steels that makes them such popular materials is the enormous range of mechanical properties that

can be obtained with only small changes in composition. A comparison of steel to other products is shown in *Table 57*. The steel wires show a wide range of strengths, which the other materials cannot match .

Before the introduction of stainless steels in dentistry (generally in the early 1930s), the only metal that was felt to have good enough corrosion resistance to allow it to be used in the mouth was gold. Stainless steel possesses a high tensile strength, and is used to form springs in removable orthodontic appliances. It is also used in fixed appliances for construction of bands,

| Table 57 A comparison of fracture, or yield strengths, of steels with other materials. | |
|---|---|
| | Fracture or yield strength (MPa) |
| Steel wire | 300–2800 |
| Bulk steel | 300–800 |
| Iron | 150–200 |
| Brass | 200–400 |
| Aluminium alloys | 200–600 |
| Copper alloys | 300–600 |
| Titanium alloys | 600–1100 |
| Glass | 50–150 |
| Carbon fibre | 2200–2800 |

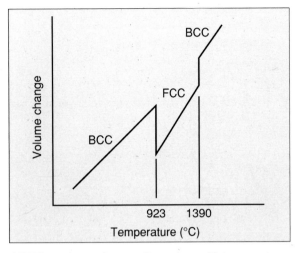

**157** The volume change of pure iron with temperature.

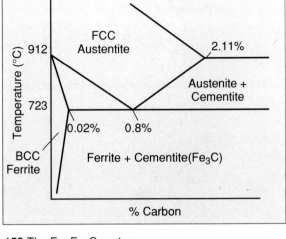

**158** The Fe–Fe₃C system.

brackets and arch wires. In fact, virtually all the components for fixed appliances used in orthodontics can be constructed out of stainless steel.

Orthodontic wire is made from what is known as austenitic stainless steel. This is a form of steel that can be readily shaped into a wire by rolling and subsequent extrusion through dies. This elongates the grains into long fibrous structures which run in the direction of the wire.

More specifically, the material used for orthodontic wires is known as a *stabilised austenitic stainless steel*. The best way of describing this material is to take the raw material, iron, and develop it, step by step, into the final product. Along the way, the different types of steel will be explored and their particular applications considered.

# Iron

Iron is an allotropic material, i.e. it undergoes two solid-state phase changes with temperature.

At room temperature, pure iron has a body-centred-cubic (BCC) structure, known as the α-phase. This structure is stable up to a temperature of 912°C, where it transforms to a face-centred-cubic (FCC) structure, the γ-phase.

At 1390°C the FCC iron reverts back to BCC, and retains this structure until it melts at 1538°C. These changes are accompanied by changes in the volume of the iron (**157**).

# Steel

Steel is an alloy of iron and carbon, where the carbon content must not exceed 2%. Iron with a carbon content greater than 2% is classified as a *cast iron* and will not be considered here.

## Carbon Steels

Carbon steel is a an alloy only of iron and carbon. In its BCC form, when small amounts of carbon are dissolved in the iron, the material is known as α-iron or *ferrite*.

The solubility of the carbon in this BCC structure is very low compared with that in the FCC structure, being a maximum of 0.02wt% at 723°C and only 0.005wt% at room temperature. This is despite the greater unoccupied volume in BCC (packing factor 68%) compared to FCC (74%).

The FCC form of the material has a considerably higher solubility of carbon, of up to 2.11%. The reason for this is that the largest interstitial holes in BCC iron (diameter 0.072 nm) are smaller than those in FCC iron (diameter 0.104 nm). This FCC form of the steel is known as *austenite*.

Both of these forms of steel are relatively soft and ductile, and, in particular, the austenite is readily shaped at elevated temperatures by hot forging and rolling operations.

When the limit of solubility for the carbon is exceeded for either of these forms of steel, the excess carbon precipitates out as $Fe_3C$ which is a hard and brittle phase, given the name *Cementite*. The various phases in the iron–cementide system are presented in the partial equilibrium phase diagram in **158**.

## Hyper- and Hypo-Eutectoid Steels

At a carbon concentration of 0.8%, the alloy shows a transformation from the single-phase austenite to a two-phase structure consisting of ferrite and cementite:

$$\gamma \downarrow \alpha + Fe_3C$$

This solid transformation is defined as a *eutectoid*, as distinct from a *eutectic*, which is a transformation of a single liquid phase directly into two solid phases.

Steels with a carbon content of exactly the eutectoid composition are called *eutectoid steels*. Those with a carbon content greater than 0.8% are *hyper-eutectoid steels*, and are used in the manufacture of burs and cutting instruments, while those with a carbon content of less than 0.8% are *hypo-eutectoid steels*, and are used in the manufacture of dental instruments such as forceps.

The eutectoid transformation is very important in the production of steels because a number of interesting things can happen when a carbon steel is cooled from its austenitic high temperature condition to room temperature.

### Slow Cooling

On slow cooling, the changes in structure for a 0.8% carbon steel are as predicted from the equilibrium phase diagram. The austenite is converted into a mixture of ferrite and cementite which is described as *pearlite* (**159**). However, cooling is not usually carried out slowly, but involves rapid-cooling by immersing the object into cold water in a process that is known as *quenching* .

### Rapid Cooling

When austenite is quenched in water, the ferrite and cementite cannot form because there is not enough time for diffusion and rearrangement of the atoms. Instead, a very rapid transformation occurs to a body-centred-tetragonal structure, which is rather like a distorted BCC. This form of

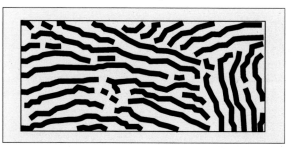

**159** The structure of pearlite which is a laminar mixture of ferrite and cementite.

steel is described as *martensite*, and is extremely hard and brittle. (In fact, it is far too hard and brittle for any practical purposes.)

Nevertheless, this transformation can be put to good use, because, by reheating to a temperature in the range of 200–450°C and then cooling rapidly, it is possible to transform the martensite into *pearlite* (ferrite + cementite). The degree of conversion can be carefully controlled by the temperature and duration of the heat treatment, a process known as *tempering* (**160**).

For cutting instruments, a hyper-eutectoid steel (carbon content > 0.8%) is generally used, because it combines the hard martensite with a large presence of the hard cementite, such that a cutting edge can be produced which does not blunt readily. For instruments such as forceps, the brittle nature of hyper-eutectoid steel would be unacceptable and a lower carbon content is present as in the hypo-eutectoid steels (carbon content < 0.8%). This allows predominantly the formation of the more ductile ferrite, while the hardness is controlled by the presence of martensite and much lower amounts of cementite.

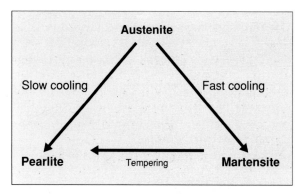

**160** Heat treatment known as tempering of martensitic steels to control the mechanical properties.

**Table 58** The three forms of stainless steel that are used in dental application.

|  | Cr (%) | Ni (%) | C (%) |
|---|---|---|---|
| Ferritic | 11.5–27 | 0 | 0.2 (max) |
| Austenitic | 16–22 | 7–22 | 0.25 |
| Martensitic | 11.5–17 | 0–2.5 | 0.15–0.25 |

# Stainless Steel

Although many other elements can be added to the basic carbon steels to improve the properties (e.g. molybdenum, silicon, cobalt, manganese), the two of greatest importance are chromium and nickel.

Stainless steel is an alloy of iron that is resistant to corrosion. It was discovered accidentally in the UK during the early part of the First World War by the Sheffield metallurgist Brearley who, at the time, was working on steels for armament construction. A rejected billet of a steel alloy was left out in the work's yard for some months, and it was subsequently observed that the billet had not rusted in the wet weather. This turned out to be due to its high chromium content.

The possibilities presented by the alloy were recognised, and it was patented in 1917. The addition of chromium to the carbon steel improves the corrosion resistance of the metal by forming a protective surface coating of chromium oxide. For this to be fully effective, the chromium content of the alloy has to exceed 11%; only then is it designated as a *stainless steel*.

# Austenitic Stainless Steel

The addition of nickel surpresses the transformation of austenite to martensite on cooling, such that the austenite becomes stable at room temperature when cooled rapidly. Slow cooling would again allow the formation of ferrite and cementite, but, since this is a diffusion controlled process, the rapid cooling by quenching prevents these phases from forming.

There are essentially three forms of stainless steel used for dental applications (see *Table 58*).

The ferritic steels are used mainly for the production of tools, whereas austenitic stainless steels have a very wide application and are used in orthodontic wires, autoclaves, table tops and cabinets. The martensitic steels are primarily used for cutting instruments.

The attraction of the austenitic stainless steel is that it is highly malleable and so can be readily shaped for a wide variety of purposes. The alloy can not be heat treated to change the properties in the way that martensitic and ferritic steels can, but it can be cold worked to improve the yield stress (although this will be at the expense of the ductility).

Nevertheless, it is this ability of austenitic stainless steel to be made with a wide variety of mechanical properties whilst maintaining its corrosion resistance in the mouth that has made it such an attractive material for orthodontic applications. In orthodontics, we are concerned almost exclusively with the austenitic variety, and the alloy most used is 18/8 stainless steel, which is composed of 18% chromium, 8% nickel and 0.2% carbon.

# Stabilised Austenitic Stainless Steel

Although it is common practice for most wrought alloys to be given a stress-relief anneal, this is not possible with the austenitic stainless steels due to structural changes that occur at the annealing temperature.

## *Formation Of Chromium Carbides*

At temperatures in excess of 500°C, chromium and carbon react to form chromium carbides which precipitate at the grain boundaries causing brittle behaviour. Also, the corrosion resistance is decreased due to depletion of the central regions of the crystals of chromium, which has migrated to the boundaries to form the carbides (**161**).

This process is known as *weld decay*, since it was first noticed as a problem when welding sheets of steel. The problem can be overcome by adding titanium to the alloy, which has the effect that the carbon preferentially reacts with the dispersed titanium such that the chromium remains where it is at its most effective. This gives what is known as *stabilised austenitic stainless steel*.

## Transformation To Ferrite And Cementite

The austenite is formed by rapid cooling from elevated temperatures to prevent the formation of cementite and ferrite. Raising the temperature allows diffusion of the atoms, such that these other phases *can* form.

This formation of other phases is an irreversible process unless the material temperature is raised above the eutectoid and then quenched to room temperature to reform austenitic steel.

However, the annealing process allows recrystallisation and the formation of the chromium carbides, which impairs the corrosion resistance.

## Recrystallisation

If the temperature is raised above the eutectoid temperature, recrystallisation of the metal takes place, and the long, fibrous grains which are produced by rolling and drawing during fabrication of the wire become transformed into large, equiaxed grains.

If this happens, the material will have softened and the springy properties of the wire will have been lost and cannot be restored. The rate at which this occurs is controlled by time and temperature.

# Properties

Austenitic stainless steels are favoured for orthodontic applications because of their excellent corrosion resistance in the biological environment, the wide range of mechanical properties available and the ease with which they can be joined by soldering or electrical resistance welding.

## Mechanical Properties

Depending upon the degree of cold working carried out by the manufacturer in forming the orthodontic wire, a range of mechanical properties are produced (see *Table 59*). It is important to select the appropriate type for the application in mind.

If little shaping, i.e. cold working by bending, is needed, a hard or extra-hard stainless steel wire can be selected. If, on the other hand, a lot of shaping is required, then one needs to start

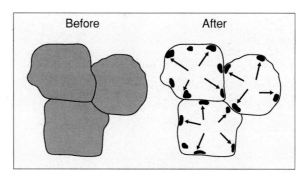

**161** Weld decay due to overheating of the alloy.

with a soft alloy, as it will work-harden on bending. If too hard a wire is selected to begin with, there is the danger that the wire will fracture on bending due to the loss of ductility.

## Soldering and Welding

Since the fabrication of appliances often requires the joining of separate components by soldering or welding, the heat produced can have an extremely detrimental effect on the properties of stainless steel. Therefore, techniques must be designed to avoid prolonged exposure of the components to high temperatures.

### Hard Soldering

Stainless steel components are generally joined by 'hard soldering' as distinct from 'soft soldering', the latter involving the use of low melting point alloys such as Sn–Pb alloys. Hard soldering may be carried out with gold or silver alloys, which are sufficiently corrosion resistant. Since gold-alloy solders must contain at least 45% gold to ensure a low enough melting temperature, on cost grounds, silver solders are preferred. The composition of silver solders used in orthodontics is approximately 50% silver, 16% each of copper, cadmium and zinc, and 3% nickel.

| **Table 59** Mechanical properties of a range of stainless steels used for orthodontic appliances. | | | |
|---|---|---|---|
| | 0.2% proof stress | Young's modulus | Elongation (%) | Hardness (BHN) |
| | (MPa) | (GPa) | | |
| Soft | 280 | 200 | 50 | 170 |
| Hard | 1050 | 200 | 6 | 250 |
| Extra-hard | 450 | 230 | 1 | 350 |

**Table 60** Relative merits of alloys for orthodontic applications.

| Material | Stiffness | Resilience | Ductility | Ease of soldering or welding |
|----------|-----------|------------|-----------|------------------------------|
| Stainless steel | High | Good | Adequate | Reasonable |
| Gold alloy | Medium | Adequate | Adequate | Easy |
| Co–Cr alloy | High | Good | Low | Difficult |
| Ni–Ti alloy | Low | Very high | Poor | Difficult |
| β-Ti alloy | Medium | High | Adequate | Difficult |

There are two basic methods of producing the heat that is necessary to melt the solder: the gas blow torch, and electrical resistance welding. Gas soldering has the advantage of requiring only low-cost equipment. The apparatus for electrical resistance soldering is considerably more expensive and requires greater skill in its use, but has the advantage that the heat is much more localised.

It is important to realise that the interface between a silver solder and stainless steel is more mechanical than alloying. An adequate amount of solder must therefore be used, and excessive finishing and polishing should be avoided as this will weaken the joint.

### Spot Welding

When an electrical current is passed through a metal it causes the metal to heat up. Spot welding involves the localised application of heat to the component to be joined by the use of a high current at low voltage. If, at the same time, pressure is applied at the point where the two parts are to be joined, recrystallisation occurs across the joint and the two parts are fused together.

Note that the metal does not melt. In fact, if the metal is excessively heated and melting occurs the joint is considerably weakened. In order to avoid this problem, as well as that of weld decay, welding time is kept to 1/50th of a second.

Basically, a welder is a set of electrodes that are bro ught together under pressure, and which are directly connected to the secondary winding of a pulse tranformer. A timer is used to limit the duration of the welding cycle.

Most of the separate components of fixed appliances are joined by spot welding, although the need for this has reduced in recent years with the introduction of complex prefabricated components. However, both spot welding and soldering are still extensively used for the repair and construction of appliances.

## Other Alloys

Other alloys that may be used for orthodontic appliances include gold alloys, Co–Cr alloys, Ni–Ti alloys and β-Ti alloys. The relative merits of these varieties of wrought alloy wires used in orthodontics are presented in *Table 60*.

The stiffness is both a function of the wire diameter and the elastic modulus of the material and determines the amount of force applied to a tooth.

For materials with a high elastic modulus, thinner wires can be used than for materials with a low elastic modulus. However, the thinner the wire the more likely it is to suffer from permanent deformation and loss of applied force to the tooth.

High stiffness is desirable when rapid large forces need to be applied to cause a tooth to move, whereas flexible wires applying a low force need to be used when slow movement of a tooth is desired.

The resilience of the wire is a measure of its ability to undergo large deflections without causing permanent deformation. It is given by the ratio of yield stress to modulus of elasticity such that a combination of low modulus and high yield strength would be ideal.

# Summary

Stainless steel is widely used for intra-oral appliances, particularly in orthodontics. The material has some limitations in that it is rapidly work-hardened and detrimental changes in properties can occur if excessive temperatures are applied.

# Further Reading

Burstone C. J. & Goldberg J. (1983) Maximum forces and deflections from orthodontic appliances. Am. J. Orthodont. **84**, 95–103

Waters N.E. (1975) Properties of wire in *Scientific Aspects of Dental Materials* Von Frauenhofer J. A. (Ed) , pp. 2–15, Butterworth, Sevenoaks.

# INDEX

234